THE UNFORTUNATE TRUTH ABOUT

VACCINES

EXPOSING THE VACCINE ORTHODOXY

LEON CANEROT, M.S., M.F.T., L.E.P.

CONTENTS

Preface xi

Introduction xiii

    Anti-Vaxxers vs. Pro-Vaxxers xix

Part I—Vaccinations: The Right to Choose 1

    Early Court Decisions. 2

    Nuremberg Trials. 3

    Institutional Racism 4

    Utilitarianism 4

    California Senate Bill 277 6

    Related Legislation 7

    National Adult Immunization Plan (NAIP) 10

    21st Century Cures Act. 11

    H.R. Bill 6666 11

        For the Greater Good 12

Part II—How Times Have Changed 15

    Evolution of Man 15

    Big Tobacco 18

    Big Pharma 19

    U.S. Childhood Statistics—Then and Now 20

    What Causes Autism?. 21

    Rates of Autism 22

    What Happened? Vaccines Happened! 24

    Vaccinated vs. Nonvaccinated Children 27

Part III—Assumptions About Vaccines **31**
   1. **Vaccines Are Safe, and Benefits Outweigh Risks**. . . **31**
      National Childhood Vaccine Injury Act (NCVIA) . . **32**
      National Vaccine Injury Compensation Program
      (NVICP)—"Vaccine Court" **34**
      Vaccine Ingredients—Aluminum, Formaldehyde,
      Thimerosal, Polysorbate 80, Squalene, Neomycin and
      Streptomycin, Monosodium Glutamate (MSG). **38**
   2. **Vaccines Are Effective and Long-Lasting** **48**
      Natural Immunity **48**
      Artificial Immunity **49**
      Herd Immunity **49**
      The Immune System. **52**
   3. **Vaccines Have Wiped Out All Major Diseases** **55**
      Diseases Associated with Poor Living Conditions. . . **56**
      Chart—U.S. Disease Mortality Rates **57**
      History of Smallpox and the Vaccine **58**
      Other Critics of Vaccinations **60**
          Mortality vs. Morbidity. **65**
   4. **No Connection Between Vaccines, Autism, and**
      Other Neurological Disorders **67**
      Vaccine Product Inserts **67**
      Evidence of Harm **69**
      Vaccine-Induced Autism. **72**
      Omnibus Autism Proceedings. **73**
      Hannah Poling Case. **74**

Part IV—The Theory Behind Vaccinations **77**
      Types of Vaccine Ingredients. **78**
          Aborted Fetuses Used in Vaccines **80**
      The Adverse Effects of Vaccines. **82**
      Demyelination. **84**
      Microbiome and Autoimmune Disorders. **85**
      Leaky Gut Syndrome **86**
      Institute of Medicine (IOM) **87**

Part V—Vaccines **89**

  Vaccine Classification 90

  Vaccine Studies 92

    Hepatitis B 92

    Diphtheria, Pertussis, Tetanus 95

    Hemophilus Influenzae Type B Meningitis 101

    Rotavirus 103

    Pneumococcal Disease 104

    Poliomyelitis (Polio) 105

    Influenza (Flu) 109

    Measles, Mumps, Rubella 111

    Chickenpox (Varicella Virus) 118

    Shingles Vaccine 119

    Human Papilloma Virus 119

      Mouse Toxicity Test 124

  Related Vaccine Induced Conditions 124

    Sudden Infant Death Syndrome (SIDS) 124

    Peanut Allergies 126

    Shaken Baby Syndrome 126

    Gulf War Syndrome 127

    Childhood and Adult Cancers 128

    Obsessive-Compulsive Behavior 129

Part VI—The Pharmaceutical Industry's Influence on Governmental Agencies, the Medical Community, Politicians, and the News Media **131**

    Centers for Disease Control and Prevention (CDC). 137

    Food and Drug Administration (FDA) 139

    American Academy of Pediatrics (AAP) 142

    Environmental Protection Agency (EPA) 144

    World Health Organization (WHO) 145

    Critics of the Pharmaceutical Industry 147

    Defenders of the Pharmaceutical Industry 155

    Edward Bernays and Propaganda 162

    Astroturf and Other Fictions 163

Vaccine Safety Science Is Flawed 165
Ethical Behavior and the Pharmaceutical
Industry 168

Part VII—Manufacturing Hysteria **169**
Virus Mania 170
Swine Flu (1976) 170
HIV/AIDS 170
Mad Cow Disease (BSE) 171
Severe Acute Respiratory Syndrome (SARS) . . . 172
Avian Flu (H5N1) 172
Swine Flu (2009) 173
Zika Virus 173
Coronavirus (SARS-Co-2) 175
Impact of Worldwide Lockdowns 178
Vaccine Effectiveness 179
Relative Risk Versus Absolute Risk 181
Adverse Reactions 182
Falsifying Data 188
Treatment Options 191
The Origins of COVID-19 194
Vaccine Passports 197
The Israeli Experiment 198
Japan's COVID-19 Vaccination Policy 200
The Great Barrington Declaration 201
The Rome Declaration 202
Misinformation, Censorship, and Coercion . . 203

**Part VIII—Medical Treatment and the Biomedical
Approach** **207**
Pasteur vs. Béchamp 207
Hippocrates 209
Conventional Medicine 209
Functional Medicine 210
Biomedical Treatment Options for Autism 211

Detoxify the Body 213
Improving the Microbiome (Gut) 214
Allergen-Free Diet 215
Bolster the Immune System with Vitamin and
  Mineral Supplementation 216

Part IX—Summary and Recommendations **219**
Highlighting Major Points 219
Personal Actions 226
Recommendations at the National and State Level . 227

Appendix
A—Unethical Human Experimentation in the
  United States 231
B—How to Report an Adverse Event to VAERS 237
C—Autoimmunity and the Immune System. 239
D—A Brief History of Polio. 245
E—How to Identify Vaccine Reactions (NVIC). 249
F—Bogus Cancer Charities. 251
G—A Brief History of the Pharmaceutical Industry's
  Influence on the Medical Field. 253
H—Pharmaceutical Settlements 259
I—How to Win the Vaccine Credibility War (Ted Kuntz) . 261
J—Censorship in Science 263
K—How to Report an Injury from COVID-19 Vaccine
  for Reimbursement. 267
L—Physicians Declaration: Global COVID Summit—
  Rome, Italy. 269

Glossary of Medical Terms. **273**

Bibliography **289**
Books 289
Videos. 292
Website Resources 293

Acknowledgments **299**

Notes **301**

Index **325**

About the Author **337**

This book is dedicated to all those who have suffered the ill-effects of vaccinations. Hopefully, their suffering will not be in vain and the world will come to realize that there are better ways to foster health than by simply injecting toxins into one's body.

PREFACE

My reason for writing this book is based on my 35 years' experience as a school psychologist, working with special-needs children at the preschool and elementary through high school, and postsecondary levels. It was during the early 1990s, while working in Head Start and later the elementary school system, that I first became aware of this unprecedented increase in autism. Prior to that time, autistic children were hard to find, with estimates of about 1 in 10,000 in 1970.[1] Today, the rate of autism in the United States continues to grow unabated, with estimates as high as 1 in 30 children in 2020.[2] This is a growing epidemic, the long-term implications of which will have a devastating impact on society.

Some in the medical field suggest that the spike in autism is not real—that it is a result of the expanded autism diagnosis. But this is in no way a credible explanation, given the unprecedented increase in cases. Autistic children do not suddenly appear because of a change in diagnosis; they immediately stand out from normally developing children. Others suggest that autism might be caused primarily by hereditary factors, but human genetic change occurs slowly, over centuries, not in a matter of a few years. Some have even theorized that fathers who are older or socially inept personality types could explain the emergence of autism, but these are not uniquely new factors that could explain a sudden explosion in autism.

The possible connection between the increasing use of vaccines during this period and the incidence of autism has been suggested, but this was thoroughly dismissed by the medical establishment; it seemed to be out of the question. But the more I investigated the varying critiques surrounding autism and vaccines by attending conferences and workshops, and researching the subject by reading books, a multitude of articles, scientific studies, opinion papers, and so on, on every side of the argument, the more it became evident to me that the connection was real.

As I attempted to talk with others in the field about the research I came across, I was surprised to find such resistance to the notion that vaccines could in any way be contributing to the increase in autism and other neurological disorders. I ran up against what can be called the "vaccine orthodoxy"[3] that holds all vaccines are safe and effective and the benefits outweigh the risks. Everyone has been taught to believe that vaccines have been the miracle cure for so many dangerous and deadly diseases such as smallpox and polio, as well as, how vaccines have greatly contributed to the health and safety of children and prevented the death of millions of lives around the world. How could anyone question what is so obvious to so many? To suggest that there are serious issues regarding vaccines was tantamount to attacking one of society's most cherished beliefs about the efficacy of vaccinations.

So, what happened? How did we go from autism being a rare condition to a worldwide epidemic in the span of 30+ years? To understand that question and many others, we must go deeper into the history of what has actually happened. As the expression goes, "The devil is in the details" and the whole topic of the pros and cons of vaccinations is no exception. There are many nuances in attempting to understand the complex nature of this topic. This book is an attempt to synthesize and simplify the voluminous information that has been covered in the many excellent books and programs on this subject. The aim here is to provide the general public with an easy-to-read summary of the essential argument that vaccines have contributed to the many adverse reactions we are seeing in children and adults today. The book contends that the medical establishment, the politicians, and the mainstream news media have failed to seriously address these concerns as a result of the undue influence of the pharmaceutical industry.

INTRODUCTION

There is a joke that goes, "What is the difference between ignorance and apathy?" The answer is "I don't know, and I don't care!" While this play on words is quite humorous, it can also be seen as quite telling. Ignorance comes from the root word, to ignore, which is to make little of or to disregard out of a lack of concern. If it comes to your attention, your reaction may be one of indifference—"Who cares?" In regard to vaccinations, if you don't know the potential adverse effects of a vaccine, the assumption is that there is nothing to worry about. Only when you or your child or someone you know personally has experienced a bad reaction from a vaccination, do you then become aware of and concerned that vaccines can pose a real risk of harm.

The expression, "People see what they want to see," exemplifies the bias that people develop as a result of the beliefs, values, attitudes, and behaviors that they have been exposed to going back to childhood. We tend to equate our beliefs with the way things really are, when in fact, they are points-of-view and not necessarily the truth. In order to question our beliefs, we must be willing to take the perspective that "There is more to the matter than what meets the eye," because our tendency is to think that what we see is all there is to see. Consciously or unconsciously, we tend to look for those things that validate our beliefs. Politics and religion are perfect examples of this, as I would contend is the case with vaccinations as well.

The American historian Daniel J. Boorstin wrote, *"The greatest obstacle to discovery is not ignorance—it is the illusion of knowledge."*[4] If one assumes to know the truth, then one ceases to question the "so-called" facts. A powerful mythology has been created around the efficacy of vaccines that is so readily and unquestioningly accepted as fact today. The vaccine orthodoxy is constantly reinforced by the medical community and the mainstream media, who cite authorities from agencies, such as the Centers for Disease Control and Prevention (CDC), the Food and Drug Administration (FDA), the American Medical Association (AMA), and the American Academy of Pediatrics (AAP). These agencies contend that there is no convincing evidence of harm due to vaccines.[5] However, this flies in the face of numerous scientific studies that show that vaccines do cause harm. Even the U.S. Supreme Court in 1986 deemed that "vaccines are unavoidably unsafe."[6] When it comes to vaccinating children, the medical community takes the unique perspective that "one size fits all." Given that vaccine reactions are unpredictable, it would seem quite problematic to assume that every child can be indiscriminately vaccinated in the same way, without regard for individual differences.

Barbara Loe Fisher, co-founder of the National Vaccine Information Center (NVIC) and mother of a vaccine-injured child, wrote:

> *People are not all the same, and we do not all respond the same way to drugs or vaccines, just like we do not all respond the same way to infectious diseases…some people are genetically, biologically, and environmentally more susceptible to suffering brain inflammation and other types of serious vaccine reactions, but doctors often do not know who will be injured or die from vaccination.[7]*

Children in the United States today lead every country in the world in both the number of vaccines given and the early age at which vaccines are introduced. One would think that all these vaccinations to protect children from diseases would create healthier outcomes, but this is clearly not the case. For example, consider the infant-mortality rate—that is, the number of infant deaths in the first year of life. In the 1950s, the United States had one of the lowest infant-mortality rates in the world; fast forward to today, and we see on the CIA website that the United States is listed 54th in infant-mortality rate, behind all developed countries in the world.[8]

The legitimate fears regarding vaccine safety have been repeatedly discounted by the medical establishment. Negative findings that are brought to light are often ignored or dismissed as being faulty in some way. Public officials are reluctant to acknowledge any problem with vaccines for fear this would discourage the public's faith in vaccinations. Denying these vaccine injuries also serves to insulate the medical community from culpability. It would seem that protecting the vaccination program at all cost supersedes any concerns for the safety of those receiving these vaccines. This is especially relevant considering all of the adverse reactions being reported that are associated with the increasing number of vaccinations being given.

By the mid-1980s, lawsuits against the pharmaceutical industry for childhood injuries caused by vaccines were becoming increasingly problematic for the drug companies because of the higher legal costs being incurred. It reached the point that the manufacturers were threatening to stop producing vaccines unless they were released from vaccine-injury liability. Consequently, the U.S. Congress was persuaded to pass the National Childhood Vaccine Injury Act (NCVIA) in 1986, removing all responsibility from the drug companies and doctors as a result of any adverse reactions from vaccines. The NCVIA states, "No vaccine manufacturer shall be liable in a civil action for damages arising from a vaccine-related injury or death." *(Public Law 99-660).*[9] Rather than address the obvious issues around vaccine safety, "Big Pharma" instead was given a free pass to push for more vaccines without fear of any penalty. Consequently, we have gone from **5 vaccine doses in 1962 to 72 vaccine doses today,** that children are scheduled to receive based on the CDC guidelines. What other industry has a product that is mandated by law while at the same time being exempt from any liability for that product?

One of the most insidious aspects of this whole controversy around vaccine safety has been the medical community's dismissive attitude toward the tens of thousands of parents who have witnessed their children regress after being vaccinated. The myopic view of those in the medical field who emphasize the importance of vaccinations while dismissing their harmful effects has distorted the public's perspective on vaccine safety. Without knowing the sheer scope of vaccine injuries, one tends to simply accept the prevailing mindset that vaccines are safe. Numerous attempts to draw attention to the neurological damage caused by these vaccines have been met with strong resistance by the medical establishment and the mainstream news media. Try to envision what the impact would be if it became widely accepted by the public that vaccines, in the long run, may actually be more harmful to children than beneficial.

In medical schools, there is rigorous and intensive study of the medical literature that covers human anatomy, pathology, biochemistry, microbiology, symptoms and diagnoses of diseases, and so on. However, when it comes to vaccines, there is a noticeable absence of information given to interns. Medical books don't discuss vaccines—it is simply taken for granted that vaccines are safe and effective because that is what students have been taught. Suzanne Humphries, Medical Doctor (MD), summarized the extent of training in this way:

> *When we participate in pediatric training, we learn that vaccines need to be given on schedule. We learn that smallpox and polio were eliminated by vaccines...We are indoctrinated with the mantra that vaccines are safe and effective—neither of which is true.*[10]

Many medical doctors don't know about vaccine research except what they have been told, and they would be hard pressed to say even what is in those vaccines that they routinely inject into their patients. They simply assume that the research done by the pharmaceutical companies is accurate and above board without questioning it, thinking that the governmental agencies like the CDC and FDA would not have approved these vaccines if there were any concerns regarding their safety. What medical doctors are not made aware of, as with the general public, is the corrupting influence of the pharmaceutical industry on government officials approving these vaccines, the medical agencies promoting vaccinations for profit, and the news media that routinely parrots misinformation about the exaggerated dangers of not being vaccinated.

Doctors and other medical officials who push vaccinations on the public often resort to intimidation by finger-pointing and ostracizing parents who resist having their children vaccinated. Doctors may become incensed when being challenged by parents who express any doubts regarding the "virtues" of vaccinations and may refuse to provide medical services if parents don't follow the doctor's orders to vaccinate their children. The medical community's focus on fear, by suggesting that children could be seriously injured or die if not vaccinated, becomes a primary tactic for pressuring parents to comply with vaccine mandates. Even the American Medical Association (AMA) has come out recently in favor of a minor as young as 12 years old being able to consent to vaccinations without a parent's approval, describing parental consent as a *barrier to vaccination.*[11] In effect, this allows doctors to circumvent parental authority by declaring that children have the maturity to make their own decisions on this matter.

Maintaining profitability by following the recommended vaccine schedule seems to be the overriding principle of the medical establishment as opposed to heeding concerns over children's safety. Pediatricians in particular receive much of their income from vaccines and the drug companies, in coordination with government, providing financial incentives to ensure that children are fully vaccinated.

There are four possible positions that parents may take regarding vaccination. Parents may choose to fully vaccinate their children based on the CDC vaccine schedule; they may choose to delay vaccines until the child is older; spread out the shots so there is less likelihood of toxic overload; or, finally, opt out of any or all vaccines. Unfortunately, the first option is increasingly becoming the only option for many under the draconian laws being passed today. As a result, when it comes to vaccinations, the right of individuals to determine what medical procedure one receives based on informed consent is being systematically undermined.

You may have come to this book already with a strong view regarding the issue of vaccinations. What is going to be presented to you in these pages may go against everything you have heard or been taught. This has become a highly charged subject, with strong opinions on both sides and a deep desire to defend one's point of view. If you happen to be in the camp that denies that vaccines are a problem, you would fall into one of three categories according to Elliott Freed, author of the book, *Vaccine Primer: An Inoculation* (2016),[12] as summarized below:

1. **The Casual Denier**—People who read in the newspaper or see on TV that scientists have proven there is no link between vaccines and autism and are satisfied that there is nothing more to the story. Freed states, *"Sadly, many doctors fit into this category. They read in some report somewhere that the science was settled and that is that."*

2. **The Studious Denier**—People who have read a lot from the point of view that vaccines are safe and effective and can quote the standard pro-vaccine position while dismissing any contrary evidence as "quackery."

3. **The Intentional Denier**—People working in governmental agencies such as the CDC and officials working in the pharmaceutical industry who know that vaccines are not safe and effective and that autism and other neurological disorders are related to vaccinations. Freed writes, *"These are the people who throw data in the trash when it shows clear correlations between vaccines and autism,"* as described by the whistleblower William Thompson, a CDC official (to be covered later).

What is being asked of you now, so you can evaluate for yourself the information presented in this book, is a willingness to withhold judgment for the time being while remaining open to the possibility that there is more to vaccines than what has been presented to the general public. There is an enormous amount of data and research that has been summarized here on credible science that is not being covered in the mainstream news media due to blatant censorship. Your willingness to put in the time to study this information will, hopefully, give you a broader and more objective perspective. The information introduced here is an attempt to present the other side of the vaccine debate rather than just accept the ongoing mantra that vaccines are safe and effective in a "one size fits all" world.

Anti-Vaxxers vs. Pro-Vaxxers

The term "anti-vaxxer" has become a derogatory word suggesting that anyone who is against vaccinations is by definition naïve, ignorant, anti-science, even irresponsible by putting others in harm's way by refusing to vaccinate their children and, as a result, are threatening the safety of other children. In contrast, "pro-vaxxers" are portrayed as responsible and informed individuals who base their information on science. But if we were to look more deeply into the research on vaccine safety, we might have a different take on the efficacy of vaccinations.

Anti-vaxxers, to a large extent, were pro-vaxxers initially, who then experienced the adverse impact that vaccines have had on their own children or themselves. Consequently, a more accurate term for anti-vaxxers might be ex-vaxxers. No longer were they blind to the possibility of harm caused by vaccines, having seen the irrefutable damage and even death caused by vaccinations. Consequently, these anti-vaxxers, who have had to come to terms with the harm done by vaccines, have as a result become intensely engaged in learning more about what went wrong. Parents, in particular, have become the strongest advocates for their children, no longer accepting the doctor's standard excuse that these injuries were "unrelated to the vaccine, just a coincidence." By researching and discovering on their own the facts about vaccines, they in effect have become authorities on the subject in their own right. It is out of their investigation that they came to realize that there was more to the matter than what they had been told by the medical establishment and the mainstream media, who continue to perpetuate the "vaccine orthodoxy," maintaining that vaccines are safe and effective and that the benefits outweigh the risks.

If we were to view anti-vaxxers and pro-vaxxers on a continuum from one end to the other, we would see that the pro-vax position is supported by the pharmaceutical and medical establishment who are staunch advocates for vaccines. On the other side, we have the anti-vax group, who hold a more skeptical view that vaccines are problematic and far from efficacious. What largely determines an individual's place on this spectrum ultimately has to do with what one has been taught to believe. If you are convinced that your doctor knows what is best, you will most likely go along with whatever vaccines are recommended. If you have been taught to question vaccines, based on what you have heard or experienced, you might be less eager to faithfully follow a doctor's orders.

Vaccination is a complex topic that raises many questions. For example: Has the science around vaccines already determined that they are safe and effective, or are there still questions that have not been answered satisfactorily? Does the science support the "one size fits all" use of vaccines? Does the medical community provide an objective look at both the pros and cons of vaccination? Do people have a choice in the matter, or is it already predetermined that vaccines should be given regardless of one's concerns? If these and other questions are not adequately addressed, is it really safe to assume that everything is fine?

There are numerous scientific studies on vaccines by researchers who have raised serious concerns regarding the assumption that all vaccines are safe and effective. Unfortunately, their voices have been largely ignored or even vilified by the medical establishment and by the mainstream media, who just parrot whatever the medical establishment says. Advocating for vaccinations seems to take a higher priority than first stopping to address the fundamental issue of vaccine safety. Why is that? After all, shouldn't the safety of our children be of paramount concern? Sadly, there is substantial evidence that the pharmaceutical interests have had a corrupting influence over organizations such as the CDC, FDA, AMA, AAP, universities relying on grant money, governmental officials, and other entities that have benefitted financially in some way. And the general public is left to come up with an informed opinion based largely on skewed information.

PART I

VACCINATIONS: THE RIGHT TO CHOOSE

A country that requires all children to receive a product—no matter how beneficial—knowing that some children will die and others' lives will be destroyed by the use of that product, risks losing all moral authority.
—James Turner, JD

In the book, *Vaccine Epidemic: How Corporate Greed, Biased Science, and Coercive Government Threaten Our Human Rights, Our Health, and Our Children,* by Louise Kuo Habakus, M.A. and Mary Holland, J.D. (2011), a convincing argument is made for vaccine choice. They contend that vaccinations, like all medical interventions, should be a choice based on free and informed consent. To deny that basic principle is to violate the fundamental human right to have control over one's body when it involves a medical procedure and, by extension, the parents' right, as guardian, over medical decisions affecting their own children.

The premise that individuals should have the right to determine what medical procedures they consent to would seem rather obvious. However, looking at the history of human rights, it is quite clear that the right to choose has been subject to the powers that be. History is replete with many examples of tragic violations of human rights, under the guise of the common good. A prime example of the horrid medical experimentation in the U.S. was the Tuskegee Experiment, which was conducted over a 40-year period, in which African-American men who contracted syphilis were purposely denied available treatment in order to chart the progression of their disease. Historically, weak and vulnerable populations including minorities and disadvantaged groups, often in institutional settings, children and adults alike, have been subjected to gruesome experiments under the guise of advancing medical research. Many examples of these atrocities, sponsored by the U.S. government and conducted by those in the medical field, over the past couple of centuries are listed in heart-wrenching detail in **Appendix A, *Unethical Human Experimentation in the United States.***

Early Court Decisions—The rationale for these experiments is grounded in the notion of eugenics, the study of hereditary improvement, especially of humans through genetic controls. In essence, it is a nice way of saying that governments have the right, even the obligation, to rid itself of certain unfit people deemed as inferior and therefore a drain on society. In the United States, the first eugenics law passed in 1895, aimed at preventing marriage for those considered inferior and unqualified to procreate, which eventually led to the involuntary and forced sterilization of as many as 70,000 individuals described as mentally deficient "imbeciles" in the early 1900s.[13]

In the 1905 case of *Jacobson vs. Massachusetts,* the U.S. Supreme Court ruled that states could force citizens to be vaccinated based on the principle that it served the greater good of the wider society. Specifically, it forced people to receive the smallpox vaccine on the flawed assumption that medical doctors could determine in advance who would be injured or die from the smallpox vaccination. Unfortunately, doctors can never accurately predict the outcome of a vaccination because of the unique characteristics of each person. This ruling was based on the utilitarian position that citizens opposed to vaccinations can be forced to get vaccinated regardless of their concerns.

This 1905 court decision had enormous implications in the 1927 Supreme Court case of *Buck vs. Bell,* when Justice Oliver Wendell

Holmes Jr., cited *Jacobson vs. Massachusetts* to justify Virginia's state rights to force the sterilization of a young woman, Carrie Buck, who was considered to be mentally retarded, like her birth mother. Carrie's foster mother, who was raising her at the time, testified that Carrie was epileptic and feebleminded and recommended that she be sterilized, in spite of the fact that Carrie had normal intelligence, was doing well in school, and did not have a seizure disorder.

The U.S. Supreme Court ruled that the Virginia Sterilization Act of 1924 did not violate the U.S. Constitution. In Justice Holmes' 1927 ruling, he infamously stated that *"three generations of imbeciles are enough,"*[14] making reference to Carrie's mom, Carrie, and her daughter, Vivian, who was the result of Carrie being raped by the foster parents' nephew. The state of Virginia went ahead and had Carrie sterilized in the name of the greater good, after which she was released from incarceration.

Nuremberg Trials—During the Nuremberg Trials after World War II, the Nazi scientists who were charged with crimes against humanity referred to America's sterilization program as a justification for their own inhumane experiments. It was in the Nuremberg Trials in 1947 that the concept of utilitarianism (the greatest good for the greatest number of people) was discredited on the grounds that this could be used to justify any behavior considered appropriate by government edict.

At the same time, the Nuremberg Trials reinforced the principle of "informed consent" as a basic human right, especially as it applies to an individual's free consent to a medical procedure without pressure, coercion, or reprisal. Even the AMA states in its Code of Medical Ethics:

> *The patient should make his or her own determination about treatment… Informed consent is a basic policy in both ethics and law that physicians must honor, unless the patient is unconscious or otherwise incapable of consenting and harm from failure to treat is imminent.*[15]

This view is quite different from what is being presented to the public today when it comes to vaccinations. Informed consent is being systematically undermined by the influence of the pharmaceutical industry on the medical community, the news media, and politicians, by attempting to mandate childhood vaccinations for all children regardless of one's objections.

Institutional Racism—In Brett Wilcox's book *Jabbed*, he devoted a chapter to how the U.S. vaccine program fostered institutional racism, in which he suggested that experiments on minorities and the disadvantaged throughout the world was not coincidental. That the ruling elite were motivated in an attempt to limit the minority population, which was seen as a "national security threat" as promoted by Frederick Osborn, and others, as cited by Wilcox, and best exemplified by the Rockefeller Foundation's Population Council:

> *Established in 1952 by John D. Rockefeller III, the purpose of the Council from the beginning was the reduction of population growth, particularly among "undesirable" humans. Rockefeller appointed Frederick Osborn, a leader of the American Eugenics Society, as the Council's first president. Among other organizations, the United Nations, World Bank, The Presidential Committee on Population and Family Planning, the Ford Foundation, and the American Assembly lent support to the Council.*[16]

Wilcox also chronicled the nefarious efforts to develop and use vaccinations under the guise of fostering birth control, when in fact, it served as a way of sterilizing women in developing countries in order to reduce the third-world population. He gives examples of how this was done in countries such as India, the Philippines, and Kenya.

Utilitarianism—The rationale for mandatory vaccinations is based on the principle of utilitarianism and if the government has the right to determine what is best for the individual regarding vaccinations, what other medical decisions can they decide are in the best interests of the individual? Utilitarianism comes from the root word, "utility," which refers to the condition or quality of being useful. The dictionary describes utilitarianism as *"the ethical theory proposed by Jeremy Bentham and John Stuart Mill that all moral, social, or political action should be directed toward achieving the greatest good for the greatest number of people."*[17] Because utilitarianism usurps the rights of the individual in order to ensure the greater good for all, it is critical that the criteria for its application should be founded on valid reasoning.

As it relates to vaccinations, do mandates make sense? Do they really justify the principle of the "greater good" if in fact, the assumptions about vaccines do not hold up? The advantages of vaccination must be shown to outweigh the great costs and suffering of those being adversely affected by vaccines. For example:

- Has the government proved that vaccines are safe, regardless of individual differences, especially when giving multiple doses at one time?
- Is it true that these contagious diseases have been eradicated by the introduction of vaccines, as opposed to improved living conditions?
- Do vaccination mandates really create "herd immunity," thereby reducing the possibility of disease?
- Do the benefits of vaccination outweigh the risk of contracting common infectious childhood diseases?
- Do vaccines create the conditions that are potentially worse than the disease?
- Is it possible that the vaccines can force the disease to mutate, causing a more virulent form of the disease that it was supposed to prevent?

These questions raise ethical concerns about the application of the utilitarian principle of "the greater good." Yet the drive to make vaccines mandatory throughout the United States continues at full speed, unabated, without any serious consideration of the "one-size-fits-all" philosophy of vaccinations. This is quite a departure from standard medical procedures that take into consideration the inherent individual differences found in children and the general public.

CA Senate Bill 277—This overreach is best exemplified by the passage of the California Senate Bill 277 in 2015, which eliminated parents' rights to personal and religious vaccine exemptions for their children, as summarized below:

- Parents no longer have the right to decide which vaccines to give their children (if any) and when to give them.
- Families that do not comply with the "one-size-fits-all" mandate lose their constitutional right for their children to receive a free and appropriate education in either a public or private school.
- The open-ended vaccine mandate allows the State of California to add any additional vaccines it deems necessary in the future.
- The only exemption available is a medical exemption that, up to now, doctors have denied in more than 99% of children.

The rationale for such legislation was the measles outbreak at Disneyland that was sensationalized in the news media and the medical community who warned of an out-of-control epidemic if swift action was not taken. Politicians, backed by the medical establishment and "Big Pharma," pushed for mandatory vaccinations because it was assumed that the unvaccinated were at fault. This led to the draconian SB277 mandatory legislation that all school children must be vaccinated in order to attend public or private school. Let's look at what really happened:

- Approximately, 150 people ended up contracting measles, out of a population of more than 300,000,000 people in the United States.

- How many people developed a severe disability or died as a direct result of the measles? Nobody! This measles outbreak did not even spread to children in the schools.
- Where did it happen? In an amusement park. Does this mean everyone should now be forced to show their vaccination record before being allowed to enter Disneyland?
- Who caused the outbreak? The unvaccinated, or could it be the vaccinated? We do not know, but what we do know is that vaccinated children are able to "shed" the live virus vaccine to others because they are contagious up to 6 weeks or more after being inoculated.
- The use of fear to conjure up the dire predictions regarding a measles outbreak became the justification for enacting SB277, causing a knee-jerk reaction that has taken away the right of parents to determine what medical procedures their children should receive.

Following the passage of the California Senate Bill 277 in 2015, authored by Senator Pan, mandating vaccinations for all children, the rate of autism in kindergarten children in 2016 jumped by **17%**.[18] Many parents who refused vaccines or were behind schedule were suddenly forced to catch up on their children's vaccinations for their children to be allowed to attend school. This sudden vaccine overload, it is argued, coincided with the increased cases of autism.

Related Legislation—In 2019, California Senator Pan introduced new legislation, SB276, under the pretense of addressing the *"proliferation of fraudulent medical exemptions"* by *"a small handful of rogue doctors,"* according to the California Medical Association President, David H. Aizuss, MD.[19] The bill signed into law by Governor Newsom essentially challenges the legitimacy of the doctor-patient relationship regarding vaccine decisions. It gives state health officials the ultimate authority over the family doctor in deciding who will have the final say as to whether an exemption is approved. This stringent legislation further curtails the few vaccine exemptions that still exist, putting at greater risk children who can no longer rely on the judgment of family doctors who know best the children's vulnerabilities, given their personal histories and circumstances.[20]

This legislation would threaten doctors' decision-making by subjecting them to unprecedented supervision and scrutiny if they write more than five exemptions per year or if a school's vaccination rate dips below 95%. Doctors could be put on probation and even lose their medical license if they do not follow these arbitrary measures that essentially nullifies a family doctor's professional judgment. Previous exemptions legally made under SB277, could be negated, and families would have to apply for exemptions again under the new legislative rules. When it comes to vaccinations, Senator Pan, who is a pediatrician, refuses to acknowledge that vaccines have contributed to autism, sudden infant death syndrome (SIDS), or any other neurodevelopmental disorder (NDD), reflecting either his bewildering lack of knowledge or his total disregard for the potential risk of injury due to vaccines. In a November 5, 2015 presentation entitled, "Child Immunization: Herding Parental Concerns" held at the University of California Berkeley campus, Senator Pan made the absurd comment that the most dangerous substance in vaccines is "water," apparently surpassing aluminum, mercury, formaldehyde, and a host of other toxins found in vaccines. When asked to clarify his comment, his illogical response was that more children died from drowning than from vaccines.

Senator Pan has had a cozy relationship with Big Pharma going back to at least 2012, when he sponsored AB2109, requiring a doctor's consultation and signature in order to approve a vaccine exemption. He has been doing the bidding of the pharmaceutical industry ever since. In the 2017–2018 election period alone, Pan received more than $400,000 in personal campaign donations from the healthcare industry.[21] The CDC reported that 21 people contracted measles in California in 2018, out of the state population of approximately 40,000,000. This is the extent to which this supposed "crisis" became the rationale for further restricting the right of parents to obtain vaccine exemptions. Other states are now following the lead of California in presenting similar bills, backed by the pharmaceutical industry, attempting to pass legislation modeled after the SB 277 law enacted in California.

In March 2019, Texas state senator, Bob Hall (R), introduced Senate Bill 2350, which would prohibit vaccines from being administered unless certain safety criteria were met. All vaccines would need to undergo multiyear, double-blind placebo studies over an extended period of testing. In addition, the vaccine manufacturers would be required to test the safety of vaccines in combination.[22] Unfortunately, SB2350 did not pass. Texas would have been the first state to take the lead in assuring the safety of vaccines, bucking the dangerous trend toward the unbridled mandate to vaccinate all children without question.

At the federal level, the House of Representatives attempted to introduce the Bill HR 2232 called the **Vaccinate All Children Act of 2015** which is essentially the federal version of SB 277. It would have eliminated informed consent for vaccinations throughout the entire country. Though this bill did not pass, a new version of the bill, **H.R. 2527 Vaccinate All Children Act of 2019,** was introduced by Congresswoman Frederica Wilson (D-Fl-24) which would prevent all states from allowing vaccine exemptions for anything except medical reasons. Religious and personal exemptions would no longer be allowed. As of now there has not been a roll call vote on the bill though it remains a potential threat. Govtrack.us, which describes the bill in positive terms, references an article by Public Health.org that presents eight *Vaccine Myths Debunked*.[23] It contends that the following assertions are all myths:

1. Vaccines cause autism;
2. Infant immune systems can't handle so many vaccines;
3. Natural immunity is better than vaccine-acquired immunity;
4. Vaccines contain unsafe toxins;
5. Better hygiene and sanitation are actually responsible for decreased infections, not vaccines;
6. Vaccines aren't worth the risk;

7. Vaccines can infect a child with the disease they're trying to prevent;
8. We don't need to vaccinate because infection rates are already so low in the United States.

In fact, all of these so-called "myths" have been validated by scientific research, yet the public continues to be bombarded with statements by the CDC, FDA, and other agencies, backed by Big Pharma's financial influence, to convince the public that vaccines are not a problem. Furthermore, there are those in the medical community who contend that parents who refuse to vaccinate their children, would be grounds for charging them with child neglect and endangerment with the potential of losing custody as a result. As a matter of fact, this has already occurred in cases across the country. It is a scary prospect when the government has the ultimate authority to remove a child from the home against parent's wishes in order to force vaccinations in spite of the real, potential risks of vaccine injury.

Adults in the healthcare profession and teachers in the schools have been given the ultimatum, "Get vaccinated or risk losing employment" and they are not the only ones being targeted for mandatory vaccinations. The requirement is expanding to other areas as well under the guise of protecting the general public. This increasing societal pressure to mandate vaccines on those who refuse to be vaccinated, regardless of one's apprehensions or disapproval, is creating a slippery slope that is limiting an individual's choice when it comes to personal medical decisions. The current attempt to force the COVID-19 vaccine program on people has only intensified this pressure to remove vaccine choice altogether. This is especially abhorrent in the current attempt by government to mandate the experimental COVID-19 vaccines to children down to the age of 6 months.

National Adult Immunization Plan (NAIP)—The medical establishment is now pushing the idea that vaccines should be mandated throughout adulthood in the same way that they are being required for children. The National Adult Immunization Plan (NAIP) developed by the U.S. Dept. of Health and Human Services (DHHS), is driving this very agenda, to mandate vaccines from birth to the grave. It is the government's attempt to increase vaccination rates among adults by 2020 and beyond, by extending mandatory childhood vaccinations into the adult population.[24] The NAIP has four primary objectives:

1. Strengthen the adult immunization infrastructure
2. Improve access to adult vaccines
3. Increase community demand for adult immunizations
4. Foster innovation in adult vaccine development and vaccine-related technologies

The assumption is that healthy adults need to be vaccinated in the same way that children are being vaccinated today. In other words, the government will decide what is best for the adult population just like it has decided what is best for children when it comes to vaccinations. How does informed consent and freedom of choice fit into this plan?

21st Century Cures Act—It gets even worse as a result of both Houses of Congress passing the **21st Century Cures Act** in December 2016, which provides billions of dollars for the NIH and FDA, in order to expedite the process by which new drugs and devices are approved.[25] In essence, the pharmaceutical industry won a major victory, by being able to bring more vaccines and drugs onto the market with fewer safeguards, thanks to the lowered standards for approval, under the pretext of a national medical emergency requiring immediate attention. The bill was largely supported by the drug companies who see this as a large windfall and opposed by consumer organizations, who fear that it will allow more dangerous drugs, vaccines, and ineffective treatments to be approved. The COVID-19 vaccines are a perfect example of how government has given the medical establishment a "green light" to push experimental vaccines on the general populace without the necessary safety testing being done first.

H.R. Bill 6666—In a related story, Representative Bobby Rush (D) of Illinois, in May 2020, sponsored House Bill 6666, called the COVID-19

Testing, Reaching, and Contacting Everyone (TRACE) Act. It would authorize the CDC to award grants, totaling $100 billion in 2020 and unlimited federal funding in future years, for testing, contact tracing, monitoring, and other activities to address COVID-19. It would create and operate a massive surveillance, testing, and tracing enforcement system at the federal level that could violate constitutional rights effecting privacy, due process, and freedom of choice.

The National Vaccine Information Center (NVIC) stated that if this bill was passed by Congress and enacted into law:

> It could lead to denial of an individal's right to appear in public spaces and travel; the right to employment and education or participation in government-funded services, and the right to receive care in a government-funded hospital or any other medical facility.[26]

Well, though Congress did not pass this legislation into law, the federal government has essentially created these same restrictions through the measures that they have taken to limit the public's freedoms under the guise of protecting Americans against the COVID-19 virus.

For the Greater Good

While it is true that vaccines can be protective for some, at least in the short term, it is also true that others can be harmed by the same vaccines. As with all vaccines, there is the potential for injury and even death for those who are biologically, genetically, or environmentally susceptible to an unpredictable adverse reaction. It would seem that forcing vaccinations on everyone in a one-size-fits-all approach without regard for individual differences is problematic, since there is no assurance that a physician can know in advance if an adverse vaccine reaction might occur. In addition, the so-called vaccine safety science is based on studies conducted by the drug companies, who have a dubious track record based on conflicts of interest, which casts doubt on the objectivity of their findings. Regrettably, the pharmaceutical industry and the medical profession are also completely insulated from all liability for harm done as a result of vaccines. As a result, the burden of responsibility falls on the family for the lifelong care of an injured child or the trauma of coming to terms with a child's death. Being forced to take a medical risk without informed consent or the right to refuse vaccination, is a violation of the basic human right to have control over one's own body. Only an individual or parent/guardian should be able to decide how, when, or whether to be vaccinated. Medical exemptions by family doctors need to be protected from intrusion from governmental officials or state medical boards, which do not have the background history or the personal connection with the child to make informed decisions.

Vaccines are licensed by the FDA, recommended by the CDC, mandated by state officials, backed by the medical establishment and the media, which are all influenced by the pharmaceutical interests. Though public officials repeatedly declare that vaccines are safe and effective, the reality is far more complex than what the public is led to believe. Injuries and deaths occur much more often than what is acknowledged by the medical establishment. The "greater good" becomes the rationale for forcing vaccinations on everyone in spite of the inherent risks. Most disturbing is the egregious censorship of information by those in authority whenever facts don't conform to the establishment's narrative. When medical decisions can be taken away from the individual, the question becomes, "What other human rights can be jeopardized under the pretense of protecting the greater society?"

PART II

HOW TIMES HAVE CHANGED

Today's very bright scientists are "Mickey Mousing around" with our genes and our environment without understanding how interconnected everything on this planet is—a course of action bound to have tragic results. —Bruce H. Litton, Ph.D.

Evolution of Man

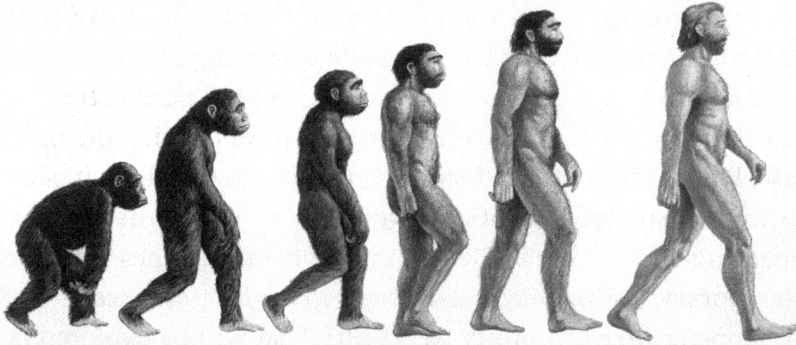

DAVID GIFFORD/SCIENCE PHOTO LIBRARY

Man evolved from primates between 6 and 7 million years ago. The early origin of man goes back approximately 2.5 million years. Modern man evolved around 1 million years ago. To put 1 million years in perspective, if Christ lived 20 centuries ago, modern man evolved over 10,000 centuries before that.

If vaccinations have been around for only roughly 2 centuries (a blip in historical terms), how is it that modern man evolved over eons of time without the benefit of vaccines and managed to survive all of these deadly diseases?

Now it is true that diseases have had a deadly effect over the centuries, such as the bubonic plague (Black Death), but less understood is the fact that diseases have also served a constructive purpose as well. Diseases actually helped mankind by challenging and strengthening the immune system naturally. This is why man has continued to survive in spite of diseases, over a long period of time and well before vaccines were ever introduced.

Vaccination is the process of inoculating numerous substances, including known toxins, such as mercury, aluminum, and formaldehyde, with the intent of fooling the immune system into reacting as though vaccines, with their artificial ingredients, are synonymous with the natural disease. Common sense would tell you that this makes no sense at all. How can something artificially made by man with toxic ingredients, as are added to a vaccine, be able to mimic the same immunizing effect as the naturally occurring disease?

Initially, when vaccines were presented to the public, they were touted as providing complete immunity from contracting the natural disease. But when that turned out to be false, we were told that booster shots were absolutely essential if we wanted to keep diseases from reappearing. The reality is that immunity from vaccines is artificial and temporary, lasting maybe 2–10 years in the best-case scenario. So, what happens after immunity wears off? That will be explored later on in considerable detail.

Attitudes toward childhood diseases have changed dramatically since the 1950s. What happened? In the 1950s, children were given few vaccines and usually at an older age, allowing their immature bodies to develop. Common diseases such as mumps, measles, and chickenpox were viewed as inconvenient but necessary childhood rites of passage. These diseases were not the fearful infectious afflictions back then that they are now portrayed in today's charged climate. The poster below, "How times are changing", showing the difference between 1955 and now, makes one wonder what happened that brought about such a change in attitudes regarding childhood diseases.

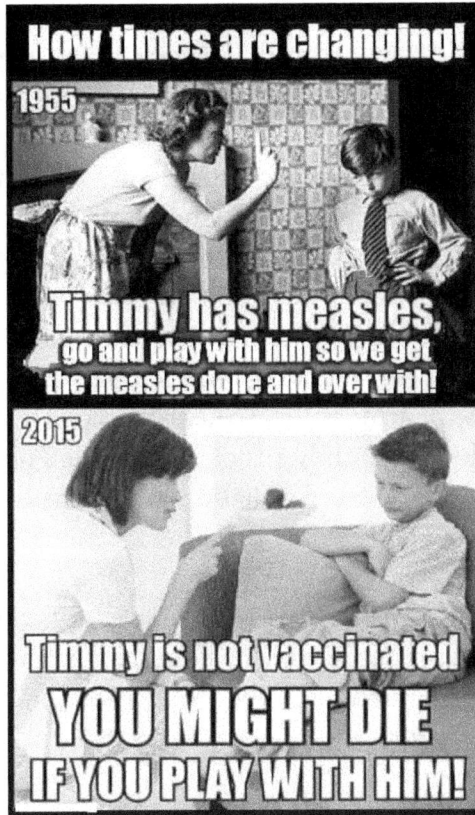

Children growing up in the 1950s were a pretty healthy group as a whole. Autism back then, for most people, was unheard of; children did not get autoimmune diseases like today, and childhood cancers like leukemia were extremely rare. Peanut allergies were not a problem; kids would bring peanut butter and jelly sandwiches to school without any thought of wondering if someone in class was going to have a life-threatening reaction. Today, children allergic to peanuts have to sit at a separate table in the school cafeteria during lunch to avoid a possible adverse reaction. In the 1980s, things started to change as more vaccines started to come onto the market. Increasingly, children were having more adverse reactions, as a result of vaccines such as the DPT shot (diphtheria-pertussis-tetanus) that combined three vaccines in one. *A Shot in the Dark*, by Harris L. Couter and Barbara Loe

Fisher, was the first book to draw attention to the potential dangers of pertussis in the DPT vaccine and gave voice to those families that were being adversely impacted. More and more, the vaccine industry was being taken to court and sued for vaccine injuries. It got so bad that, by the mid-1980s, the drug companies were actually threatening to get out of the vaccine business if the government didn't provide legal protection. This eventually came in the form of legislation passed by Congress in 1986, called the National Childhood Vaccine Injury Act (NCVIA), as previously noted, which removed all drug company liability for any adverse reaction from vaccinations.

How were the pharmaceutical interests able to wield such power? To find out, lets look at both Big Tobacco and Big Pharma to see how these industries worked hand in hand with the medical community and the news media.

Big Tobacco—Big Tobacco denied that smoking cigarettes caused lung cancer for more than 40 years before the medical research could no longer be denied. But back in the 1950s, magazine advertisements showed medical doctors smoking cigarettes while praising the health benefits of smoking.

Some Cigarette advertising examples from the 1950s include:

- Camel cigarettes assert that "NOT ONE SINGLE CASE OF THROAT IRRITATION due to smoking CAMELS!"
- L&M cigarettes advertised, "Leading doctors in the field of cancer research insist …CIGARETTES DO NOT CAUSE CANCER!"
- Ronald Reagan told us, "I'M SENDING CHESTERFIELDS to all my friends. That's the merriest Christmas any smoker can have—Chesterfield mildness plus no unpleasant after-taste."

While that may all seem pretty absurd now given what we know, back in the 1950s, these messages were generally accepted without question. The tobacco industry used doctors and celebrities in their advertisements to convey that cigarettes were healthy and desirable. The influence of money perpetuated this myth for decades until the evidence of harm from cigarette smoking became overwhelming. Nevertheless, as late as 1994, seven chief executives of the tobacco industry went before Congress stating one after the other, under oath, that cigarettes did not cause lung cancer based on "tobacco science," that is "science" manipulated by the tobacco companies to show that cigarettes are safe.[27]

Big Pharma—Today, the pharmaceutical industry denies that vaccines cause autism and other neurodevelopmental disorders. The problem is that Big Pharma is backed by the medical establishment and they're both involved in perpetuating the "vaccine orthodoxy." One area of difference between Big Tobacco and Big Pharma is the fact that the public can sue tobacco companies in court, but they have no recourse when it comes to suing the pharmaceutical industry for vaccine injuries.

Evidence of the vaccine–autism connection has been documented by Mary Holland and Lou Conte who reviewed Vaccine Court cases, in which they found that financial payments have been made to 83 families of children who developed autism as a result of *"vaccine-induced brain damage."*[28] Yet, the CDC website perpetuates the false claim that *"vaccines do not cause autism,"* when in fact, it knew quite well that there was an obvious link between the two. While continuing to dismiss any connection between vaccines and autism, the CDC continues to fall back on genetics as the primary explanation for autism. A study published in the journal *JAMA Psychiatry,* concludes:

> *Based on the data, about 80% of their risk of developing the condition [autism] was due to genetics, with the remainder of the risk tied to as-yet-unidentified environmental causes… we are not yet able to identify a specific genetic cause for autism in many children.*[29]

The fact that tens of thousands of parents have witnessed their children regress into autism after being vaccinated is dismissed outright by the "experts," and viewed as simply anecdotal, less than scientific, therefore not to be taken seriously.

U.S. Childhood Statistics—Then and Now—In 1950, the United States had the third lowest infant-mortality rate in the world. That is the number of infant deaths in the first year of life. By 1960, the U.S. infant mortality slipped to 12th and by 2005, it was 30th. Today, the U.S. ranks 54th in infant mortality, behind all other **'developed'** countries in the world, according to the Central Intelligence Agency (CIA) website.[30]

Now, more than half of the children in the nation have some type of chronic condition: autism, asthma, allergies, attention deficit disorder, childhood cancers, learning and language disabilities, mental retardation, motor delays, autoimmune diseases, seizures, obesity, and so on. This is based on a 2011–12 National Survey of Children's Health study conducted by the U.S. DHHS, involving 96,000 children between birth and 17 years old; **54%** of the children surveyed had at least 1 out of 20 chronic illnesses.[31] Comparing these recent statistics with the 1994 estimates of 12.8% chronic illnesses, it shows a dramatic 4-fold increase in childhood disorders in less than 20 years, as reflected in some of the data highlighted below:

- **Asthma**—Back in 1980, asthma occurred in 1 out of 27 children. According to the CDC, it is up to 1 in 13 today, more than a twofold increase, meaning that approximately 8.7% of children have an asthmatic condition.[32] In another study, 17.7% of 5.5-year-olds had been classified as having asthma.[33]
- **Learning disabilities**—In 1976, 1 in 30 children were classified as having a learning disability; today, it is 1 in 5 children when including attention issues that also affect learning.[34]
- **Attention deficit/hyperactive disorder (ADHD)** has increased 400% in a 30-year period between 1985 and 2015. In one study, as many as 16% of children were classified as having a hyperactive disorder.[35]
- **Food allergies** have also increased by 400% between 1985 and 2015, with milk, eggs, shellfish, wheat, yeast, and nuts,

being the most common. Today, 5–10% of U.S. children have some form of food sensitivities, with peanut allergies affecting up to 3% of children.[36]

- **Seizure disorders** have increased dramatically with as many as 1 in 20 children under the age of 5 having been diagnosed with some form of epilepsy. That is 5% of all children in this age group.[37]

- **Autism** in the United States, by any statistical measure, is at epidemic levels, going from 1 in 10,000 in 1970 to 1 in 36 in 2018.[38] In New Jersey, the rate of autism in boys alone was as high as **1 in 20** in 2016.[39] Some estimates put the current percentage of children in the U.S. with autism at 3 percent.[40] In 2020, it was estimated that *"close to a hundred thousand American children per year are being diagnosed with ASD."*[41]

- **Childhood cancers,** like leukemia, occur most often between 1 and 4 years of age, around the same time that children are being given numerous vaccinations. Before 1960, cancers in children were an anomaly, but not today. In January 2020, the American Cancer Society (ACS) stated, *"After accidents, cancer is the second leading cause of death in children ages 1 to 14."*[42]

What happened to create such an historic increase in these childhood disorders? For sure, environmental causes are at play here. There are thousands of chemicals that can contribute to developmental neurotoxicity, such as PCB's, solvents, lead, mercury, and arsenic which have been associated with autism and other neurodevelopmental disorders. Vaccines alone contain over 60 chemicals, many of which are toxic, that must also be considered when one takes into account the numerous vaccines that children receive today. In fact, there is a direct correlation between the increasing number of vaccines given, starting in the late 1980s and the early 1990s, and the dramatic rise in autism and other disorders.

What Causes Autism?—The answer depends on where you get your information. On the CDC website, the following risk factors for autism are listed: genes, genetic or chromosomal conditions, children who have a sibling with ASD, prescription drugs taken during pregnancy like valproic acid and thalidomide, critical periods before, during, and immediately after birth, and children born to older parents.[43] But, when it comes to addressing vaccines as a possible cause, the CDC unequivocally states that there is no connection. Unfortunately, there are numerous scientific studies that dispute such persistent denials. While it is true that a genetic predisposition has been associated with autism, the toxic ingredients in vaccines are the primary triggers that have been shown in laboratory studies to cause neurotoxicity. For example, toxins in vaccines have been shown to damage the myelin sheath, the protective coating that surrounds the nerve fibers in the brain, optic nerves, and spinal cord. This is referred to as demyelination, in which the nerve cells that facilitate the passing along of electrical impulses in the CNS are damaged, causing neurological problems.

Beldeu Singh, Panjab University professor in India, completed a comprehensive review of 205 vaccine studies showing the neurotoxic effects of vaccine ingredients, namely mercury and aluminum, which can precipitate neurodevelopmental disorders (NDD) including autism. He emphasized that this is especially critical when vaccinating infants in the first 6 months of life, before the immune system is allowed to mature, which *"makes the CNS especially vulnerable to toxic agents."*[44] The body's inability to detoxify these poisonous substances further weakens the immune system that can contribute to the onset of autistic behaviors. Even drugs such as acetaminophen (Tylenol), in combination with vaccines, has been shown to deplete glutathione, an antioxidant that helps to eliminate heavy metals from the body, *"increasing the risk for autism."*[45] The role of vaccinations in causing a whole range of neurodevelopmental disorders and autoimmune conditions will be discussed in greater detail in Parts III, IV, and V.

Rates of Autism—Autism showed a dramatic increase starting around 1990, at the same time that hepatitis B, Hib, and an additional measles and DTaP were added to the vaccine schedule. In 1970, the autism rate was approximately 1 in 10,000; as of 2020, autism is up to 1 in 30 children in the U.S., as the chart below indicates.[46] (*Treffert et al., CDC*)

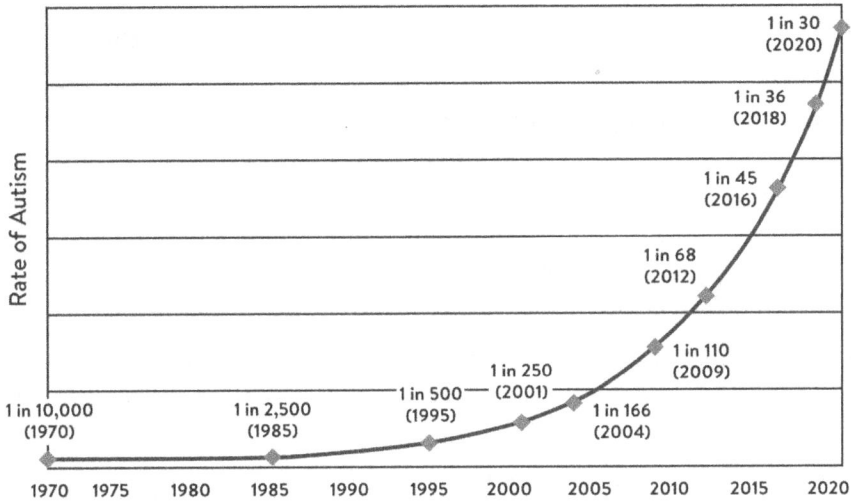

Dr. Stephanie Seneff, a senior research scientist at the Massachusetts Institute of Technology (MIT), predicted that, if the current trend continues, the autism rate could reach one in every two boys by 2032.[47] The prospect of so many children becoming autistic by that time would be catastrophic, overwhelming the educational system, confounding healthcare services, and placing an enormous strain on the family, both emotionally and financially. Predicting this rate of autism in the not-too-distant future might seem outlandish, but if someone had suggested back in 1970 that a rare condition like autism would go from 1 in 10,000 to less than 1 in 40 children today, it would have been viewed as inconceivable.

On December 2, 2021, the CDC released the latest estimates for autism based on data from the Autism and Developmental Disabilities Monitoring (ADDM) Network. The report indicated that California surpassed New Jersey for the highest rates of autism among 8-year-old boys, with 6.4% having an autism spectrum disorder (ASD). The report also showed that "autism prevalence has increased continuously over twenty years in the U.S. and that autism affects as many as 4%

of children born in 2010." The overall rate of ASD has increased 23% in just the past 2 years.[48]

What Happened? Vaccines Happened!—In the 1950s, if the parents were so inclined, children may have received four to seven vaccine doses at the most, by the time they were **6 years old.** Fast-forward to today, when children are given as many as 26 vaccines doses by the time that they are **6 months old,** based on the recommended CDC vaccine schedule. This doesn't include what vaccines the child may have been exposed to via the mother while in utero, which also carries potential risks for the developing fetus.

A few hours after birth, an 8-pound baby receives 250 micrograms (mcg) of aluminum in the hepatitis B vaccine; that exceeds roughly 14 times the amount of aluminum that is FDA-approved.[49] The newborn also receives the vitamin K shot, which contains a number of toxins including sodium acetate anhydrous, aluminum, benzyl alcohol, propylene glycol, and polysorbate 80. Vitamin K is supposed to prevent the possibility of bleeding problems in which the blood is unable to clot, a condition which is extremely rare in newborns, yet for which a vaccine is routinely given.

The remaining shots given to infants in the first 6 months of life, as recommended by the CDC, are listed below:

- At 2 months old, infants receive 8 vaccines:
  Diphtheria, Tetanus, Pertussis (DTaP), Inactivated polio (IPV), Rotavirus, Hemophilus Influenzae Type B Meningitis (Hib), Pneumococcal Conjugate (PCV 13), and Hepatitis B (HepB).
- At 4 months old, they are given 7 more vaccines:
  DTaP (3 in 1), IPV, Rotavirus, PCV 13, Hib.
- At 6 months old, 9 more vaccines:
  DTaP (3 in 1), IPV, Rotavirus, Hib, PCV 13, HepB, and influenza (Flu).
- By 18 months old, babies will have received 36 vaccine doses.

The following graph lists the number of vaccines given to children up to the age of 6, according to country. One can easily see that the United States has the most, however, this chart does not tell the complete story. In 2019, the CDC schedule had children receiving 49 vaccine doses by the time they are 6, if parents were to follow the recommended immunizations.

(*Source: CDC Recommended Immunizations for Children from Birth Through 6 Years Old*).

Number of Vaccines ≤ 6 Years Old

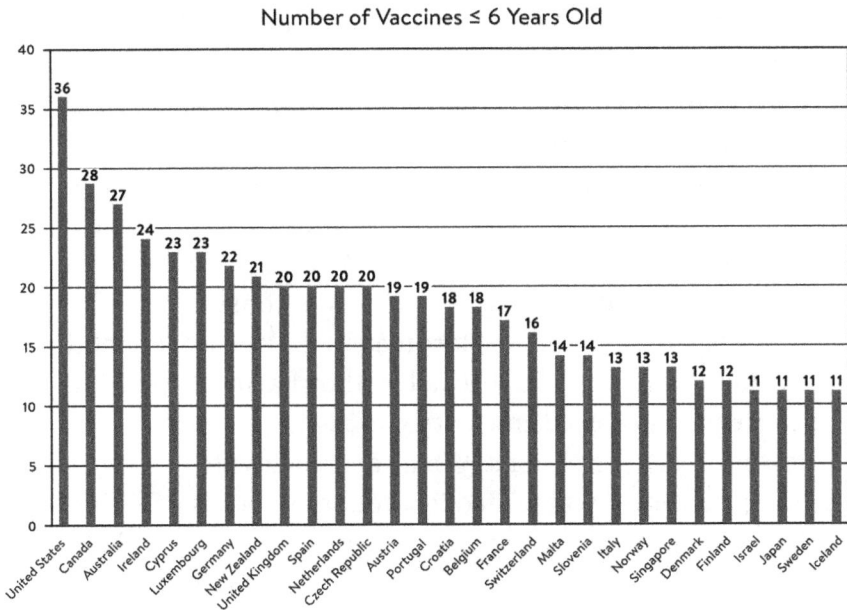

To put this in perspective, children in Japan are some of the least vaccinated children in the developed countries of the world, while having one of the healthiest outcomes based on life expectancy. Back in 1975, when Japan first raised its minimum vaccination age to 2 years, its overall infant-mortality rate went from 17th place to the lowest infant mortality rate in the world. Though the Japanese 2002 vaccine schedule changed to nine vaccines being recommended in the first 2 years of life, nevertheless Japan still has one of the lowest rates of infant mortality in the first year of life. In contrast, the United States has roughly three times as many infant deaths in the same period of time.[50]

In 1994, Japan made the decision that vaccinations should be voluntary instead of mandatory. Consequently, there is no vaccine requirement for Japanese children entering preschool or elementary school. Infants do not receive the hepatitis B vaccine at birth unless the mother tests positive for hepatitis which occurs in significantly less than 1% of all pregnancies. Japan does not vaccinate pregnant mothers or infants with the flu shot. The Tdap vaccine is also not given to expectant mothers. The measles-rubella vaccine (MR) excludes the mumps vaccine and the human papillomavirus vaccine (HPV) is no longer recommended as a result of serious adverse reactions that have prompted numerous lawsuits.[51]

The following chart by *LearnTheRisk.com* reflects the explosion in mandated vaccines over approximately the past 50 years. All of these vaccines contain a multitude of toxins that have overloaded children to such an extent that it has caused detrimental consequences based on numerous scientific studies. Unfortunately, the medical establishment and the mainstream media, backed by the pharmaceutical industry, have conveniently avoided any serious discussion of research that shows the downside of vaccinations. What we are left with is the failure of the U.S. government and related institutions to protect children, who are the most vulnerable recipients of these vaccines.

VACCINES DOSES for U.S. CHILDREN

1962	1983	2018	
TOTAL DOSES: 5	**TOTAL DOSES: 24**	**TOTAL DOSES: 72**	
Polio	DTP (2 months)	Influenza (pregnancy)	Influenza (18 months)
Smallpox	OPV (2 months)	DTaP (pregnancy)	Hep A (18 months)
DTP	DTP (4 months)	Hep B (birth)	Influenza (30 months)
	OPV (4 months)	Hep B (2 months)	Influenza (42 months)
	DTP (6 months)	Rotavirus (2 months)	DTaP (4 years)
	MMR (15 months)	DTaP (2 months)	IPV (4 years)
	DTP (18 months)	HIB (2 months)	MMR (4 years)
	OPV (18 months)	PCV (2 months)	Varicella (4 years)
	DTP (4 years)	IPV (2 months)	Influenza (5 years)
	OPV (4 years)	Rotavirus (4 months)	Influenza (6 years)
	Td (15 years)	DTaP (4 months)	Influenza (7 years)
		HIB (4 months)	Influenza (8 years)
		PCV (4 months)	Influenza (9 years)
		IPV (4 months)	HPV (9 years)
		Hep B (6 months)	Influenza (10 years)
		Rotavirus (6 months)	HPV (10 years)
		DTaP (6 months)	Influenza (11 years)
		HIB (6 months)	HPV (11 years)
		PCV (6 months)	DTaP (12 years)
		IPV (6 months)	Influenza (12 years)
		Influenza (6 months)	Meningococcal (12 years)
		Influenza (7 months)	Influenza (13 years)
		HIB (12 months)	Influenza (14 years)
		PCV (12 months)	Influenza (15 years)
		MMR (12 months)	Influenza (16 years)
		Varicella (12 months)	Meningococcal (16 years)
		Hep A (12 months)	Influenza (17 years)
		DTaP (18 months)	Influenza (18 years)

*In 1986, pharmaceutical companies producing vaccines were given full federal protection from lawsuits resulting from vaccine injury or death via the Childhood Vaccine Injury Act passed by Congress. If vaccines are so safe, why did they need a law to protect from liability?

After this law, vaccines became HIGHLY profitable. There are almost 300 vaccines in development, and mandatory vaccine laws for children — and ADULTS — being pushed in most states.

The US gives 2-3x more vaccines to children than most developed countries, yet we have skyrocketing rates of childhood issues that are NOT seen in other countries. Things like asthma, childhood diabetes, food allergies, childhood leukemia, developmental delays, tics, ADHD, autism, lupus, arthritis, eczema, epilepsy, Alzheimers, brain damage, etc. . . It's NOT a coincidence.

Vaccines contain toxic chemicals that do NOT belong in our bodies, such as aluminum (known to cause brain and developmental damage even in small doses), polysorbate 80, MSG and formaldehyde (known to cause cancer in humans). .

LEARN THE RISK.ORG
Knowledge • Action • Health

Vaccinated vs. Unvaccinated Children—The logical way to evaluate the effectiveness of vaccines would be to look at the comparison between vaccinated and unvaccinated children. Yet the CDC has refused to study the differences under the spurious premise that it would be unethical to withhold vaccinations from children. What might be another reason for avoiding such a study? Could it be that the findings might show that vaccines aren't as efficacious as they are portrayed? Well, fortunately we do have independent studies that have investigated the differences between these two groups of children.

Glanz and Newcomer (2013), who analyzed more than 300,000 cases of children under 2 years, concluded,

> *Children who were under-vaccinated because of parental choice had significantly lower utilization rates of the emergency department and outpatient settings than children who were vaccinated on time.*[52]

In a 2017 study highlighted below, Anthony R. Mawson et al., compared the health outcomes of 6- to 12-year-old vaccinated children versus the unvaccinated, based on the results of a parent survey. The researchers found that

> *The vaccinated were less likely than the unvaccinated to have been diagnosed with chickenpox and pertussis, but more likely to have been diagnosed with pneumonia, otitis media, allergies and NDD...While vaccination remained significantly associated with NDD after controlling for other factors, preterm birth coupled with vaccination was associated with an apparent synergistic increase in the odds of NDD.*[53]

[NDD: Neurodevelopmental disorders include learning disabilities, attention deficit hyperactive disorder (ADHD), and autism spectrum disorder (ASD)].

The chart below shows the results of the parent survey indicating that vaccinated children had 2.4 x's chronic diseases, 2.9 x's eczema, 3.7 x's neurodevelopmental disorders, 4.2 x's autism, 4.2 x's ADHD, 5.2 x's learning disabilities, and 30.1 x's allergic rhinitis (hay fever), when compared to the unvaccinated children.

A new groundbreaking survey of hundreds of homeschooled American children found that, compared to the UNVACCINATED children, the VACCINATED children had higher odds of developing the following conditions.

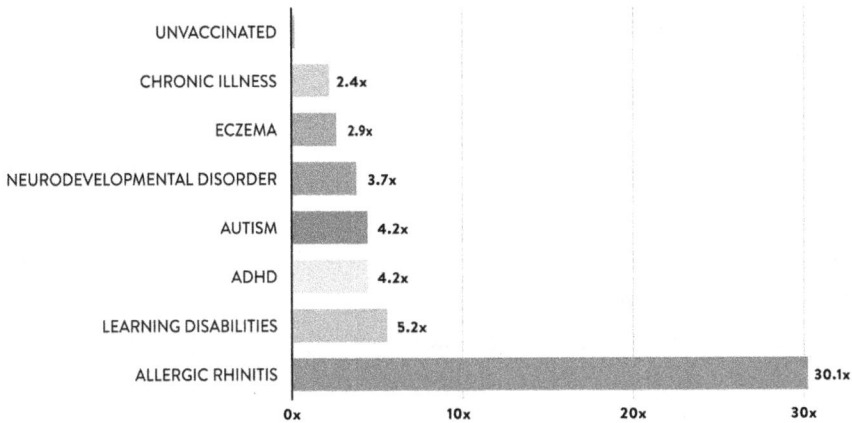

UNVACCINATED	
CHRONIC ILLNESS	2.4x
ECZEMA	2.9x
NEURODEVELOPMENTAL DISORDER	3.7x
AUTISM	4.2x
ADHD	4.2x
LEARNING DISABILITIES	5.2x
ALLERGIC RHINITIS	30.1x

0x   10x   20x   30x

Above graph courtesy of the Children's Medical Safety Research Institute (CMSRI) showing the research findings from Mawson, et al.

In a June 2021 paper by Hooker and Miller, entitled *"Health effects in vaccinated versus unvaccinated children, covariates for breastfeeding status and type of birth,"* the parents of 1565 children from 3 pediatric medical practices were interviewed, in order to compare fully vaccinated, partially vaccinated, and unvaccinated children. Again, the results confirmed that the unvaccinated had less severe allergies, autism, gastrointestinal disorders, asthma, ADD/ADHD, and chronic ear infections.

> *Results from the analysis of relationships between vaccination and breastfeeding status showed that the lowest percentages of adverse diagnosis were observed for unvaccinated and breastfed children; the highest were observed for vaccinated and not breastfed children.*[54]

This points to the importance of breastfeeding in helping to pass on the protective immunity to children from their mothers, as opposed to the artificial baby formulas advanced by monetary considerations that serve to undermine the natural and superior protection of breastfeeding.

Another source highlighting the differences between vaccinated and unvaccinated children is the movie sequel, *VAXXED II.* Through family interviews, the film shows in dramatic and vivid detail how the unvaccinated children were much healthier with fewer hospitalizations and medical interventions required than the vaccinated. The parents reported that their children got sick less often, were less likely to use antibiotics, and had fewer allergies, asthma, and other health issues.

A Harvard immunologist, Dr. Obukhanych, wrote an open letter in 2020 to federal legislators to correct several misperceptions about vaccines, asserting that unvaccinated children do not pose a threat to others. She concluded by stating:

> *In summary, a person who is not vaccinated with IPV, DTaP, HepB, and Hib vaccines due to reasons of conscience poses no extra danger to the public than a person who is. No discrimination is warranted...Taken together, these data make it apparent that elimination of vaccine exemptions, currently only utilized by a small percentage of families anyway, will neither solve the problem of disease resurgence nor prevent re-importation and outbreaks of previously eliminated diseases.*[55]

PART III

ASSUMPTIONS ABOUT VACCINES

"Are vaccines protecting people, or do we just think they are?" —Cynthia Cournoyer, *What About Immunizations?*

- **Four Major Assumptions About Vaccines:**

1. Vaccines are safe and the benefits of vaccines far outweigh any risks.
2. Vaccines are effective and long lasting—they are necessary to keep diseases from returning.
3. Vaccines have wiped out all the major diseases like smallpox and polio.
4. There is no connection between vaccines and autism or any other neurodevelopmental disabilities.

Assumption 1—Vaccines Are Safe, and Benefits Outweigh the Risks

Today, the notion that vaccines are safe and that the benefits far outweigh any risks permeates society at every level beginning in early childhood and continuing into adulthood. It is reinforced in the schools, praised in the media, backed by the medical community, and confirmed by public officials who simply parrot the vaccine orthodoxy. In essence, vaccines have become the "sacred cow" of medicine, not to be questioned but instead accepted as indisputably beneficial;

those who dare to question the efficacy of vaccines are seen not only as naïve and uninformed but also a threat to the safety of children. In the mainstream media, these parents are summarily discredited and labeled as stupid and met with disdain. Government officials, backed by the medical establishment, have increasingly responded by pushing vaccine mandates, while viewing those who dissent as unaware and irresponsible, in spite of the fact that vaccine skeptics tend to be highly educated and well versed on the subject of vaccine research.

National Childhood Vaccine Injury Act (NCVIA)—It was during the 1980s that parents started expressing their concerns based on vaccine injuries that resulted in numerous lawsuits being filed against the pharmaceutical industry. It was becoming increasingly problematic for the drug companies owing to the high legal costs being incurred. So much so that, as indicated previously, the manufacturers threatened to stop producing vaccines unless they were released from all liability. Consequently the U.S. Congress passed the National Childhood Vaccine Injury Act (NCVIA) which removed all responsibility from the vaccine manufacturers, as well as doctors, for any adverse vaccine reactions. It would stand to reason that if the drug companies were threatening to stop making vaccines altogether because of numerous lawsuits claiming injuries, vaccines couldn't be that safe, could they?

A report from the Dept. of Health and Human Services (DHHS) indicated that, between 1988 and 2015, 15,747 people filed petitions for compensation through the **National Vaccine Injury Compensation Program (NVICP)** based on vaccine injuries. The **Vaccine Adverse Event Reporting System (VAERS)** was set up to record all such injuries; however, the number actually reported is considered a small fraction of the total figure because parents, doctors, and the drug companies were not given clear guidelines for data to be collected. Many parents and doctors were not even aware of a reporting system to begin with, and if they were, the criteria for reporting adverse reactions were left vague. For almost 3 decades, the CDC did nothing to correct this "passive surveillance system" in spite of its own acknowledgment that *"…determining causal associations between vaccines and adverse events is usually not possible."*[56]

The DHHS finally sponsored a $1 million study through Harvard Medical School to create an automated reporting system to more accurately identify adverse reactions from vaccinations, given that *"Fewer than 1% of vaccine adverse events are reported,"*[57] based on the VAERS passive reporting system. To be clear, that means more than 99% of vaccine injuries were not being reported, according to the government's own sponsored study. Harvard Pilgrim Healthcare collected data from 2006 to 2009 on 376,452 patients who were given 1.4 million vaccine doses and 35,570 possible adverse reactions ended up being reported over the 3-year period. Vaccine injuries occurred in 1 out of 39 vaccinations or 2.6% of the children. This is a far cry from the typical claims made by the medical community that vaccine injuries are "one in a million."[58] But the CDC conveniently ignored the results of the Harvard study that was charged with upgrading the vaccine safety surveillance system. Why? Because it contradicted the CDC's claim that side effects from vaccines are exceedingly rare. Once again, we see that anything that goes up against the "vaccine orthodoxy" is censored accordingly.

Instead of addressing the obvious concerns regarding vaccine injuries and how to make a safer product, the pharmaceutical industry has essentially been given the green light to push for more vaccines without fear of any penalty, providing Big Pharma with an ongoing stream of vaccine mandates with no end in sight.

It is instructive to note that, since the 1950s, the CDC has taken numerous vaccines off the market for one reason or another, which raises the question, What was so wrong with those vaccines that they were discontinued? If vaccines were described as "safe and effective," why would so many be replaced by a newer and apparently better version? That would suggest that vaccines are not always as effective and risk free as they are purported to be. What reassurance does the public have that these "new and improved" vaccines won't also be supplanted by yet another vaccine deemed to be better still? For example, Tripedia, the diphtheria and tetanus toxoids and acellular pertussis vaccine, was taken off the market in 2012 by Sanofi Pasteur, owing to adverse events being reported. The manufacturer listed the following adverse reactions in its vaccine product insert:

> *Idiopathic thrombocytopenic purpura, SIDS, anaphylactic reaction, cellulitis, **autism,** convulsion/grand mal convulsion, encephalopathy, hypotonia, neuropathy, somnolence and apnea. Events were included in this list because of the seriousness or frequency of reporting.*

Then the following caveat was added:

> *Because these events are reported voluntarily from a population of uncertain size, it is not always possible to reliably estimate their frequencies or to establish a causal relationship to components of Tripedia vaccine.*[59]

This is a convenient way to dismiss those who have reported these adverse events, as being ostensibly unreliable sources.

The National Vaccine Injury Compensation Program (NVICP) that was established in 1988, as part of the NCVIA, is summarized as follows. It is also referred to as the "Vaccine Court," though it isn't really a court in the traditional sense.

- In the Vaccine Court, there is no standard legal process with a judge, jury, or open court proceedings.
- Parents are unable to sue pharmaceutical companies because they have been exempted from any liability in the case of a vaccine injury, whereas parents could sue in the case of any type of prescription-drug injury.
- Families have to petition the DHHS and argue their case before a Special Master, who is a political appointee by the Dept. of Justice (DOJ) who presides over a private hearing and issues a ruling without reporters being present.

- Because the Special Master is an agent of the government and a defendant in the Vaccine Court, his role is seen as adversarial. The burden of proof falls on the family and their attorney to get the court to admit that the vaccine caused their child's injury and to seek compensation for the child's care.
- The Vaccine Court relies on thorough medical records while conversely discounting parental reports of injury as being circumstantial and less than scientific.
- The Vaccine Court is not obligated to make data available, and the DOJ stipulates that all records are kept confidential so the public has no way to confirm the rationale for decisions made.
- Because the petitioner has no subpoena power, the vaccine maker does not have to participate in the proceedings and incriminating documents held by the vaccine manufacturers can remain hidden. In addition, most doctors are reluctant to testify at the hearing for fear of self-incrimination.
- Many families may simply not know that there is a program for compensation because the Vaccine Court is not readily publicized by doctors, government officials, and others.
- There is a 3-year time frame within which an injury must be reported. Initially parents may not understand the cause of these injuries due to a delayed vaccine reaction. By the time they attempt to file for compensation, the 3-year time frame may have passed, preventing them from receiving any reparations.
- Cases can often drag on for years, with the average settlement taking more than 3 years, causing a financial hardship for the families seeking compensation. Plaintiff lawyers have waited as much as a decade or more (the longest being 14 years) before being paid for their services. Consequently, some families end up being left without legal representation.

- Two thirds of all injury claims are rejected outright, and, of those cases that are adjudicated, compensation is capped at $250,000, even if the child dies as a result of the vaccine. The actual cost for the care of an autistic child over a lifetime is estimated to start around $2.5 million and increase substantially from there, depending on the severity of the child's condition.
- Since 1986, DHHS was supposed to study vaccine injuries and report to Congress every two years on working to improve vaccine safety standards, but in the last **30 years,** not one report has ever been submitted to Congress.[60]

[An excellent YouTube video narrated by Rob Schneider called, *"Do Vaccines Cause Autism?"* explains the Vaccine Court process in greater detail.]

Refer to **Appendix B** to get information on **How to Report an Adverse Event to VAERS** (Vaccine Adverse Event Reporting System).

As noted previously, Mary Holland, a legal scholar trained at Harvard and Columbia Universities, and Lou Conte, both parents of autistic children, studied 150 cases of children compensated through the NVICP and found that 83 of them qualified as being autistic. However, the vaccine court would not compensate children with an autism diagnosis, so the term "encephalopathy" had to be used in order to receive compensation from the Vaccine Court. Encephalopathy is a generalized term that refers to any disease or disorder affecting the brain.

In this January 2011 study, published in the *Pace Environmental Law Review*, Holland et al. concluded:

> *While there are likely many routes to "autism," including prenatal neurological insults and toxic post-natal exposures, this preliminary analysis of VICP-compensated cases suggest that autism is often associated with vaccine-induced*

brain damage… Based on this preliminary assessment,
there may be no meaningful distinction between the cases
of encephalopathy and residual seizure disorder that the
VICP compensated over the last 20 years and the cases of
"autism" that the VICP has denied.[61]

Robert F, Kennedy Jr., founder of the Children's Health Defense (CHD), has been one of the most vocal advocates for vaccine safety and one of the most knowledgeable individuals on the scientific and political implications regarding the issues surrounding vaccination. Unfortunately, he has been intentionally blacklisted from the mainstream media after Big Pharma's threat to stop funding news organizations that allow any dissenting views to be aired that would dare to challenge the "vaccine orthodoxy."

In a March 13, 2018 article from the CHD, entitled, *Congress Receives Vaccine Safety Project Details, Including Actions Needed for Sound Science and Transparency*, Kennedy wrote:

Insistence on fully-informed consent and individual rights
to refuse a vaccination become imperative given the lack of
long-term follow-up and surveillance; only 1% of adverse
events are captured and reported; vaccine recommendations
are tainted by financial conflicts of interest of regulators;
the current childhood vaccine schedule was not approved
using evidence-based science and policy; the childhood
vaccine schedule has never been tested on fully vaccinated
vs. unvaccinated; and there is sparse research into which
patients are likely to experience an adverse event.[62]

Given the sheer number of vaccines that infants receive today, there should be cause for concern because it is virtually impossible to predict one's susceptibility to an adverse reaction, owing to the toxic overload of vaccine ingredients that accumulate in the body over time. There is an abundance of scientific research that shows that the more vaccines given at one time, the greater the probability of children requiring hospitalization and a greater likelihood of dying.[63]

What is clear from analyzing the vaccination schedules of 34 developed nations is that the United States has the worst infant-mortality rate of all these countries, while at the same time, it administers the most childhood vaccines.[64] In spite of reassurances by the vaccine makers, the medical community, such as the AMA and AAP, and various government agencies, such as the CDC, FDA, and National Institute of Health (NIH), that vaccines are safe and pose little or no risk, the scientific literature tells a different story. This is especially apparent when considering what is put into these vaccines.

Vaccine Ingredients—There are more than 60 chemicals in vaccines, many of which have been proven toxic to the human body. To make matters worse, the damage caused when these ingredients are combined magnifies the deleterious effects. The major toxins found in vaccines are summarized as follows:

- **Aluminum** is a heavy metal used in vaccines that has been linked to symptoms associated with inflammation of the brain, autoimmune disorders and neurological diseases, including chronic fatigue, dementia, autism, macrophagic myofasciitis, Alzheimer's, Lou Gehrig's disease (amyotrophic lateral sclerosis [ALS]), lupus, multiple sclerosis (MS), and Parkinson's disease.[65]

  In the 1970s, children got only four vaccines containing aluminum in the first 18 months of life. Today, children get 17 vaccines with aluminum in that same period of time. A 2018 study published in the *Journal of Trace Elements in Medicine and Biology* showed that the CDC vaccine schedule exceeded the FDA safety level for aluminum by **17 times** for infants on the first day of life when adjusted for body weight.[66] Aluminum has been shown to kill brain cells based on research from animal studies. It is considered too toxic to study in humans, especially in the developing brain of infants. When aluminum is injected into the body, a certain amount can end up in a person's bones, brain, and various other tissues, especially when given in large amounts from multiple vaccines at one time. In the first 6 months of life alone, infants can receive up to 1475 micrograms of aluminum at each of the 2-, 4-, and 6-month vaccine scheduled appointments, damaging the nervous system and causing autoimmune disorders.[67]

When aluminum is combined with other vaccine toxins, such as thimerosal, lead, fluoride, formaldehyde, phenoxyethanol, and polysorbate 80, there is a synergistic effect that is much more toxic than any one ingredient alone.[68]

In a 2017 study entitled, *Short Review of Aluminum Hydroxide Related Lesions in Preclinical Studies and Their Relevance*, by Nils Warfving, et al, it stated:

> *aluminum is a well-demonstrated toxin in biological systems and its specific impacts on the nervous system have been widely documented...It must also be recognized that aluminum compounds may vary in their toxic potential depending on the specific route of administration. Mice **fed** with aluminum hydroxide...did not reveal neurodevelopmental damage, while **parenteral (injected)** administration of aluminum chloride in rats...caused material deaths, embryo lethality, growth retardation, and fetal abnormalities.[69]*

This study highlights how aluminum when orally ingested is allowed to pass through the gastrointestinal tract and be eliminated from the body with less than 1% being absorbed. In contrast, when aluminum is injected directly into the body via vaccination, the absorption is nearly 100%. This illustrates the inherent problem with equating the oral ingestion of chemicals, such as aluminum, with the injection of vaccines. The vaccine ingredients are absorbed into the circulatory system, where they can accumulate in different organs of the body, with no clear path for elimination.

An example of the toxic effects of aluminum adjuvants in vaccines is macrophagic myofasciitis (MMF), a muscle disease causing joint pain and stiffness that was first identified in 1993. The researchers concluded that

> *the MMF lesion is secondary to intramuscular injection of aluminum hydroxide-containing vaccines, shows both long-term persistence of aluminum hydroxide and an ongoing local immune reaction, and is detected in patients with systemic symptoms which appeared subsequently to vaccination.*[70]

Sealey et al. studied environmental factors affecting autism, stating,

> *A comprehensive literature search has implicated several environmental factors associated with the development of ASD. These include pesticides, phthalates, polychlorinated biphenyls, solvents, air pollutants, fragrances, glyphosate, and heavy metals, **especially aluminum used in vaccines as adjuvants**.*[71]

Aluminum is used in the DTaP, HepA, HepB, Hib, HPV, Meningococcal, Polio, and Prevnar vaccines.

- **Formaldehyde** is a human carcinogen that poses a significant danger to human health because of its toxicity and volatility, according to the *U.S. National Toxicology Program* (2011).[72] It is used in embalming corpses and has been implicated in childhood cancers like leukemia and in adult disorders like Alzheimer's disease. In vaccines, it is used as a preservative. According to the *National Research Council,* it is estimated that formaldehyde is able to trigger an allergic reaction in roughly 10%–20% of the general population.[73] Though the FDA states, *"There is no evidence linking cancer to infrequent exposure to tiny amounts of formaldehyde via injection as occurs with vaccines,"*[74] it does not consider the combined level of exposure when given multiple doses of vaccines containing formaldehyde at one time. Formaldehyde is used in the following vaccines: HepB, DTaP, polio (IPV), Hib, influenza, and HepA, which would result in the child receiving a total of 1,795 micrograms (mcg) by the time he or she is 5 years old.[75]

Challenging the immature immune system of an infant with high levels of formaldehyde injected directly into the body is not the same as the relatively small amounts of formaldehyde from indirect environmental sources, such as cigarette smoke, car-exhaust fumes, flame-retardant chemicals, polyester fibers, and personal-care products. Nevertheless, more than 100 adverse effects from environmental formaldehyde exposure have been identified as causing damage to various organs in the body, including the brain and central nervous system (CNS). Curiously, studies done on formaldehyde have been based only on the toxic effects from **inhalation or ingestion,** according to the *Environmental Defense Fund.* No studies have ever been done to determine the safety of **injecting** formaldehyde directly into the immature bodies of newborn infants and children, who are exposed to much higher levels of formaldehyde.[76]

- **Thimerosal (Ethylmercury)** is a toxic heavy metal that is 49.55% mercury by weight and is considered the second most poisonous element on Earth after the radioactive element uranium and its derivatives. In spite of that, thimerosal is used as a preservative and an adjuvant in vaccines. Though thimerosal has been used since roughly 1930, safety testing has been woefully absent. Studies initially performed on animals as well as humans have had deadly results, yet the Eli Lilly drug company declared thimerosal to be safe enough to be used in vaccines. In 1935, 5 years after thimerosal was initially added to vaccines, the vaccine manufacturer, Pittman-Moore, stated that "Merthioiate [thimerosal] is unsatisfactory as preservative for serum intended for use on dogs." Then, in 1982, an FDA panel recommended that mercury-based preservatives be removed from over-the-counter topical products because of safety concerns. In 1991, the FDA even considered taking thimerosal out of dog vaccines because of its toxicity. But evidently, the pharmaceutical industry has no concerns with the high concentrations of thimerosal that are being injected into newborn infants.[77]

In May 2003, after a 3-year investigation, the Subcommittee on Human Rights and Wellness, headed by Representative Dan Burton, concluded that:

> *Thimerosal used as a preservative in vaccines is likely related to the autism epidemic...Our public health agencies' failure to act is indicative of institutional malfeasance for self-protection and misplaced protectionism of the pharmaceutical industry.*[78]

While the CDC has long claimed that ethylmercury in vaccines is not toxic to humans, a 2017 study confirmed its toxicity when given to babies and pregnant women. Both methylmercury and ethylmercury

> *significantly disrupt central nervous system development and function...The ethylmercury in thimerosal*

does not leave the body quickly, as the CDC once claimed, but is metabolized into highly neurotoxic forms.[79]

Though the FDA warns pregnant women about the methylmercury in fish, there is a noticeable silence regarding the high levels of ethylmercury found in vaccines. Injecting ethylmercury into the body and bloodstream, where it is allowed to accumulate in parts of the body including the brain, is quite different from eating fish containing methylmercury that goes through the digestive tract and is then eliminated from the body.

Brian Hooker, Janet Kern et al. reviewed more than 165 studies showing the harmful effects of thimerosal, dispelling the CDC's claim that mercury in vaccines was safe based on a review of six flawed studies that were funded by the CDC. They reported that the CDC withheld important results from *their* final publication and drew conclusions that contradicted numerous studies that showed the adverse effects of thimerosal.[80]

Similarly, in the book *Thimerosal: Let the Science Speak* (2014), Robert F. Kennedy, Jr. reviewed the unfounded claims made by the Institute of Medicine that there was no causal link between thimerosal and autism based on the skewed epidemiological studies sponsored by the CDC. In a 2018 interview, Kennedy talked about having reviewed 321 studies, citing **240** that showed the toxic effects of thimerosal causing brain injury, ADD/ADHD, and speech and language delays. He also reported on **81 studies** alone that showed an association between thimerosal and autism.[81]

Researchers have discovered that boys are more likely to become autistic by an approximate ratio of 4 to 1 when compared to girls. The apparent reason being that testosterone in males increases the toxicity of thimerosal whereas estrogen in girls seems to be more protective due to the increased "*glutathione antioxidant capacity in females.*"[82]

The Material Safety Data Sheet (MSDS) is a document published by the Occupational Safety and Health Administration (OSHA) that reviewed hazardous materials. Thimerosal was found to be mutagenic, affecting genetic material; it damages the kidneys, liver, spleen, bone marrow, and CNS. It reduces fertility and can cause birth defects.[83]

Vaccines labeled "thimerosal free" may still contain up to 300 parts per billion (ppb) of mercury. The EPA states that 200 ppb of mercury in water and food is considered toxic. Yet these amounts of thimerasol in vaccines are viewed as safe according to the FDA and CDC, in spite of EPA safety limits. The authors emphasize that there is *sufficient evidence to show that low-level exposure to Hg [mercury] can be hazardous to vulnerable populations, particularly developing fetuses, infants, and children.*[84]

Though thimerosal was taken out of many of the vaccines back in the early 2000s, it is still used to prevent bacterial growth, as in the multi-dose vials used in the influenza shot. In other vaccines, thimerosal is used in trace amounts as part of the vaccine-development process, which does not have to be disclosed because it is considered inconsequential. However, there are studies showing that even trace amounts of thimerosal are considered toxic, especially when combined with other toxins, such as aluminum, creating a more potent synergistic effect.[85]

Numerous studies have shown an association between the regressive form of autism and the effects of mercury poisoning, as summarized in an article entitled, "*Autism: A Novel Form of Mercury Poisoning,*" in the journal *Medical Hypotheses (2001).*[86] Common traits noted in both mercury poisoning and autistic behaviors include: social withdrawal, repetitive and perseverative behaviors, mood swings, flat affect, temper tantrums, lack of eye contact, loss of speech, delayed language, speech-comprehension deficits, echolalia, sound and touch sensitivities, rocking and arm flapping, toe walking, head banging, borderline cognitive abilities, poor concentration, inability to understand abstract ideas, agitation, unprovoked crying, and sleeping difficulties.

• **Polysorbate 80** is a preservative that acts as an emulsifier used in prescription drugs because of its ability to cross the blood brain barrier (BBB) to cause the intended drug reaction. However, when used in vaccines, Polysorbate 80 has the unwanted effect of transferring heavy metals, such as mercury and aluminum, across the BBB as well, where they can then accumulate in the brain. This is particularly critical during infancy and early childhood when the BBB is considered more porous, especially during the first 6 months of life, thereby facilitating the greater inclusion of toxins into the child's brain, as well as other organs of the body. Polysorbate 80 used in animal studies can cause infertility in rats, genetic mutations, cancer, and cardiac anomalies. The use of Polysorbate 80, raises serious questions regarding what impact this may have on human studies, especially considering the synergistic effect of multiple vaccines given at one time.[87]

Clinical studies have implicated Polysorbate 80 in an increased risk of

> *serious side effects (e.g., blood clots, stroke, heart attack, heart failure), and death in some cases. It has also been shown to shorten overall survival and/or increase the risk of tumor growth or recurrence in patients with certain types of cancer.*[88]

Vaccines with Polysorbate 80 include DTaP, Hep B, Influenza, Prevnar13, Rotavirus, Meningococcal, and Gardasil.

- **Squalene** is an oil-based adjuvant used in vaccines that causes an autoimmune response when injected into the body that is quite different from squalene consumed as in olive oil and shark liver oil; the latter use has a positive effect on the body similar to omega-3 fatty acids. However, animal experiments have shown that, when injected, squalene triggers inflammatory and severe autoimmune reactions that include encephalomyelitis, resulting in damage to the myelin sheath; neuritis, inflammation of the nerves that can cause paralysis, and other autoimmune disorders.[89] This oil-based adjuvant *"can disable the immune system to the degree that it loses its ability to distinguish what is self from what is foreign,"* thus causing the conditions for autoimmunity."[90]

  The anthrax vaccine administered to soldiers during the Gulf War contained squalene, which has been linked to severe autoimmune diseases referred to as the Gulf War Syndrome (GWS). Symptoms included arthritis, rashes, fibromyalgia, chronic fatigue and headaches, abnormal hair loss, skin lesions, narcolepsy, ulcers, memory loss, seizures, mood disorders, lupus, MS, and neuropsychiatric problems.[91]

- **Neomycin and streptomycin** are antibiotics used in vaccines to prevent the growth of bacteria. These are two of several antibiotics that are contraindicated for pregnant women and nursing mothers according to the drug manufacturers. This is especially so when two antibiotics are combined in one vaccine (e.g., Fluvirin) yet the CDC still recommends its use in spite of drug company warnings.[92] Antibiotics destroy bacteria indiscriminately that can affect both the good and bad microorganisms in the gut. The general overuse of antibiotics today has led to diseases mutating so that some antibiotics no longer work. Regarding antibiotics used in vaccines, we don't know the long-term impact this might have during this critical stage of early child development. Antibiotics are found in MMR, Chickenpox, Polio, HepA, Meningococcal, and influenza vaccines.

- **Monosodium glutamate (MSG)**—Another neurotoxin that can cause damage to nerve cells and contribute to seizures. MSG is found in yeast extracts used in vaccines and has been implicated in disorders such as migraine headaches, asthma, irritable bowel syndrome, diabetes, seizures, anaphylactic shock, Alzheimer's, and Lou Gehrig's disease. Dr. Russell Blalock, a neurosurgeon who has written extensively on excitotoxins, states that MSG is an excitotoxin that overstimulates cell receptors in the brain, causing them to function abnormally and contribute to seizures.[93] In a study by Kamal Niaz et al., the toxic effects of MSG included *"CNS disorder, obesity, disruptions in adipose tissue physiology, hepatic damage, CRS (Chinese restaurant syndrome), and reproductive malfunctions."*[94] In 1978, MSG was banned from baby foods for children less than 1 year old because of its toxicity, according to the AAP and the National Academy of Sciences.

As a side note, many of the ingredients that are used to make vaccines in the U.S. come out of China, where there is little oversight or supervision regarding safety standards. For example, a 2018 CNN article by Westcott and Wang entitled, *Number of faulty children's vaccines in China surges more than 900,000,* found that nearly one million vaccines given to Chinese children were found to be faulty; the study led to Chinese demonstrations. 400,000 doses of the DPT vaccine found to be defective were produced at the Wuhan Institute.[95]

Assumption 2—Vaccines Are Effective and Long-Lasting

> *"While herd immunity may not exist, herd mentality most definitely does. Health authorities, media commentators, and schools and their parent-teacher associations waste no opportunity in perpetuating this myth."* —Gretchen DuBeau, Esq.

The effectiveness of vaccines is based primarily on their ability to provide immunity from diseases. When vaccines for smallpox, pertussis, and measles were first introduced, it was believed that they would provide lifelong immunity from diseases. When this turned out to be false, booster shots were then recommended by the vaccine industry in order to prolong protection, as previously mentioned. But vaccination is not the same as immunization even though they are often used interchangeably. Natural immunity from disease is complex and cannot be replicated by the artificial stimulation of antibodies via vaccination. Major differences between natural and artificial immunity are clarified below:

Natural Immunity
- Natural immunity occurs only after recovering from the actual disease.
- It usually confers lifelong immunity from the disease.
- Natural diseases challenge the immune system, thereby enhancing the body's ability to fight infections. Contrary to the general perception that all diseases are a scourge and something to fear, diseases actually serve an important function in helping to strengthen the immune system.
- Immunity can be transferred from the mother to the fetus. If the mother contracts a disease as a child, she will then be able to pass on her naturally acquired immunity

to the fetus through the placenta and later through breast feeding the infant.

Artificial Immunity from Vaccinations

- Vaccines actually interfere with and suppress the body's natural immune process from occurring, no longer allowing children to contract these common childhood diseases naturally.
- Immunity from vaccines ends up being temporary, lasting anywhere between roughly 2 and 10 years, prompting the need today for more and more booster shots.
- In many cases, the disease is contracted later in life when temporary immunity wears off, creating a significantly more serious reaction as in the case of chickenpox, measles, and mumps.
- As children receive additional inoculations, the effectiveness of the booster shots decreases progressively, while at the same time increasing the likelihood of an adverse reaction from the cumulative effect of toxins being stored in the body.
- Artificial immunity cannot be passed on from the mother to the fetus.

Herd Immunity

- Herd immunity originally referred to the protection from an infectious disease when a certain percentage of the population becomes immune as a result of previously contracting the natural disease. This makes it less likely for those without immunity to be exposed to the natural virus.
- Originally, the theory of herd immunity was based on the work of Dr. A.W. Hedrich, who from 1900 to 1931 documented annual measles rates from the naturally acquired disease. In 1933, he published his study showing that, when

68% of children became immune to measles by contracting the actual disease, the measles epidemic ceased, which he referred to as "herd immunity."

- Health officials ended up adopting the term "herd immunity" to also mean immunity as a result of vaccinations. But as indicated above, artificial immunity provides only temporary protection, therefore requiring additional booster shots that, in turn, wane with each additional shot, making herd immunity even more unattainable.

- In October 2020, the WHO attempted to define herd immunity as the result of vaccination, without reference to immunity through natural infection. Due to public backlash, WHO revised its definition to include natural infection, but then added that vaccination is preferred over acquiring natural immunity, in order to avoid being exposed to the pathogen that causes the disease. What is not acknowledged are the points made above, highlighting the superiority of natural immunity over artificial means.

- If all children in the United States were 100% vaccine compliant, they would still make up only a small percentage of the population, leaving the majority of adults who make up the biggest percentage nowhere near the vaccination rate needed to create herd immunity. This serves to further highlight the flawed notion that herd immunity is achievable through vaccination of children.

- In addition, children who receive the live virus vaccines are able to "shed" the virus to others, for weeks or even months after being inoculated. Shedding can occur when the vaccine virus is transmitted to others through fecal matter, urine, saliva, and air-borne transmission of the infection.

- Back in 1963, it was theorized that 56% of children needed to be vaccinated in order to eliminate measles, but that was changed to 70%, then 75%, 80%, 85%, and now the CDC argues that up to 96% vaccine compliance is needed, and yet herd immunity through vaccination has still not been achieved.

- The increasing number of mumps outbreaks today in highly vaccinated populations, such as on college campuses, reaching as high as 99.8% vaccination compliance, proves that herd immunity is based on the flawed assumption that you can eliminate the spread of diseases if enough people get vaccinated.

- Public health officials use herd immunity today as an argument to pressure parents into vaccinating their children in order to prevent the spread of disease to others. Unfortunately, disease outbreaks, such as mumps, measles, whooping cough, and chickenpox are occurring largely in those who have been fully vaccinated.

- Finally, if vaccines are truly effective, it would stand to reason that vaccinated children would be protected from those children who are not vaccinated.

In the book, *What About Immunizations? Exposing the Vaccine Philosophy*, Cynthia Cournoyer talks about natural immunity and its connection to one's tolerance for substances over a period of time. Using the example of smoking a cigarette for the first time, the initial experience causes a person to cough, and feel sick and nauseated. But as the body adapts to smoking, one is able to increase their tolerance for cigarettes without any obvious outward signs of harm. But eventually, the chronic smoker will be at a high risk for developing emphysema, lung cancer and the like, as a result of the cigarette's toxic effects. In a similar fashion, the toxic ingredients in vaccines may not manifest in the short term. But in time, the toxins that accumulate in the body gradually weaken the immune system's ability to fend off infection. Contracting the natural disease causes the immune system to attack the **acute** infection itself whereas the artificial immunity from vaccines causes the body to adapt to or tolerate the buildup of toxins, as in the case of smoking, laying the groundwork for a **chronic** degenerative condition over time.

The Immune System—A more detailed discussion of the immune system is crucial to understanding the problem with vaccinations. In *Vaccines, Autoimmunity, and the Changing Nature of Childhood Illness,* Thomas Cowan, MD, (2018) presented an argument for why vaccines ultimately impede the natural immune process that has evolved over millions of years. The increasing use of vaccines has created unintended consequences including the explosion in autoimmune diseases that is being seen today. What follows is a brief summary of how this extremely complex, and not totally understood, immune system works.

The immune system is made up of cells, tissues, and molecules that protect the body from disease-causing microbes and toxins in the environment. The body's defense against these invaders falls into two categories: innate immunity and adaptive immunity.

Innate immunity provides the first line of defense against infection from viruses, bacteria, parasites, and the like. This includes: physical barriers, like the skin; the gastrointestinal and respiratory tracts; protective fluids, such as secretions, mucus, and saliva; and general immune-system responses, such as inflammation that is part of the healing process.

Adaptive immunity, also called acquired immunity, is activated against pathogens when the innate immune response is insufficient. It is composed of cell-mediated immunity and humoral immunity.

Cell-mediated immune system, which operates within the cells, functions by sending white blood cells to areas of the body that have been invaded by a foreign substance, like a virus, bacteria, or toxin, as in the case of mercury or aluminum used in vaccines.

Humoral immune system functions outside the cells involving any fluid-like substances that circulate in the body, such as blood, bodily secretions, and other fluids. The humoral response to an invading antigen is to release antibodies that provide a secondary defense when the first defense, cell-mediated immunity, is unable to contain the intruder. Together, they work hand-in-hand to defeat foreign substances.

The cell-mediated immune system creates the bodily experience of sickness in the form of a fever, rash, mucus, or a cough that is the body's attempt to rid itself of the disease and to restore health. Cowan argued that the typical medical approach to illnesses is to address the symptoms by reducing a child's fever, for example, through the use of medicines, such as acetaminophen or ibuprofen. In this way, the cell-mediated response is thwarted, as in the case of vaccines that interfere with the child's exposure to the natural virus. A perfect example of this is the chickenpox vaccine that has been effective initially in preventing children from contracting the natural chickenpox virus. Although this seems to be an appropriate goal in theory, in practice the unintended consequences create greater problems down the road. Because the chickenpox vaccine is a live virus vaccine, those who get it can spread the vaccine-strain varicella zoster virus to others through shedding, causing severe cases of shingles. In the past, shingles was a disease associated with the elderly, but today we are seeing it even in young children as a result of the shedding effects of the chickenpox vaccine itself. In addition, the vaccine-induced immunity is temporary so that, later on, when the child becomes a young adult, for example, there is an increased risk of contracting the varicella virus at an age when much more serious and deadly complications can occur. Consequently, the chickenpox vaccine now poses a greater risk for children developing shingles at a young age, while at an older age people may catch chickenpox as immunity wears off. Contrast that with the generally mild natural chickenpox virus that children contracted before the vaccine came out in 1995. The natural disease provided lifelong immunity to children and helped to keep shingles in check, due to the adult's exposure to the children's chickenpox virus that inhibits the reactivation of the varicella zoster virus. There is also clear evidence that contracting the natural virus has the additional advantage of helping to strengthen the child's immune system.

This natural evolutionary immune process has developed over millions of years and now is being upended by the increasing use of vaccines that have regrettable consequences. Cowan wrote:

Unfortunately, the practice of medicine over the course of the last century is a story of reckless interference with our immune system and, in particular, interference with our cell-mediated immune response.[96]

Cell-mediated immunity is being bypassed by an artificially generated immune response that is temporary and distinctively different from the naturally occurring disease. The problem is that vaccines rely too much on humoral immunity, which has the effect of overstimulating antibody production caused by antigens from vaccines being injected into the body. As a result, the increased antibodies attack not only the invading viruses but also the body's own tissues. Consequently, vaccines disrupt the immune process by amplifying humoral immunity while obstructing cell-mediated immunity, laying the foundation for increased autoimmune diseases as a result of giving too many vaccines one after the other and over a prolonged period of time. Japanese researchers from Kobe University studied the effects of overstimulating the humoral immune response and concluded:

Systemic autoimmunity appears to be the inevitable consequence of over-stimulating the host's immune system by repeated immunization with antigen, to the levels that surpass the system's self-organized criticality.[97]

The vaccinologists who think they can imitate the natural immune system by injecting toxic chemicals into people in order to create an artificial antibody reaction, at best, will provide only temporary immunity. And so, as the vaccines wane, the medical authorities push for additional booster shots with more toxic substances that cause further disruption to the immune system, increasing the risk of harm with each additional shot. Thus, the more vaccines given, the greater the number of injuries and deaths based on numerous studies highlighted in this book. The obsession with vaccines as the only real solution to the eradication of diseases, undermines the body's innate ability to heal through healthy lifestyle choices that strengthen the immune system naturally.

Assumption 3—Vaccines Have Wiped Out All Major Diseases

"To give vaccines credit for global reduction in disease is like giving a band-aid credit for healing a wound that was already closing." —Brian Rogers, Researcher

To better understand the assumed impact that vaccines have had in wiping out diseases like smallpox, it is helpful to look at the evidence of such claims from an historical perspective. In Suzanne Humphries, MD, and Roman Bystrianyk's highly informative book, *Dissolving Illusions: Disease, Vaccines, and the Forgotten History* (2013), they reviewed the history of diseases and vaccines, showing that vaccinations were not the reason for the sharp decline in many diseases. In vivid detail, they chronicled the history of diseases in the past, showing how these diseases were largely the result of poor living conditions that caused widespread infections. Industrialization in the 1800s created overcrowding in large cities, producing poverty, hunger, and sickness. They wrote:

> *Infectious diseases were a constant terror during the 1800s. With increasingly dense populations, wars, and abject poverty, diseases of all varieties exacted a horrendous toll. The poverty-stricken masses carried the brunt of the relentless assaults of these diseases, yet no class was spared. Periodic epidemics and pandemics swept across the globe, wreaking havoc and killing millions, rivaling the horrors of war. Abysmal sanitation, hygiene, nutrition, and working and living conditions combined with a sense of utter hopelessness, laid the foundation for the devastation.*[98]

The working poor lived in crowded dwellings without running water or toilets. Sewage would seep into local water supplies, creating the conditions for disease. Garbage was left in the streets, and rats and other vermin along with disease-spreading insects became rampant. Food was of poor quality, often contaminated, and government safety standards were non-existent. Diseases that were associated with poor living conditions started to disappear as the quality of life improved moving into the 20th century.

Diseases Associated with Poor Living Conditions—Below are some of these diseases associated with poor living conditions that dissipated before the advent of vaccines and antibiotics.

- **Typhoid fever** is caused by the salmonella bacteria in feces that contaminate the food and water supply.
- **Cholera** is a bacterial infection of the small intestine caused by poor sanitation that leads to diarrhea and dehydration, requiring copious amounts of water to hydrate the body.
- **Dysentery** is an inflammation of the intestine caused by bacteria brought by fecal contamination of food and water. Hydration is critical, owing to the loss of body fluids from diarrhea.
- **Typhus fever** is a bacterium transmitted by lice, fleas, ticks and other insects, related to conditions of overcrowding, poor hygiene, and lack of sanitation.
- **Scarlet fever** is a bacterial infection caused by streptococcus producing a fever and sore throat characterized by a red rash.
- **Tuberculosis (TB)** is a bacterial infection that affects the lungs and is common in areas where malnutrition is prevalent. It is spread through airborne droplets from coughing or sneezing.
- **Yellow fever** is a viral disease transmitted by infected mosquitoes, causing jaundice.

Although these deadly diseases have largely disappeared in developed countries today, they continue to be a major source of devastation in areas of the world where poor living conditions still exist.

Chart—U.S. Disease Mortality Rates—The following chart, *Vital Statistics of the United States,* maintained by the U.S. government, shows the mortality rates of these various diseases: measles, scarlet fever, typhoid, whooping cough, and diphtheria from 1900 up to the 1960s. The dramatic decrease in these diseases was the result of improved living conditions *"due to improvement in sanitation, nutrition, and medical care."*

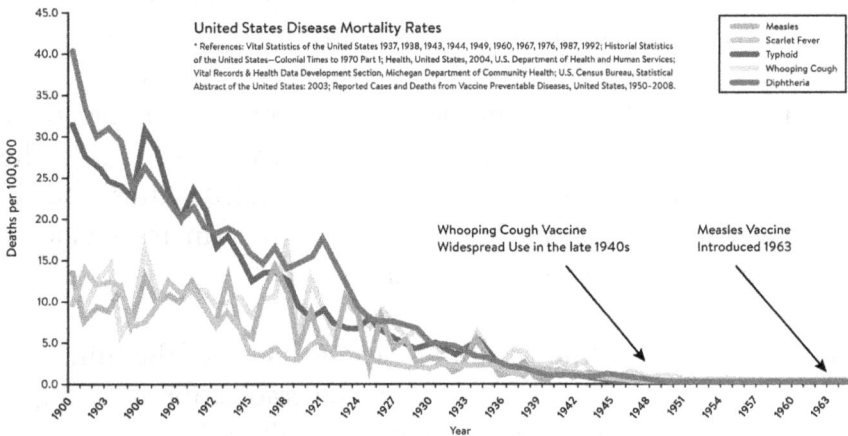

United States Disease Mortality Rates

Many attribute the low rate of death from infectious disease in the modern age to vaccination alone. History shows these diseases were in decline long before widespread vaccination due to improvement in sanitation, nutrition, and medical care. *Figure courtesy of Roman Bystrianyk.*

- The vaccine for whooping cough came out in the late 1940s, as did the widely used diphtheria vaccine. The chart shows that the mortality rate for these diseases essentially went down to zero before the vaccines were introduced.
- The measles vaccine didn't come out until 1963, and you can see, looking at this chart, that mortality was essentially down to nothing by the time the measles vaccine was introduced.
- Then, there were other diseases like scarlet fever and typhoid, for which a vaccine was never developed. These diseases faded away with time as living conditions improved.

Pediatrics is the journal published by the AAP. In its Dec. 2000, *Annual Summary of Vital Statistics: Trends in the Health of Americans During the 20th Century,* it stated:

> *Thus, vaccination does not account for the impressive declines in mortality seen in the first half of the century...nearly 90% of the decline in infectious-disease mortality among U.S. children occurred before 1940, when few antibiotics or vaccines were available.*[99]

The AAP explicitly acknowledged that improved living conditions were the real source of declining mortality from diseases. This is a rather obvious contradiction from the repeated claims made by the medical establishment that vaccines are the primary reason for the decline in diseases in the 20th century.

The History of Smallpox and the Vaccine—One of the things the medical community prides itself in is the eradication of smallpox thanks to vaccination. If we look at history a little closer, we see that this is not actually the case.

The term, "vaccine" came from the Latin word, "vacca", meaning "cow." It was originally coined by Edward Jenner (1796), who theorized that cowpox derived from cows was essentially the same as smallpox and, if it were placed in an open cut on the arm, the body would respond by protecting the individual from contracting the smallpox disease. Initially, Jenner's new vaccine efforts were met with disdain. But he eventually convinced the Royal College of Physicians and the British Parliament that his inoculation was safe and effective, as well as profitable. Increasingly, vaccines became more widely accepted by the medical establishment and the governments that stood to gain financially from this "cash cow."

Many of the European countries during the latter part of the 19th century were making vaccinations compulsory despite a growing number of deaths as a result of the smallpox vaccine itself. Nevertheless, with rare exceptions, the smallpox vaccine continued to be defended by the medical community and government agencies.

In March 1885, the outrage over forced vaccinations reached a boiling point when the citizens of Leicester, England, protested in the streets against the law enforcing smallpox vaccinations under penalty of fines or imprisonment. In spite of mandatory smallpox vaccinations, outbreaks of smallpox increased, resulting in more vaccine-induced injuries and deaths.

Dr. Hadwen, MD, in his book, *The Case Against Vaccination* (1896), he wrote:

> *Since the passage of the United Kingdom Compulsory Vaccination Act of 1853, we've had no less than three distinct epidemics. In 1857 to 59, we had more than 14,000 deaths from smallpox. In 1863 to 65, the epidemic reached 20,000 deaths, and, between 1871 and 72, there were 44,800 deaths. Stricter enforcement led to the highest vaccination rate ever achieved in England in 1871.*[100]

All of these people were dying from smallpox, even though there was a 97.5% vaccine compliance rate that coincided with England's worst smallpox epidemic. In other words, the smallpox vaccine did not work and actually caused more deaths than the disease itself. What did make a difference was the improvement in sanitation and the isolation of those infected.

There was a satirical poem about vaccinations that was circulated in 1876 called, "*The Doctors.*" It read:

> *Try revaccination—it never will hurt you,*
> *For revaccination has this one great virtue:*
> *Should it injure or kill you whenever you receive it,*
> *We all stand prepared to refuse to believe it.*[101]

- In the late 1800s, Dr. Hadwen quoted Dr. Drutt, who wrote: *"You may just as well try and stop a smallpox epidemic by vaccination, as to prevent a thunderstorm with an umbrella."*[102]

Other Critics of Vaccinations:
- Alfred Russell Wallace was a British naturalist, explorer, geographer, biologist, and anthropologist, who was best known for independently formalizing the theory of evolution at the same time as Charles Darwin.
  He wrote in 1898,

> *Vaccination is a gigantic delusion ... it has never saved a single life; but that it has been the cause of so much disease, so many deaths, such a vast amount of utterly needless and altogether undeserved suffering, that it will be classed by the coming generation among the greatest errors of an ignorant and prejudiced age, and its penal enforcement the foulest blot on the generally beneficent course of legislation during our century.*[103]

- J.T. Biggs, Sanitary Engineer for Leicester (1912), wrote:

> *There is but little vaccination in Leicester now, no smallpox, and the death rate from these seven principal zymotics* has fallen in 1908–10 ...What has achieved this astounding revolution? Certainly, not vaccination. It is the direct outcome of active, persistent, and solid progress in sanitation, which in its broadest sense, covers the entire exclusion of absolutely insanitary and disease-diffusing practice of cow-poxing.*[104]

[* Seven principal zymotic (contagious) diseases included: Smallpox, Measles, Scarlet Fever, Diphtheria, Whooping Cough, Fevers, Diarrhea.]

- Mahatma Gandhi expressed his view about vaccinations in 1921, by writing:

  Vaccination is a barbarous practice and one of the most fatal of all the delusions current in our time. Conscientious objectors to vaccination should stand alone, if need be, against the whole world, in defense of their conviction.[105]

- Dr. William Howard Hays spoke in June of 1937 about the worst smallpox epidemic that had ever occurred in the Philippines after 8 million people received more than 24 million vaccine doses, resulting in the **death rate quadrupling.** He wrote:

  It is nonsense to think that you can inject pus and it is usually from the pustule of the dead smallpox victim; that is the basis of it; we used to think it was from cowpox, but the manufacturers deny that and say the most reliable form originates in the pustule of someone who had died from smallpox—it is unthinkable that you can inject that into a little child and in any way improve its health.[106]

- Doctor Charles Cyril Okell wrote in *The Lancet* in 1938:

  Without propaganda there can, of course, be no large-scale immunization but how perilous it is to mix propaganda with scientific fact. If we baldly told the whole truth, it is doubtful whether the public would submit to immunization.[107]

- R.B. Pearson, the author of *Pasteur: Plagiarist, Imposter, The Germ Theory Exploded* (1942), wrote:

  Note that those immigrants from countries having compulsory vaccination die off at a rate three to four times higher than immigrants from countries not having compulsory vaccination. There is no doubt that there are other causes to be considered, such as sanitation, living conditions, diet, and that the relative vitality of the different races may vary, so why should these death rates seem to divide simply on their vaccination status?[108]

- George Bernard Shaw stated in 1944:

  At present, intelligent people do not have their children vaccinated, nor does the law now compel them to. The result is not, as the Jennerians prophesized, the extermination of the human race by smallpox; on the contrary more people are now killed by vaccination than by smallpox.[109]

- In 1973, Nobel Prize winner Dr. R.R. Porter wrote:

  The major contributing factor toward improved health over the past 200 years has been improved nutrition. Nearly 90% of the total decline in the death rate in children between 1860 and 1965 due to whooping cough, scarlet fever, diphtheria and measles occurred before the introduction of antibiotics and widespread immunization against diphtheria.[110]

- Richard Moskowitz, M.D., author of *"Vaccines: A Reappraisal"* (2017), wrote:

*The public is surely entitled to convincing proof,
beyond all reasonable doubt, that artificial immunization is in fact a safe and effective procedure,
in no way injurious to health, and that the threat
of the corresponding natural diseases remains sufficiently clear and urgent to warrant mass inoculation of everyone, even against their will if necessary.
Unfortunately, such proof has never been given.
Journal of the American Institute of Homeopathy,
March 1983.*[111]

- Dr. Albert Sabin M.D., creator of the oral polio vaccine,
  stated in a 1985 lecture in Italy:

  *Official data have shown that the large-scale vacci-
  nations undertaken in the U.S. have failed to obtain
  any significant improvement over the diseases against
  which they were supposed to provide protection.*[112]

- Dr. Glen Dettman, an Australian pathologist, stated in
  1992:

  *I don't know that the safety of vaccines has ever really
  been proven. We don't know the long-term effects of
  vaccines. It will take several generations before we
  see some genetic alterations that are going to occur
  quite obviously.*[113]

- Dr. Boyd Haley, professor and chair of the Dept. of
  Chemistry at University of Kentucky (2001), stated: *"A
  single vaccine given to a six-pound newborn is the equivalent of giving a 180-pound-adult, 30 vaccinations on the
  same day."*[114]

- Gerhard Buchwald MD, a German medical doctor specializing in internal medicine, who wrote, "Vaccination Nonsense" (2005), stated:

  Vaccinating against measles is not just useless, but harmful. In the past, infants would get protection from their mothers who used to have measles themselves. Mothers who were vaccinated against measles cannot pass on the protection to their infants, so infants now get measles.[115]

- Dr. Russell Blaylock, a neurosurgeon and author, who has been critical of a number of vaccines, asserted in 2013:

  Tetanus vaccine is probably one of the most ridiculous vaccines ever. Your chances of getting Tetanus are about the same as walking outta here and getting hit by a meteor. If you get a cut or puncture wound and you put peroxide on it, your chances of getting tetanus are zero because the tetanus organism is anaerobic. It cannot live in oxygen. Tetanus comes from the bowels of animals; as long as you don't have a sheep or a cow in your house, I don't think you're in any danger.[116]

- Robert Mendelsohn, an outspoken and respected pediatrician for more than 30 years, was highly critical of medical practices that he viewed as often more dangerous than the diseases they were designed to treat. In his book, *How to Raise a Healthy Child...In Spite of Your Doctor* (1984), Mendelsohn expressed his objection to vaccines as summarized below:[117]

- "There is no convincing scientific evidence that mass inoculations can be credited with eliminating any childhood disease."
- While the Salk vaccine is credited with eliminating the polio epidemic in the U.S., the polio epidemic ended in Europe without any major vaccine program.
- "There are significant risks associated with every immunization and numerous contraindications that may make it dangerous for the shots to be given to your child."
- "No one knows the long-term consequences of injecting foreign proteins into the body of your child."
- "There is growing suspicion that immunization against relatively harmless childhood diseases may be responsible for the dramatic increase in autoimmune diseases since mass inoculations were introduced."

To a large degree, Mendelsohn foretold the difficulties with vaccinations that we are seeing today, as in the case of autoimmune diseases. In this all-encompassing effort now to eradicate generally mild infectious diseases through the use of numerous vaccines with toxic chemicals given at early stages in an infant's development, we have inadvertently created an array of pervasive diseases and disabilities that are crippling a significant number of vulnerable children.

Mortality Versus Morbidity

"Mortality" comes from the root word, "mortal," meaning one who is subject to death. Mortality refers to the number of deaths in proportion to a population, the death rate. "Morbidity" comes from the root word, "morbid," relating to or caused by disease. Morbidity has to do with the rate of disease in a population. There is a tendency to equate the two terms as equivalent when discussing vaccinations. The medical community will refer to morbidity to emphasize the degree of disease occurring in the population as a result of the level of vaccinations given. So increased diseases are seen as a reflection of the lowered vaccination rate. The assumption is that this is a bad thing, therefore the need to ensure higher vaccination rates. Mortality on the other hand, is much more serious given that this is the rate of death due to diseases.

From the perspective of the immune system, allowing diseases to occur naturally, as in the past regarding measles, mumps, chickenpox, and so forth, the body is able to respond in a way that strengthened one's immunity not for a few years but essentially for a lifetime. So, in this context, "morbidity" does not have the negative connotation associated with "mortality." Unfortunately, the medical establishment uses morbidity to alarm the public in order to justify the need to vaccinate, when in fact the immune system benefits from contracting these common childhood diseases.

Assumption 4—No Connection Between Vaccines, Autism, and Other Neurological Disorders

"It is difficult to get a man to understand something when his salary depends upon his not understanding it."
—Upton Sinclair

Numerous independent scientific studies have shown a correlation between vaccines and autism, along with other adverse neurodevelopmental reactions. Yet the CDC continues to deny any connection, despite the pharmaceutical industry itself listing adverse events associated with each vaccine.

Vaccine Product Inserts—The pharmaceutical companies publish a list of possible adverse reactions in their "vaccine product inserts" included with each vaccine. The paper insert is large with tiny print that is difficult to read, listing vaccine ingredients that are difficult to find, and containing medical jargon that makes it hard for lay people to understand. The unfortunate consequences associated with vaccinations has been compiled by the Children's Health Defense which listed 217 adverse medical reactions on the vaccine product inserts for the prevention of 13 illnesses.[118]

To put this in greater perspective, an excerpt from the hepatitis B product insert for the Engerix-B vaccine produced by GlaxoSmithKline (GSK) is included here. The infant receives a series of 3 doses, the first given a few hours after the newborn comes out of the womb, then again between the first and second month of life, and a third time at 6 months. All trial subjects were monitored for only 4 days post-administration. Here are the risk factors from just this one vaccine as listed in the vaccine product insert:

**ENGERIX-B [Hepatitis B Vaccine (Recombinant)]—GlaxoSmithKline.
Postmarketing adverse reactions reported: Infections and Infestations:**

Herpes zoster, meningitis. **Blood and Lymphatic System Disorders:** Thrombocytopenia. **Immune System Disorders:** Allergic reaction, anaphylactoid reaction, anaphylaxis. An apparent hypersensitivity syndrome (serum sickness-like) of delayed onset has been reported days to weeks after vaccination, including: arthralgia/arthritis (usually transient), fever, and dermatologic reactions such as urticaria, erythema multiforme, ecchymoses, and erythema nodosum. **Nervous System Disorders:** Encephalitis; encephalopathy; migraine; multiple sclerosis; neuritis; neuropathy including hypoesthesia, paresthesia, Guillain-Barré syndrome and Bell's palsy; optic neuritis; paralysis; paresis; seizures; syncope; transverse myelitis. **Eye Disorders:** Conjunctivitis, keratitis, visual disturbances. **Ear and Labyrinth Disorders:** Earache, tinnitus, vertigo. Cardiac Disorders: Palpitations, tachycardia. **Vascular Disorders:** Vasculitis. **Respiratory, Thoracic, and Mediastinal Disorders:** Apnea, bronchospasm including asthma-like symptoms. **Gastrointestinal Disorders:** Dyspepsia. Skin and Subcutaneous Tissue Disorders: arthritis, muscular weakness. **General Disorders and Administration Site Conditions:** Injection site reaction. **Investigations:** Abnormal liver function tests. **Source: www.immunize.org/packageinserts**

All of the vaccine product inserts also acknowledge that:

- Vaccines have been tested only individually, never in combination.
- Vaccines have never been tested for safety involving pregnant women.
- Vaccines have never been tested to rule out the possibility of mutations.
- Vaccines have never been tested to rule out carcinogenic susceptibility.
- Vaccinated children are contagious and can shed the live virus to other children whether they are vaccinated or unvaccinated.

Increasingly, as children receive more and more vaccines, adverse reactions become more prevalent. Far from keeping diseases from returning, vaccinations have quite the opposite effect, showing that diseases in the United States are on the rise in highly vaccinated populations, reflecting the waning effects of vaccines. Vaccines also have the ability to mutate, thereby losing whatever ability they initially had to provide protection. For example, the pertussis vaccine has actually increased cases of whooping cough via a mutated form of the *Bordetella pertussis* strain *(Bordetella parapertussis)*. The vaccine has no effect on this more virulent form, which causes more hospitalizations and deaths as a result.[119]

What gets presented in the mainstream media is that the unvaccinated are to blame for disease outbreaks such as whooping cough, measles, mumps, and so on. Consequently, they are viewed with contempt by the largely uninformed medical community, government officials, and the public. What goes unnoticed for the most part is that unvaccinated children tend to be healthier than vaccinated children. For example, autism is essentially nonexistent or extremely rare in those communities where vaccines are generally not given, as with the Amish community, Orthodox Jews, Mennonites, and home-schooled children.

Evidence of Harm—The book *Evidence of Harm—Mercury in Vaccines and the Autism Epidemic: A Medical Controversy,* by David Kirby (2005), is a comprehensive look into the controversy around autism that often reads like a mystery novel attempting to unravel the origins of the autism epidemic. It focuses on mercury (thimerosal) in vaccines along with other toxins affecting child development. It chronicles the close and questionable ties among Big Pharma, government agencies, and the medical establishment. This is most evident in Kirby's account of the **Simpsonwood Conference** that was held in Georgia in 2000, where high-level officials from the Centers for Disease Control (CDC), the Food and Drug Administration (FDA), and the World Health Organization (WHO), met with representatives from the all the major vaccine manufacturers, including GSK, Merck, Wyeth, and Aventis Pasteur, in a private meeting away from public scrutiny.

The reason the conference was held in such a secretive manner had to do with the research findings of Tom Verstraeten, an epidemiologist from the CDC, who analyzed the Vaccine Safety Datalink (VSD) database. He compiled the medical records of 100,000 children maintained by the CDC and the FDA. Unexpectedly, Verstraeten found that there was a high correlation among mercury (thimerosal), autism, and other neurologic developmental impairment. This was not the news that most attendees were anticipating. After some discussion, during this 2-day conference, it was decided that this report should be withheld from the public because of the concern that this would discourage vaccinations. Then, over the next 3 years, the data was reworked on 4 more occasions, in order to make the link between thimerosal and vaccine injuries go away. It was only through the Freedom of Information Act (FOIA) that the CDC's unpublished Verstraeten study was obtained showing a 7.6-fold increase in autism, a 5-fold increase in sleep disorders, 2.1-fold increase in speech disorders, and a 1.8-fold increase in neurodevelopmental disorders when comparing one-month-old vaccinated versus unvaccinated children.[120] The CDC even went so far as to hand the giant database of vaccine records over to a private British company making it off-limits to researchers until the public got access to this data through the FOIA.

Kirby's book also reports on some of the most relevant vaccine research that helps to shed light on the connection among vaccines, autism, and other disorders as summarized below:

- Dr. Vijendra Singh, a neuroimmunologist from the University of Michigan, said that autism was an autoimmune disorder linked to the live virus exposure from the MMR vaccine (1998).
- Dr. Wakefield, a pediatric gastroenterologist from London, noted that severe gastrointestinal distress and leaky gut syndrome was caused by the MMR vaccine (1998).

- In 1999, the WHO stated that more than 200 mcg. of mercury in a fetus or infant could cause moderate to severe brain damage that would result in a rise in learning impaired children.
- Dr. David Baskin, professor of neurosurgery at Baylor College of Medicine in Houston demonstrated how thimerosal destroys brain cells even in trace amounts (2000).
- Jill James, professor of pediatrics at the University of Arkansas for Medical Sciences, showed how autistic children lacked glutathione, an antioxidant that prevents cell damage caused by heavy metals, thereby preventing the body from excreting mercury (2003).
- Jeffery Bradstreet, MD, described autistic children as having severe gastrointestinal distress, extremely poor food absorption, and a disorder known as *"leaky gut syndrome."* His study on chelation showed how autistic children excreted 500% more mercury than control subjects. (2001)
- Dr. Amy Holmes, a Virginia pediatrician and a mother of an autistic child, found that the use of chelation therapy was most effective with children 1–5 years old with 74% showing marked or moderate improvement. In the 6-to-12-year-olds, one third made marked or moderate gains, and above 12 years the gains were minimal (2001).
- William J. Walsh, a biochemist and chief scientist at the Pfeiffer Treatment Center in Illinois, suggested based on his research that autistic children were depleted in metallothionein (MT), a sulfur-based protein that was responsible for binding with mercury and other metals in order to excrete them from the body. Based on his analysis, **99%** of his autistic subjects exhibited an MT metabolism disorder (2003).
- Numerous studies have shown that the toxins in vaccines cause demyelination, which is the breakdown of the myelin sheath of nerve fibers, causing loss of sensation, coordination, and power in specific areas of the body. It affects

the nerves of the CNS comprising the brain and spinal cord. Patches of demyelination are the prime feature of MS, causing blurred vision, muscle weakness, and loss of coordination.

- Demyelination is also associated with an allergy-like reaction following immunization. It has been tied to numerous autoimmune and other neurological disorders such as: arthritis, diabetes, lupus, allergies, chronic fatigue syndrome (CFS), autism, cancer, miscarriages, MS, and Alzheimer's disease.

Vaccine-Induced Autism—In J.B. Handley's book, *How to End the Autism Epidemic* (2018), the author who is co-founder of Generation Rescue and father of an autistic child, summarized 11 scientific studies starting in 2004 that have demonstrated how autism is vaccine-induced by what is called "*immune activation events*" in the brain during critical periods of brain development. These more recent studies demonstrate how autism can be triggered by aluminum adjuvants that create an ongoing inflammation of the brain. This can occur *in utero* when the state of the pregnant mother's immune system is able to alter the fetal brain as well as after the infant's birth. Though aluminum adjuvants in vaccines are specifically used to provoke an immune response, unfortunately the increased number of vaccines containing aluminum hyperstimulate the immune system, triggering immune activation that has been shown to produce social, communicative, and motor deficits in rats and rhesus monkeys that closely replicates the kinds of difficulties seen in children with autism.

Handley noted that the amount of aluminum being injected into infants increased dramatically in the early 1990s, owing to the increased number of vaccines containing aluminum and the higher rates of vaccination among children, going from roughly **50%** in the 1980s to more than **90%** compliance today.

Aluminum's ability to trigger immune activation events is particularly problematic during this critical stage of infant brain development. The problem is compounded by the fact that the aluminum adjuvants are recognized as a foreign substance that, once injected into the body, end up being stored in the body, in areas such as the brain, for an indefinite period of time. This overstimulation by increased vaccinations caused a continual state of inflammation as observed in autistic children's "swollen" brains. This would help to explain the typical head banging behavior seen in autistic children who are clearly in physical distress. In summary, these recent scientific discoveries cited by J.B. Handley provide concrete evidence that autism can be vaccine-induced by aluminum adjuvants alone.

Similarly, Russell Blaylock, MD, has written about how vaccines can activate the microglia, the primary immune cells of the brain and spinal cord that can secrete immune chemicals, called cytokines and chemokines, producing free radicals that are designed to attack and kill invading organisms. Microglia also secrete other chemicals, called excitotoxins, that can be destructive to the brain and the immune system overall. Blaylock summarized his findings by stating:

> *The realization that CNS microglia can be activated by stimulation of the systemic immune system is of great concern both in terms of natural disease and attempts to protect against disease by vaccination. It appears that not only the intensity of the immune stimulation is important, but also how closely spaced apart it occurs. Closely spaced, repetitive immune stimulation maximizes CNS innate immune activation and immunoexcitotoxicity.*[121]

In other words, the excessive inoculation of vaccines at one time and over a long period, can put the brain's immune system into a constant state of activation that can cause a number of neurodegenerative diseases in children, including autism, language problems, behavioral dysfunction, and in adults, diseases, such as ALS, Alzheimer's disease, MS, dementia, and Parkinson's disease.

Omnibus Autism Proceeding (OAP)—J.B. Handley's book also recounts the deluge of claims by parents alleging that their children's vaccine injuries caused autism. By 2002, the Vaccine Court was overwhelmed with approximately 5,500 claims arising from vaccine injury. The court's solution was to lump all autism cases into a single group that would ultimately be determined based on the outcome of **three test cases.** The final judgment by the Vaccine Court's special master did not occur until 2009, 7 years after the formation of the Omnibus Autism Proceeding (OAP).[122]

Dr. Andrew Zimmerman, a pediatric neurologist from the Kennedy Krieger Institute at Johns Hopkins University, who had been the government's top expert witness in the vaccine/autism debate, had previously taken the position that vaccines did not cause autism. Later he reversed his opinion indicating that vaccines, in fact, could be a cause of autism. However, the Vaccine Court used Dr. Zimmerman's early written testimony claiming no association between vaccines and autism to justify denying all claims. And so, with the final judgment based on three cases that were denied, all 5,500 autism claims were summarily rejected through a convoluted and corrupt legal process that favored the pharmaceutical industry, the medical establishment, and government officials who were quick to dismiss any association between vaccines and autism.

Hannah Poling Case—Hannah was a 19-month-old who regressed into autism after receiving nine vaccines during an office visit in 2000. Her father, Jon Poling, at the time was a young doctor working at the highly acclaimed Kennedy Krieger Institute, where Dr. Zimmerman was the director of medical research. Dr. Zimmerman and Jon Poling, along with other specialists at the clinic were investigating what had gone wrong in Hannah's case. Dr. Zimmermann came to the realization that the vaccine overload was the probable cause of Hannah's autism, which was a dramatic shift from his previously held position. Dr. Zimmerman wrote:

> *The cause for regressive encephalopathy in Hannah at age 19 months was underlying mitochondrial dysfunction,*

exacerbated by vaccine-induced fever and immune stimulation that exceeded metabolic energy reserves. This acute expenditure of metabolic reserves led to permanent irreversible brain injury.[123]

Dr. Zimmerman's new assessment created quite a stir within the scientific community, especially at the CDC and the DOJ because of the financial implications that vaccines could be a cause of autism. Consequently, he was abruptly fired from his position as lead expert witness for the government. Then the officials attempted to minimize any connection by stating this was a "unique" case with little bearing on the discussion regarding vaccines and autism. However, as previously stated, independent investigators who reviewed the VAERS data, were able to identify 83 children who were diagnosed with autism and ended up receiving compensation for "vaccine-induced brain damage."[124]

In a study published in the *Journal of Autism and Developmental Disorders* in March 2020, Nevison and Parker assessed the data collected by the California Dept. of Developmental Services (CDDS), considered to be the *"most reliable long-term record of autism prevalence trends in the United States."* They looked at data from different counties in the state for the birth years 1993–2013. They found that autism increased among all children from 1993 to 2000, but leveled off or declined between 2000 and 2013 among white children from the wealthier counties in California. In contrast, the lower income counties, with higher numbers of Hispanic and Black children, had autism rates that increased throughout the period from 1993 to 2013. The authors concluded:

> *The results suggest that the most wealthy and educated parents, starting around birth year 2000, began either to opt out of DDS in favor of private services and/or to make choices and access options that lowered their children's likelihood of being diagnosed with the severe forms of ASD historically served by DDS.*[125]

Put simply, those families who became better informed by 2000, realizing the potential risk of vaccines, either opted out of all or some vaccines or delayed vaccinations until their children were older and less vulnerable.

PART IV

THE THEORY BEHIND VACCINATIONS

"Nobody—not even the most educated immunologists— understands or can describe the complete cascade of events that occurs after injecting a vaccine." —Suzanne Humphries, M.D.

The theory behind inoculation, commonly referred to as vaccination, is an attempt to achieve immunity to a specific disease by exposing the body to an assumed harmless form of the disease by introducing an antigen, which can be a toxin, a weakened or dead bacteria or virus, or another foreign substance that facilitates the immune system to produce antibodies in order to weaken or destroy the naturally occurring disease if contracted later on. It is presumed that the antibodies activated by the vaccine will recognize the natural disease and intervene in order to prevent the disease from taking hold.

Part of the theory around vaccines is that injecting antigens will mimic the natural disease that will in turn produce antibodies that will create immunity. But there is mounting evidence that antibodies alone do not guarantee immunity. In Brandon Turbeville's article, *"The Antibody Deception,"* he detailed a growing number of studies that suggested, *"that it is quite possible that antibodies play no legitimate role whatsoever in preventing or fighting off infections."* He concluded by stating,

"In short, neither vaccination nor antibody response equals immunity."[126]

Similarly, Jeremy R. Hammond wrote:

> *Just because someone has a high antibody titer doesn't mean that they are immune. Cell-mediated immunity and mucosal immunity—or both—may also—or instead—be required to provide adequate protection against disease.*

Hammond goes on to say:

> *The immunity conferred by natural infection is superior to that conferred by the vaccine...Indeed, the conclusion seems inescapable that the FDA's use of antibody titers as a surrogate measure of immunity for the purposes of vaccine licensure amounts to scientific fraud.*[127]

Types of Vaccine Ingredients—In addition to the antigen, vaccine ingredients fall under the category of excipients, which include adjuvants, preservatives, stabilizers, antibiotics, and cultured media. What follows is a brief description of an extremely complex array of substances and processes used in the development of vaccines.

- **Excipient**—Refers to ingredients in vaccines formulated with an active ingredient, an antigen, in order to facilitate drug absorption, and prolong and enhance the immune effect.
- **Adjuvant**—This is a substance like aluminum, the most widely used adjuvant in vaccines today which provokes a strong immune response by increasing the production of antibodies. It is combined with a specific antigen, used to mimic a weakened form of the disease, in order to produce a more robust immune response that is longer lasting and minimizes the dose of antigens needed in a vaccine.
- **Antibodies** or immunoglobulins are blood proteins produced by the body that help fight against foreign

substances such as bacteria, viruses, and foreign bodies called "antigens."

- **Antigen**—Antigens can be bacteria, viruses, or fungi, as well as toxins and chemicals that invade the body, all of which can stimulate the immune system to produce antibodies as a response to fight off diseases. Vaccines contain antigens either derived from a pathogen or produced synthetically, to induce an immune response to provide protection, when subsequently exposed to an infection or pathogen. A cold virus is an example of a natural antigen that causes the body to produce antibodies that help to prevent a person from getting sick.

- **Preservative**—A substance that prevents the contamination or growth of germs as in the case of thimerosal, which is used primarily in multi-dose vials. Other preservatives include phenol and 2-phenoxyethanol.

- **Stabilizer**—An additive that is used to protect vaccines from being altered by adverse conditions such as exposure to heat, light, acidity, or humidity. Some examples include MSG, gelatin, and Polysorbate 80.

- **Antibiotic**—Used to prevent contamination by bacteria during production and storage of the vaccine. Neomycin, polymyxin B, gentamicin, and streptomycin are antibiotics commonly used in vaccines.

- **Cell culture media**—Refers to the environment in which to grow an organism, such as a virus or bacterium, during the manufacturing production of a vaccine. The cultured media is derived from the cells of animal parts such as fetal bovine serum, monkey kidneys, chicken eggs, pig blood, and rabbit brains, etc.

  Fetal cells are also procured from human aborted fetuses (e.g., WI-38, MRC-5 cells), since viruses need cells to grow and tend to grow better in cells from humans rather than from animals. At least 23 vaccines have human DNA from aborted infants and blood protein that are injected into infants.

In the normal course of digestion, the body is able to break down foods such as meat and eggs into amino acids that the body can then utilize. However, when these foreign proteins from vaccines are injected directly into the bloodstream, they bypass the gastrointestinal tract and end up being stored in the body, which can later trigger an auto-immune reaction. This helps to explain the sharp rise in food allergies associated with vaccines from the inclusion of peanut oil, egg, gelatin, yeast, and milk proteins that can precipitate an unpredictable allergic reaction. For example, children allergic to eggs can have a serious reaction to vaccines containing egg proteins, since parents would have no idea which vaccines might contain these proteins.

Combining the various ingredients in a vaccine is a complex process that assumes all children will benefit from this "one-size-fits-all" approach. This can be quite problematic in that reactions from these vaccine formulations are unforeseeable in vulnerable children. Dr. Peter Patriarca, Director of the Viral Products Division of the FDA Center of Biologics Evaluation and Research (CBER), confirmed this unpredictability by stating:

> *One of the important things is that the technology used to make these vaccines actually exceeds the science and technology to understand how these vaccines work and to predict how they will work...So this has the potential for ending up in a situation...of unforeseen and unpredictable vaccine outcomes.*[128]

Aborted Fetuses Used in Vaccines

Dr. Leonard Hayflick from the Wistar Institute in Pennsylvania, started using cell strains from aborted babies back in the 1960s that were obtained from Sweden since abortion was illegal in the U.S. at that time. The aborted cells provided a medium for the growth of viruses that could then be used to make live virus vaccines. Because cell strains from fetal tissue

---

can be reproduced repeatedly for years from just one aborted baby, it became economically advantageous over cell cultures from animals that had to be housed, fed, maintained and bred.

The organs from the legally aborted fetuses in Sweden had to be quickly collected and delivered to the U.S. under sterile conditions in order to assure the preservation of the live tissue. Hayflick was able to successfully develop a cell line from the lungs of an aborted female 3-month-old fetus in 1962. It was called WI-38, referring to the 38th fetus used at the Wistar Institute.

Another cell line was developed in 1966 by the British Medical Research Council from the lungs of a male fetus, named MRC-5, referring to the 5th aborted fetus used in the development of vaccines. Other aborted fetuses are being developed for the eventual replacements for WI-38 and MRC-5.

On October 6, 2021, a whistleblower at Pfizer, with the help of Project Veritas, revealed that information was being withheld from the public, regarding the use of human fetal tissue in testing of the COVID vaccine. The cell line involved was HEK293, which was originally derived from human embryonic kidney cells from a female aborted fetus. Through the FOIA, it was discovered that in order to harvest usable body parts, the baby had to be removed from the womb alive, by cesarean section. Then the kidney was cut out of the body without anesthesia, in order to ensure the viability of the organ, thereby killing the infant in the process.

Human fetal cells that are currently used in numerous vaccines include: chickenpox, MMR II, Pentacel (DTP, Polio, HIB), shingles, rabies, and hepatitis A. Alternative vaccines produced in Japan that use animal sources are not available in the U.S.

The Adverse Effects of Vaccines—A major problem with vaccines today is that they contain a lot of ingredients, many of which are toxic at levels never experienced before, which can cause adverse reactions. Vaccine makers are experimenting with a highly complex immune system without fully understanding the long-term implications of their actions. What follows is a brief summary of some of the unintended consequences of vaccinations.

1. The natural immune system, which relies to a large extent on the mucous membranes of the body and the gastrointestinal tract, is being bypassed when vaccines are injected directly into a muscle, quickly exposing the body's immune system to toxins, viruses, bacteria, and other substances that cannot be easily neutralized and expelled from the body. As a consequence, these substances can end up being stored in parts of the body indefinitely, including the brain and other organs.

2. The toxins in vaccines, such as thimerosal, aluminum, and formaldehyde have been shown to damage the myelin sheath surrounding the nerves of the brain and spinal cord, referred to as demyelination, which can lead to an array of neurological problems.

3. Vaccines can actually suppress the immune system, interfering with the body's natural ability to fight diseases, thereby weakening the immune response so that individuals become more susceptible to illnesses. For example, annual flu shots have been shown to reduce the protective immunity against more virulent influenza strains contracted afterwards.

4. Vaccines can alter DNA, causing a form of genetic engineering in which foreign DNA from various animal cells and aborted human fetal tissue recombined with our body's cells which can create a vaccine-induced genetic mutation, the long-term implications of which are not fully understood.

5. The individual becomes susceptible to a much more serious reaction later on, after the vaccine's temporary immunity wears off, as in the case of teens and adults contracting diseases, such as measles, mumps, and chicken pox.

6. Children receiving live-virus vaccinations (MMR, chickenpox, influenza, rotavirus, shingles, etc.) can shed and transmit the live virus from the vaccine through close contact with others through fecal matter, urine, saliva, and breast milk of infected persons for weeks or even months after inoculation.

7. Vaccines can cause the exact condition that they are supposed to prevent. For example, Hemophilus Influenzae Type B Meningitis (Hib) has actually been shown to cause more cases of meningitis than it prevents.

8. The heavy metals in vaccines, such as thimerosal, are able to destroy glutathione, an antioxidant that prevents cell damage, as well as depletes metallothionein (MT),[129] a protein that binds with the heavy metals in order to excrete them from the body, thus making children more vulnerable to these toxins.

9. Infants and children today are more vulnerable to infection at an early age, since mothers today, who were vaccinated as children, no longer contract the natural infectious diseases of childhood that protected them for life and were then able to transfer that protection to their offspring.

10. The antigens in vaccines injected into the body are used to overstimulate the body's immune response, in order to provoke antibodies, referred to as **immunogenicity.** If the overstimulation becomes excessive, it can cause an autoimmune response that creates a chronic condition in which the body attacks and damages its own tissues, as in the case of food allergies that can lead to anaphylaxis,* a potentially life-threatening allergic reaction. This is particularly problematic when infants and children are exposed to multiple vaccinations at one time.

[*The term "Anaphylaxis" was originally coined by Dr. Charles Richet, who was able to create the condition by injecting dogs with a toxin, thinking that it would create a certain amount of immunity. However, the dogs became extremely hypersensitive, and, when given a second, smaller dose, the dogs had a violent reaction that quickly killed them.]

[*Miller's Review of Critical Vaccine Studies* (2016) lists more than 400 scientific studies (438 to be exact) related to the adverse effects of vaccinations.]

Infectious childhood illnesses, such as measles, mumps, and chickenpox, cause an inflammatory response (fever, mucus, rash, etc.) that serves to strengthen the immune system so that children become more resistant to future infections. This is in contrast to vaccines, which can interfere with the immune process. For example, studies have shown that contracting the natural measles virus can protect against heart disease,[130] allergies,[131] and autoimmune diseases.[132] Though it is true that contracting the measles virus is not without risks, because it can cause ear infections, pneumonia, and in rare cases, encephalitis (inflammation of the brain), vaccines can also cause these same conditions. However, by being exposed to these natural infectious diseases, the body develops lifelong immunity to the virus in most cases and, at the same time, strengthens the immune system naturally.

Demyelination—Myelin is the protective coating around the nerve cells of the CNS, consisting of the brain, optic nerves, and spinal cord. The myelin sheath is analogous to the protective plastic coating around electrical wiring. It forms an electrically insulating layer that increases the efficiency of nerve-impulse conduction, which is essential to the proper functioning of the nervous system. When the myelin is damaged, disrupting this electrical nerve conduction, it can result in a number of neuro-degenerative diseases. For example, MS is a form of demyelination in which patches of the myelin sheath are damaged, disrupting the ability of the nervous system to function effectively which can cause multiple symptoms including fatigue, vision problems, lack of motor coordination, and cognitive issues involving memory and concentration. Demyelination is usually caused by some form of inflammation that attacks and destroys myelin, as a result of a virus, infection, lack of oxygen, autoimmune condition, or toxins, including those found in vaccines.

A lack of nerve-impulse conduction, as a result of demyelination, has been linked to autism and may help to explain the kinds of behaviors one sees in autistic children who become disconnected from others, regress in cognitive and language abilities, cannot control motor function, display erratic behaviors, like head banging, rocking back and forth, and so on. This is especially problematic, given all of the vaccines that infants receive today, since research has shown that it takes **2 years** for the myelin sheath to completely finish its growth process in order to fully protect nerve cells.[133]

Microbiome and Autoimmune Disorders—The human microbiome is an internal complex ecosystem composed of trillions of microbial cells and genetic material from bacteria, fungi, and viruses that are on and in the body, including the nose, throat, gastrointestinal, and urogenital tracts and skin. How the microbiome, viruses, and bacteria interact helps to determine what role they play in keeping us healthy or making us sick. It is estimated that there are **more than 100 trillion** microbes that help govern nearly every function of the human body. They affect most metabolic functions, with the capacity to protect against pathogens, balance hormones, support the immune system, detoxify the gut, and so on. The gut has even been referred to as the **second brain,**[134] due to its ability to communicate with the brain through neurons and neurotransmitters, affecting everything from anxiety, depression, fatigue, autoimmunity, chronic diseases, skin conditions, digestive problems, and so on. Some researchers suggest that up to **90%** of all diseases can be traced back to the gut and to the health of the microbiome. For example, autoimmune diseases can be triggered by the gut or gastrointestinal tract, the channel through which food travels.

One way to treat autoimmunity is by restoring the microbiome through the use of probiotics, avoiding sugar, reducing stress, limiting antibiotics, regular exercise, adequate sleep, avoiding smoking, and following a healthy diet. However, when there is a microbial imbalance of the microbiome, called **dysbiosis,** it can precipitate numerous chronic and inflammatory diseases, as a result of toxins, antibiotics, poor diet, illness, stress, aging, the poisons sprayed on crops, such as glyphosate, and the reliance on baby formulas instead of the mother's own breast milk.

The purpose of the immune system is to protect the body from invading microorganisms by producing antibodies that will recognize and destroy these foreign agents. Autoimmunity occurs when these antibodies end up attacking the body's own cells and tissues, causing a variety of autoimmune disorders. In the past few decades, there has been a dramatic rise in autoimmune disorders, as exemplified by the 151 diseases identified by the American Autoimmune Related Diseases Association (AARDA) including encephalomyelitis, rheumatoid arthritis, Type 1 diabetes, lupus, multiple sclerosis (MS), inflammatory bowel disease (such as Crohn's disease and colitis), celiac disease, fibromyalgia, GBS, Kawasaki disease, narcolepsy, psoriasis, Parkinson's disease, asthma, and various food allergies to name a few.

The exact way in which autoimmunity is triggered is not totally clear but bacteria, viruses, and drugs definitely play a role. It has also been established that autoimmune disorders run in the family because of a genetic predisposition, and that these diseases can be precipitated by environmental factors, such as an infection whether from a natural disease or environmental toxins. Recently, a new autoimmune syndrome has been identified called **ASIA,** which stands for **autoimmune/inflammatory syndrome induced by adjuvants.**[135] This refers to a spectrum of immune-mediated diseases triggered by an adjuvant stimulus, as in the case of aluminum used in vaccines, in order to trigger an antibody response.

Leaky Gut Syndrome—In 2000, Dr. Alessio Fasano, a leading authority in the field of immunology, discovered that intestinal hyperpermeability or "leaky gut" is another key factor in autoimmunity. This refers to perforations in the intestinal wall allowing microorganisms, pathogens, toxins, bacteria, viruses, and food particles to leak across the intestinal wall into the bloodstream causing "leaky gut syndrome."[136] This creates an excessive inflammatory response in the body that can cause gastrointestinal tract problems, such as chronic diarrhea, constipation, and abdominal discomfort; autoimmune diseases; mood disorders; food allergies; skin conditions such as eczema and psoriasis; thyroid disorders; celiac disease caused by gluten; and nutritional deficiencies, such as low levels of vitamin B12, digestive enzymes, and magnesium. In response, the body reacts by developing antibodies that end up mistakenly attacking the body's own cells, causing inflammation that then triggers autoimmunity. If the inflammation occurs in the joints, the individual can develop rheumatoid arthritis; if the pancreas is inflamed, pancreatitis can result; if the lining of the lungs is inflamed, asthma can develop.

Institute of Medicine—In 1996, the Institute of Medicine (IOM) acknowledged that vaccines can and do cause brain damage and immune-system dysfunction. What follows are some of the adverse reactions to vaccines that IOM identified or were unable to reject based on inadequate evidence.[137]

- Diphtheria, tetanus toxoid, and pertussis vaccine (DTP) has been associated with acute encephalopathy, shock, anaphylaxis, GBS, and brachial neuritis.
- The MMR vaccine has also been implicated in thrombocytopenia (abnormal bleeding in the body), acute and chronic arthritis, anaphylaxis, encephalopathy, GBS, aseptic meningitis, and SIDS.
- The oral polio vaccine (OPV) has been associated with increased cases of poliomyelitis (polio), GBS, and death from polio-vaccine-strain viral infection.
- Hib vaccine has been correlated to greater susceptibility in contracting the Hemophilus influenzae type B meningitis disease itself.

- Hepatitis B vaccine has been associated with GBS, demyelinating diseases of the CNS, arthritis, anaphylaxis, and SIDS.

In 2001, the IOM suggested that further study was needed to better understand the adverse effects of vaccines. It also emphasized the importance of each person's unique immune system in determining the potential risk for an adverse vaccine reaction. The IOM (now called the **Health and Medicine Division of the National Academies of Sciences, Engineering, and Medicine**), endorsed the hypothesis that *"exposure to thimerosal-containing vaccines could be associated with neurodevelopmental disorders."* However, in 2004 IOM curiously reversed its position, contending that

> *"The potential biological mechanisms for vaccine-induced autism"* was seen as *"only theoretical."* The report concluded, *"From a public health perspective, the committee does not consider a significant investment in studies of the theoretical vaccine-autism connection to be useful at this time."*[138]

Mind you, this apparent lack of interest in pursuing any association between vaccines and autism coincided with the dramatic rise in autism during this same period.

Given the complexity of the immune system and the uncertainty of vaccine reactions based on the health of the child at the time; the hereditary differences among people; the state of one's immune system, and poor health conditions related to premature birth, immunocompromised conditions, neurological diseases, and the like, one would think that maybe we should be taking a more cautious approach to the current medical practice of indiscriminately vaccinating all children in the same way. This vaccine overload, especially in infants, can trigger a reactogenic response that causes excessive inflammation, leading to a more severe adverse reaction, beyond a simple fever or sore arm at the injection site. It is worth repeating that the developed nations that require the most vaccinations have the highest infant-mortality rates.[139]

Refer to Appendix C, *Autoimmunity and the Immune System* for a summary of autoimmunity and how it affects the immune system.

PART V

VACCINES

In our zeal to eradicate a few infectious diseases, we have traded typically mild illnesses of childhood, such as chickenpox, mumps, and measles, for a lifetime of poor health and drugs. —Sherri Tenpenny, DO

Prior to our discussion of vaccines, it is revealing to note the increasing cost of vaccinations over approximately the past 30 years. In 1990, the cost for vaccinating a child from birth to 18 years of age was $70. By 2000, the cost was $370, by 2012 it was $1,712, and today, it's up to $2200, based on current CDC data. That's more than 30 times the price that parents paid 30 years ago. Undoubtedly, vaccines have become big business today with the pharmaceutical industry bringing in billions of dollars each year in the U.S. alone. Unfortunately, the statistics on neurodevelopmental problems in children today clearly suggest that kids are not as healthy as in the past. This raises the question, "Are we any better off as a result of this onslaught of vaccinations that children receive today?"

Before we discuss the commonly administered vaccines, it is important to get a sense of the technology behind the different types of vaccines that have been developed. This part is probably more technical than what most people want to know, but it is useful in getting a sense of how complex and convoluted this vaccine process can be.

Vaccine Classification—Vaccines are used as a preventative measure; they are not used as a cure for an existing condition. They are designed to boost the immune system in order to prevent life-threatening diseases through the use of antibodies that are activated by the vaccine itself. The components used in vaccines determine how each vaccine works. It is important to understand that each type of vaccine has certain properties that indicate its apparent benefits as well as its contraindications. There are roughly five major categories of vaccines: live attenuated (or weakened) vaccines; inactivated vaccines; subunit vaccines, mRNA vaccines, and viral vector vaccines that are all briefly summarized below.

1. **Live attenuated vaccines** use a weakened form of the virus that causes disease. Assumed to be similar in form to the natural infection, it attempts to create a strong and longer-lasting immune response. However, it raises some safety concerns since it contains living organisms that may adversely affect people who are elderly or have a weakened immune system or other health issues. Additionally, refrigeration is critical in protecting the vaccine while being transported. Live vaccines include: MMR, chickenpox, rotavirus, oral polio, and yellow fever.

2. **Inactivated vaccines are** derived by destroying the viruses or bacteria through a process using heat, radiation, or chemicals, such as formaldehyde. In this way, the pathogens are unable to replicate. This vaccine is generally considered safe when given to a person with an impaired immune system. However, since inactivated vaccines produce a weaker response, adjuvants and booster shots are usually required to provide a more robust immune response. Inactivated vaccines include: hepatitis A, pertussis, inactivated polio, flu shot, and rabies.

3. **Subunit vaccines** are also referred to as **acellular,** meaning they do not contain any whole cells. They contain fragments of a pathogen (bacteria or virus) used to trigger an immune response and stimulate acquired immunity against the pathogen from which it is made. Though these vaccines are considered safer and easier to produce, they usually require an adjuvant to elicit a stronger immune response. There are a number of vaccines that fall into this category:

    A. **Toxoid vaccines** are derived from a specific toxin produced by certain bacteria, such as tetanus or diphtheria, which are responsible for the symptoms of the disease. The inactivated toxin is turned into a harmless form, called toxoid, and used as a vaccine antigen to create an immune response. Examples include: diphtheria and tetanus.

    B. **Conjugate vaccines** attach a weak antigen with a stronger antigen in order to increase the immune response. Haemophilus influenzae type b vaccine (Hib) is an example of a conjugate vaccine.

    C. **Recombinant vaccines** are made by combining at least two strands of DNA (referred to as recombinant DNA) in order to stimulate an immune response. For example, part of the DNA from the hepatitis B virus is put in the DNA of yeast cells. The HPV vaccine is another recombinant vaccine.

4. **Messenger RNA vaccines (mRNA)** direct cells to produce copies of a protein known as the spike protein which triggers an immune response, designed to recognize and neutralize the real virus when exposed to it. The Pfizer-BioNTech and the Moderna COVID-19 vaccines use mRNA.

5. **Viral vector vaccine** uses the genetic material from the COVID-19 virus that is placed in a modified version of a different virus, viral vector, that goes into the cells with instructions to make copies of the spike protein so when later infected with the COVID-19 virus, the antibodies will attack the virus. AstraZeneca and Johnson & Johnson are vector vaccines.

The complex nature of the vaccine-developmental process, as highlighted above, assumes that the various types of vaccines will be equally effective regardless of who receives them. Yet, the CDC has acknowledged that 66 vaccines in the U.S. have been taken off the market as of May 2019, due to issues with vaccine safety.[140] The current rush to market the COVID-19 vaccines in a matter of a few months, as opposed to years, is especially worrisome given the experimental nature of this new vaccine technology. The customary animal studies, done as a precautionary step, have been bypassed without any serious consideration of the long-term effects on the human population.

Vaccines are an enormous topic for discussion that is covered in greater detail in many of the references noted in the bibliography of this book. Studies done on vaccines that have been on the market for years, prior to the COVID phenomenon, indicate that there are still considerable questions about their own efficacy. Given these concerns, one can only wonder what issues are going to arise over time with the less understood COVID vaccines. What follows is a brief review of studies conducted on these primary vaccines.

Vaccine Studies
Hepatitis B—an inflammatory liver disease caused by the hepatitis B virus causing fever, body fatigue, nausea, vomiting, abdominal and joint pain, and jaundice. It is transmitted primarily through sex-related infections or by needle sharing among drug addicts. In rare cases, the disease can be passed on by an infected mother to her newborn. Regardless of whether the mother is infected by the virus, all infants still receive this

vaccine on the first day of life a few hours after coming out of the womb. In 1991, the CDC recommended that all infants receive the hepatitis B vaccine even though this disease occurs in adults primarily. The CDC acknowledged *"fewer than 1% of all reported hepatitis B cases occur in people younger than 15 years old."*[141]

- After the hepatitis B vaccine was introduced, the adverse reactions from the vaccine were enormous. Jane Orient, MD, Executive Director of the *Association of American Physicians and Surgeons*, stated in a 1999 Congressional testimonial:

  VAERS contains 25,000 reports related to hepatitis B vaccine, about one-third of which were serious enough to lead to an emergency room visit, hospitalization, or death...Public policy regarding vaccines is fundamentally flawed. It is permeated by conflicts of interest. It is based on poor scientific methodology (including studies that are too small, too short, and too limited in populations represented), which is, moreover, insulated from independent criticism.[143]

- There were no long-term studies on the hepatitis B vaccine and fewer than 150 children were monitored for **only 5 days,** before the vaccine was approved by the Advisory Board of the FDA. No studies were conducted to determine whether pregnant women, developing fetuses, or infants were at risk of injury. In addition, hep B has not been evaluated for its carcinogenic or mutagenic potential, or its ability to impair fertility.[142]

- Because the hepatitis B vaccine provides immunity for only maybe 5–10 years, what is the rationale for giving this vaccine to an infant? After all, this is a disease that is spread primarily through sexually promiscuous behavior or needle sharing among addicts. Consequently, the argument for vaccinating infants to protect the teen or adult population is ridiculous. Nevertheless, the CDC recommended that all newborns should receive the hep B vaccine not because they were at risk of infection but instead because the attempts at vaccinating the adult population failed. Therefore, the CDC reasoned that, *"Universal infant vaccination would eliminate the need for vaccinating adolescents and high-risk adults."*[144]

- A doctor's survey indicated that up to 87% of pediatricians and family practitioners did not believe that infants needed the hepatitis B vaccine.[145]

- Between 1990 and 1998, *"There were 24,775 adverse reactions to the [hep B] vaccine in all age groups. Of these, 9,673 were serious enough for hospitalization, life-threatening health problems or disabilities, and 439 people died."*[146]

- In 1996, VAERS received complaints of adverse reactions to the vaccine **20 times more** than from actual cases of the disease in infants in the first year of life.[147]

- In 1998, France suspended the hepatitis B vaccine after reports of chronic arthritis, MS, and other health issues. MS cases rose by 65% following the national campaign to increase hep B vaccination rates in France.[148]

- Cases of demyelination, serious autoimmune diseases, MS, arthritis, optic nerve damage, lupus, vasculitis, and thrombocytopenia have also been reported as a result of the hepatitis B vaccine.[149]

- A large series of autoimmune conditions have been reported following the hep B vaccination showing significant increases in MS (5.2x's), optic neuritis (14x's), vasculitis (2.6x's), arthritis (2x's), alopecia [loss of hair] (7.2x's), lupus erythematosus (9.1x's), rheumatoid arthritis (18x's), and thrombocytopenia (2.3x's).[150]

- GBS occurred in 9% of cases after the hepatitis B vaccination and 27% of cases occurred after receiving multiple vaccines.[151] GBS is a severe immune disorder that damages the myelin sheath of the nervous system, which can cause muscle weakness, paralysis, and even death.

- A 2008 study in the *Journal of Toxicology and Environmental Health* by Gallagher and Goodman showed that based on parental reports, boys aged 1–9 years who received three doses of the hepatitis B vaccine with mercury (thimerosal) were **8.63 times** more likely than unvaccinated boys to become developmentally disabled.[152]
- Another study by Gallagher and Goodman in 2010, determined that *"Boys vaccinated as neonates had threefold greater odds for autism diagnosis compared to boys never vaccinated or vaccinated after the first month of life."*[153]
- According to the FDA's Code of Federal Regulations, the maximum FDA allowance for parenteral [injected] aluminum is 25 micrograms per day, even though the amount of aluminum in HepB alone is roughly **14 times more** than the maximum dosage allowed for an 8-pound-newborn infant.[154] This does not include the large doses of aluminum found in both the Hib and DTaP vaccines, in addition.

Diphtheria, Pertussis, Tetanus (DPT/DTaP)—The "three shots in one" vaccine makes it more potent and potentially more toxic than if given separately. These vaccines have never been tested for safety in combination. Numerous adverse reactions have been reported in scientific research studies and by the pharmaceutical companies themselves as indicated in the "vaccine product inserts." These include medical issues such as convulsions, encephalitis (inflammation of the brain), meningitis, GBS (severe paralytic disease), anaphylactic shock (severe allergic reaction to an injection), seizures, mental retardation, diabetes, MS, leukemia, and SIDS.

- In the mid-1940s, diphtheria was combined with the pertussis and tetanus components to form the DPT vaccine. Initially, the DPT vaccine was touted as providing lifelong immunity but when that turned out to be false, a total of six booster shots ended up being included in the vaccine schedule.

- There was a 400% increase in meningitis cases between 1946 and 1986 that coincided with the widespread use of the DPT vaccine.[155]
- Today, children are given the DTaP vaccine at 2, 4, 6, and 18 months, and then again prior to entering public school. In 2005, another booster shot was recommended between the ages of 11 and 64 because of the waning immunity with each additional vaccination.[156]
- A 1987 study showed a **7-fold increase** in SIDS cases within 3 days of the DPT vaccine, and a third of the SIDS deaths occurred within 24 hours of the DPT vaccine being given.[157]
- DTaP replaced DPT in 1996 because of the severe adverse reactions from the DPT shot. The DTaP was supposed to be an improved version with a new acellular pertussis (aP) vaccine added to the original diphtheria and tetanus vaccines. However, the DTaP vaccine caused severe reactions as well, suggesting that the pertussis component of the vaccine may be at fault.[158]
- A 2000 study in the *Journal of Manipulative and Physiological Therapeutics, by* Hurwitz & Morgenstern, showed that children who were given the DPT vaccine had more than twice the rate of asthma and other related respiratory diseases compared to unvaccinated children.[159]
- Additional DTaP vaccines should be discontinued if there is an adverse reaction from a previous shot, such as: hives, difficulty breathing from swelling of the mouth or throat, high-pitched screaming or a prolonged crying spell, high fever, vomiting, and convulsions. However, this vaccine is routinely given to children with little regard for previous reactions.
- The DTaP vaccine, Tripedia, was taken off the market in 2011 as a result of adverse reactions listed by the drug manufacturer, Sanofi Pasteur, including **autism,** anaphylactic shock, and SIDS. Later the FDA stated, *"There's no credible evidence linking vaccination to autism or other*

developmental disorders," which raises the question, Why then was the vaccine taken off the market?[160]

- In 2017, Mogensen et al. reviewed a study in Guinea-Bissau, Africa, in which baby girls, ages 3 to 5 months old, died at **10 times** the rate of the unvaccinated girls after receiving the DTP vaccine. Infant boys of the same age, died at 4 times the rate of the unvaccinated boys.[161]

Diphtheria—an acute bacterial illness that causes a lack of energy, sore throat, headache, nausea, fever, and swollen glands. Swelling of the throat and larynx in severe cases can cut off one's ability to breathe. Antibiotics such as penicillin are effective in the treatment of diphtheria.

- In the past, diphtheria was a serious disease owing to poor living conditions associated with a lack of sanitation, poor hygiene, and poverty. *"In the United States, deaths from diphtheria had declined 98 percent from the year 1900 up to the mid-1940s before the DTP vaccine was introduced."*[162]
- Robert Mendelsohn, M.D., in his book *How to Raise a Healthy Child in Spite of Your Doctor* (1984) stated:

  Today your child has about as much chance of contracting diphtheria as he does of being bitten by a cobra. Yet millions of children are immunized against it with repeated injections at 2, 4, 6, and 18 months and then given a booster shot when they enter school.[163]

- In the United States, there were 2 cases of diphtheria reported between 2004 and 2015, according to CDC records. Because diphtheria is extremely rare in the States today and the bacterial disease is easily treated with antibiotics, it raises the question as to why children need to keep taking a vaccine that is not responsible for the decline of this disease to begin with.[164] In 2015, there were no confirmed cases of diphtheria in the United States out of a population of more than 300,000,000.

Pertussis (Whooping Cough)—a contagious bacterial respiratory tract infection that is usually transmitted through the air by an infected person. It starts off similar to a common cold, but as it progresses, a severe hacking cough develops, causing a whooping sound. Symptoms include runny nose, fever, and coughing that can lead to exhaustion. More than half of the cases occur in children younger than 2 years old, with the most severe reactions in infants.

- In the past, whooping cough was caused by poor living conditions—lack of sanitation, poor hygiene, contaminated water, and malnutrition. As a result of improved living conditions, there was a 99% decline in deaths from pertussis before the vaccine's widespread use in the late 1940s.[165]
- Of the three vaccines, pertussis is considered the primary cause of most adverse reactions, especially in infants. In the book *DPT: A Shot in the Dark* (1985), Coulter and Fisher noted that there was a much greater risk of dying from the pertussis vaccine than there was from the disease itself. They calculated that the risk of death from the vaccine was **94 times greater** than from whooping cough disease.[166]
- There are a number of severe reactions associated with the pertussis vaccine including high fever, high-pitched scream-ing, lethargy, collapse/shock, convulsions, anaphylactic shock, brain inflammation (encephalopathy), and death.[167]
- In animal experiments, researchers use the pertussis vac-cine specifically to **induce** encephalomyelitis, which is the inflammation of the brain and spinal cord. Yet, when it comes to humans, the vaccinators have no misgivings about inoculating infants with that same vaccine. Steinman, et al. stated:

> *Local, systemic and neurological complications have*
> *been observed following pertussis vaccination in*

children...The neurological syndrome ranges from minor irritability to convulsions, coma, and, on rare occasions, death.[168]

- In July 1994, the *New England Journal of Medicine,* reported on a study by Celia Christie, et al, in which **74%** of children between 19 months and 12 years old who contracted whooping cough had received four or five doses of the DPT vaccine. In conclusion, they stated, "the whole-cell pertussis vaccine failed to give full protection against the disease."[169]

- The new strains of pertussis (*Bordetella parapertussis*) have now replaced old strains of the disease (*Bordetella pertussis*), causing a more lethal reaction that has resulted in more hospitalizations and deaths. *Miller's Review of Critical Vaccine Studies* cited **more than 20 scientific studies** in which the pertussis vaccine caused virulent vaccine-resistant strains to emerge since it does not control all strains that cause whooping cough, enabling the bacterium to adapt and survive in humans.[170]

- Vitamin C in adequate doses has been shown to be more effective than antibiotics in reducing whooping cough symptoms. A 2003 study by A.E. Tozzi et al. showed that antibiotic-treated children had a longer recovery time than those who went untreated.[171]

- A 2011 study at Kaiser Medical Center headed by an infectious disease expert discovered that the whooping-cough vaccine lost its effectiveness within 3 years so that the vaccinated become more susceptible at a later age and *"could help to explain a recent series of outbreaks in the U.S. among children who were fully vaccinated."*[172]

- Hegerle, et al. noted that the pertussis vaccine became less effective by causing strains of the disease to mutate, shifting whooping-cough cases from children to adolescents and adults.[173]

- The CDC admitted that cases of whooping cough were increasing in spite of high vaccination rates, reflecting the failure of the vaccine to prevent the disease.[174] Unfortunately, the CDC's solution to a vaccine's waning effect on infants is to give pregnant women the Tdap vaccine during their pregnancy, despite the fact that the Tdap vaccine has never been tested to determine its safety when given to pregnant women.[175]
- In a 2016 article, Barbara Loe Fisher stated that DTaP vaccine provides only 2–5 years of temporary immunity and that:

> *Millions of vaccinated children and adults are silently infected with pertussis in the U.S. every year and show few or no symptoms but spread whooping cough to vaccinated and unvaccinated children.*[176]

Nevertheless, the unvaccinated are still being blamed for the rise in pertussis cases today.

- The NVIC reported that between 1990 and 2019, there have been:

> *160,672 serious adverse events reported to the Vaccine Adverse Events Reporting System (VAERS) in connection with pertussis-containing vaccines…Half of those serious pertussis vaccine-related adverse events occurred in children younger than 3 years old. Of these pertussis-vaccine related adverse events reported to VAERS, 3,082 were deaths, with nearly 90% of the deaths occurring in children younger than three years old.*[177]

Tetanus (lockjaw)—a disease of the central nervous system (CNS) caused by a bacterial infection that creates painful muscle spasms, often referred to as lockjaw. Other symptoms include head and body aches, difficulty swallowing, fever, seizures, sweating, and increased heart rate. The bacteria are found in the soil, dust, or fecal matter from animals. Tetanus results from the bacteria entering a cut or other wound. It is prevalent in third-world countries with poor sanitary conditions, while it is quite rare in the United States. Tetanus is **not** a contagious disease that can spread from person to person; the vaccine is intended to provide only personal protection.

- According to the CDC, there were a total of 233 cases of tetanus in the United States over a 7-year period from 2001 to 2008, with deaths averaging only 4 per year in a population of more than 300,000,000.[178]
- Tetanus in infants is essentially nonexistent, yet we vaccinate children at 2, 4, 6, and 18 months of age as part of the DTaP vaccine. *"Neonatal tetanus is rare in the United States, with only two cases reported since 1989."*[179]
- It is questionable whether the tetanus vaccine actually prevents tetanus, but it has been shown to cause severe reactions. According to the CDC,

  > *Serious reported side effects following tetanus toxoid vaccination include anaphylaxis, brachial neuritis, Guillain-Barré syndrome, acute disseminated encephalomyelitis (ADEM), arthritis, and myocarditis.*[180]

- Good wound care is the most effective way to prevent infection from tetanus without having to vaccinate because the bacteria cannot survive when exposed to air.[181]
- The National Vaccine Information Center (NVIC) raised the question, *"How can the tetanus vaccine induce immunity, when contracting the disease naturally does not give immunity?"*

Hemophilus Influenzae Type B Meningitis (Hib)—a bacterial infection that can cause severe illnesses in children based on inflammation of the membranes (meninges) that cover the brain and spinal cord. Hib is transmitted through respiratory droplets passed on from one person to another by sneezing or coughing. There are two types: **viral meningitis** (also called aseptic meningitis), which is fairly common and less severe, with no specific treatment, and **bacterial meningitis** that can cause severe reactions, such as hearing loss, neurological disorders, GBS, seizures, fever, pneumonia, and even death, if not treated promptly.

- In a Finland study of 100,000 children, the vaccine was found to have no efficacy under the age of 18 months, though today U.S. infants receive the meningitis vaccine at 2, 4, 6, and 12 months of age.[182]
- In 1988, the *Journal of the American Medical Association* reported that the Hib vaccine (PRP) was actually causing more cases of meningitis than it was preventing. Since the vaccine does not target all strains of the disease, the vaccine induces the emergence of other strains that become more virulent.[183]
- In the journal *Pediatrics*, a study showed a **1.8 to 6.4–fold increase** in meningitis one week after vaccination compared to unvaccinated children.[184]
- Before the Hib vaccine was introduced, 65% of all cases were the "b" strain. After the Hib vaccination, 84% of all cases are now caused by other strains, like Hia, and other non-b strains, thereby negating the vaccine's effectiveness.[185]
- Research indicated a link between the Hib vaccine and type 1 diabetes following a mass vaccination effort with a 26% increase in diabetes after getting four doses of the Hib vaccine. The editor of the *British Medical Journal* wrote that "*the data support a causal relation... Furthermore, the potential risk of the vaccine exceeds the potential benefit.*"[186] A similar rise in cases of type 1 diabetes was noted in Finland, New Zealand, England, Italy, Sweden, and Denmark.

- Adverse vaccine reactions reported include: GBS, transverse myelitis, aseptic meningitis, invasive pneumococcal disease, thrombocytopenia, erythema multiforme, fever, rash, hives, vomiting, diarrhea, seizures, convulsions, and sudden infant death syndrome.[187]
- Adults and, in particular, the elderly became more susceptible to contracting Hib, causing increased hospitalizations and death as a result of the Hib vaccination of children.

> *The epidemiological characteristics of invasive H. influenzae disease have changed from a disease that predominantly affects children and is dominated by type b to a disease that predominantly affects adults and is dominated by non-typeable strains.*[188]

- VAERS received 29,747 complaints regarding the Hib vaccine between 1990 and 2013, with 5,179 serious injuries (17%) and **896 deaths** (3%). SIDS was identified in 384 cases of the 749 deaths (51%). Given the total number of deaths associated with the Hib vaccine, Moro et al. came to the rather curious conclusion, *"Review of VAERS reports did not identify any new or unexpected safety concerns for Hib vaccines."*[189]

Rotavirus—a virus first identified in 1973 that causes diarrhea and is generally mild and self-limiting. Common symptoms include diarrhea, fever, cold-like symptoms, vomiting, and abdominal pain. The biggest concern is dehydration, which can be easily addressed by re-hydrating the infant. It is most prevalent between 3 and 36 months of age. Infants develop antibodies from the virus that provide immunity or a milder case if reinfected. The majority of cases occur in poor countries where children are malnourished and have limited access to medical care.

- In 1998, the Rotashield vaccine was introduced and after 11 months it was taken off the market because of cases of intussusception, in which one part of the intestine telescopes inside of another, causing severe abdominal pain as a result of intestinal blockage. The obstruction can cause intestinal injury that can lead to death if not promptly addressed.[190]

- According to the CDC, babies who got the vaccine were **30 times** more likely to develop intussusception than those not vaccinated.[191]
- In 2007, RotaTeq, a new version of the vaccine, was put on the market and caused the same problem of intussusception. Serious adverse reactions were reported in 803 cases out of 34,035 vaccine recipients (2.4%) with 24 deaths.[192]
- Additional adverse reactions from the RotaTeq vaccine have been reported by the CDC, including fever, seizures, diarrhea, vomiting, otitis media, and SIDS.[193]

Pneumococcal Disease (PCV7/PCV13/PPSV23)—a serious bacterial illness that can cause ear infections, blood infections, pneumonia, and meningitis. Though the Prevnar vaccines are supposed to protect against pneumonia and otitis media in 7 and 13 strains, there are more than 90 strains of the disease, most of which are not covered by these vaccines. The pneumococcal polysaccharide vaccine (PPSV23) was licensed in 1983, covering 23 strains; it is generally recommended for adults older than 65 years old.

- According to the 2007 *Physicians Desk Reference (PDR)*, both pneumonia and otitis media are actual side effects of the Prevnar vaccine itself.[194]
- The PCV7 vaccine came out in 2000, targeting only 7 of these strains, and, in 2010, the PCV13 was approved, this time targeting 13 of these strains. Unfortunately, the nonvaccine strains quickly replaced the strains targeted by the vaccine that ended up being more virulent. In *Miller's Review of Critical Vaccine Studies,* **15 studies** are cited, each highlighting the rapid replacement of strains

not included in the PCV7 and PCV13 vaccines that were quickly rendered inadequate.[195]

- *The American Journal of Medical Science* reported on new vaccine-induced strains that significantly increased the risk of pneumococcal disease in children and adults and have become resistant to antibiotics.[196]
- Two years after PCV13 came on the market, 94% of all pneumococcal strains of the disease were strains not targeted by the vaccine itself, according to a study in the *Pediatric Infectious Disease Journal*.[197]
- The vaccine manufacturer Pfizer lists the following adverse reactions in the Prevnar 13 vaccine product insert: muscle and joint pain, fever, vomiting, seizures, pneumonia, apnea, hypotonia, diabetes, ear infections, anaphylactic shock, and SIDS.[198]

Poliomyelitis (Polio)—referred to as infantile paralysis, polio spreads to others primarily through food or water contaminated by fecal matter. Those exposed to the viral infection usually develop immunity. Even in undeveloped countries with poor sanitation, most children develop antibodies to the infection as infants. A small number of infections can lead to paralytic polio affecting the gray matter of the spinal cord and brain. Generallly, polio is a benign disease as acknowledged by the CDC.

- In 2013, the CDC wrote:

> *Approximately 95% of persons infected with polio will have no symptoms. About 4–8% of infected persons have minor symptoms, such as fever, fatigue, nausea, headache, flu-like symptoms, stiffness in the neck and back, and pain in the limbs, which often resolve completely. Fewer than 1% of polio cases result in permanent paralysis of the limbs (usually the legs). Of those paralyzed, 5–10% of that 1% die when the paralysis strikes the respiratory muscles.*[199]

- The common perception portrayed in the media that paralytic polio was widespread and particularly crippling runs counter to the CDC's description of the disease. The public has been indoctrinated in the belief that cases of polio would result in paralysis, if people did not get vaccinated. Polio became synonymous with severe paralysis. The campaign by the March of Dimes, showing children in braces, wheelchairs, and the iron lung machine, instilled fear in the minds of the general public. The dogmatic belief regarding the efficacy of the polio vaccine has been so deeply ingrained in the public consciousness that to question this orthodoxy is considered ludicrous by most people.

- After the polio vaccine was introduced, the criteria for diagnosis became more stringent, making it seem like the vaccine was eliminating polio. Before 1954, doctors diagnosed polio if the paralysis lasted for only a short period of time, which was often the case with polio. After the introduction of the vaccine, the criteria for diagnosis were changed to 60 days, so that any paralysis lasting less than 60 days was no longer classified as polio. In this way, the number of polio cases reported decreased dramatically, creating the perception that the vaccine was the reason why.[200]

- In Suzanne Humphries' book *Dissolving Illusions: Disease, Vaccines, and the Forgotten History,* she devoted a lengthy chapter to the history of polio and the vaccine. She pointed out that in June 1955, the polio vaccine was approved in **only 2 hours,** in spite of objections by some members of the committee reviewing the vaccine.[201] The dubious vaccine was put on the market and resulted in 40,000 children contracting polio, leaving 164 severely paralyzed, and 10 dead. This was called the *"Cutter Incident"* after the Cutter Laboratories that produced the vaccine.[202]

- Eleanor McBean, in *The Poisoned Needle: Suppressed Facts about Vaccinations (1957),* reported on numerous incidences in which children were given the Salk vaccine, but results showed more cases of polio than prior to the vaccine, causing many states to halt vaccinations all together.

- Monkey kidneys were used in the manufacture of the polio vaccine that ended up containing a carcinogenic monkey virus called Simian Virus number 40 (SV40) in which 98 million doses were given to U.S. children between 1955 and 1963. It subsequently resulted in cancers, not seen until years later, causing tumors of the brain, bone, breast, colon, and kidneys.[203]

- Prior to 1954, polio was incorrectly over-reported by health officials based on a number of conditions that created polio-like paralytic diseases, including: DDT and arsenic toxicity, congenital syphilis, transverse myelitis, GBS, limb paralysis based on a variety of vaccines, lead poisoning, and enteroviruses, such as Coxsackie and ECHO (enteric cytopathic human orphan) viruses.[204]

- Initially, insects and, in particular, flies, were considered the cause of spreading the polio virus and DDT was used generously to eliminate the supposed carriers. It was sprayed on children, sprinkled on food, used on fruit and vegetable crops, put in the water supply, and so on because it was assumed to be safe and effective. Well, it wasn't, and the exposure to DDT induced the polio-like symptoms. Not surprisingly, in the 1960s, around the same time that DDT was phased out in the U.S., the incidences of polio decreased correspondingly.[205]

- Another widely used poison in the past was arsenic, also known to cause polio-like symptoms. It was sprayed on the sugarcane fields starting in 1913, to kill the weeds that made harvesting sugarcane difficult. The sudden rise of polio between 1916 and 1918 coincided with the spraying of sugarcane with arsenic.[206]

- Arsenic was also sprayed on fruits and vegetables, prescribed by doctors to treat asthma, added to tobacco for smoking, used to destroy cholera, and applied to decayed teeth in order to kill nerve endings.[207]
- The treatments used with paralytic victims actually exacerbated the condition by cutting children's tendons, straightening their legs and placing them in a plaster cast, where they would be immobilized from a few months up to two years, causing atrophy of the limbs. Sister Elizabeth Kenny was a nurse from Australia who effectively treated polio victims with the use of hot packs and physical therapy to correct the injurious conventional treatments of that time that exacerbated the paralysis.[208]
- In 1963, Albert Sabin's oral "live-virus" polio vaccine replaced Salk's "killed-virus" vaccine, but this caused even more cases of polio, and eventually the medical authorities reverted back to the inactivated vaccine.[209]
- In a 1977 congressional hearing, Jonas Salk stated, "the only cases of polio since 1961 were most likely the result of the live-virus polio vaccine." He added:

> *Live virus vaccines against paralytic polio, for example, may in each instance produce the disease it is intended to prevent; the live virus vaccines against measles and mumps may produce such side effects as encephalitis. Both of these problems are due to the inherent difficulty of controlling live viruses once they are placed in a live person.*[210]

- In a Dec. 7, 1985 lecture to Italian doctors in Piacenze, Italy, Albert Sabin, M.D., stated, *"Official data have shown that the large-scale vaccinations undertaken in the U.S. have failed to obtain any significant improvement over the diseases against which they were supposed to provide protection."*[211]

- In India today, while the wild poliovirus has declined, as a result of the oral polio vaccination program, the related acute flaccid paralysis (AFP) has exploded and is twice as deadly as the wild-virus polio. The *Indian Journal of Medical Ethics* stated:

  > *While India has been polio-free for a year, there has been a huge increase in non-polio acute flaccid paralysis. In 2011, there were an extra 47,500 new cases of non-polio acute flaccid paralysis (NPAFD). Clinically indistinguishable from polio paralysis, the incidence of NPAFD was directly proportional to the doses of oral polio received.*[212, 213]

  Appendix D, *A Brief History of Polio*, discusses polio in more detail.

Influenza (Flu)—a contagious disease caused by influenza virus that can cause fever, cough, sore throat, headache, muscle aches, and fatigue. The elderly, infants, and those with chronic diseases are most at risk. The vaccine can contain a number of ingredients including mercury, aluminum, formaldehyde, phenol, and ethylene glycol.

- The vaccine was developed in the 1940s to protect military personnel and was later recommended in 1960 for adults older than 65 years. In 2005, the flu shot was recommended for children starting at 6 months of age even though the journal *The Lancet* conducted an analysis of **24 studies** that found no evidence that the vaccine prevented the flu in children younger than 2 years old.[214]
- The flu vaccine went from 32 million doses in 1990 to 170 million in the 2015–16 flu season. The recommended annual vaccination against common strains of influenza interferes with and reduces the protective immunity against more dangerous strains of the disease.[215]

- The flu shot for the elderly has had no effect on the death rate over the unvaccinated; no correlation was found with increased vaccinations. Simonsen, et al. concluded that the *"observational studies substantially over-estimate vaccination benefit."*[216]
- In 2005, the Cochrane Collaboration, reviewed **51 studies** involving more than 260,000 children that concluded that there was no evidence that injecting children 6–23 months of age with flu vaccines is any more effective than the placebo.[217]
- Today, the CDC recommends the flu shot for pregnant women in any trimester, though this is contraindicated by the vaccine manufacturer and is not supported by scientific research. Pregnant women who were vaccinated were **4 times** more likely to be hospitalized for a flu-like illness than their unvaccinated counterparts.[218]
- In 2009, the swine flu (H1N1) was hyped up by Big Pharma and medical officials in order to prevent another "pandemic" and was approved by the CDC for children and pregnant women after only 5 weeks. In 2010, the European Union investigated the WHO for engineering a false swine flu epidemic, calling it *"one of the greatest medical scandals of the century."*[219]
- Pregnant women vaccinated against the flu and swine flu have higher rates of spontaneous abortions. In 2011, there was a **4350% increase in fetal deaths** resulting from the flu vaccine based on the VAERS database.[220]
- Children who got the flu shot were **4.4 times** more likely than those getting the placebo shot to develop respiratory virus infections. Contracting the natural influenza virus created greater immunity protection against other respiratory infections.[221]
- Dr. J. Anthony Morris, former FDA Chief Vaccine Control Officer, stated:

There is no evidence that any influenza vaccine thus far developed is effective in mitigating any attack of influenza. The producers of these vaccines know that they are worthless, but they go on selling them anyway.[222]

- According to GlaxoSmithKline's vaccine product insert, of the possible adverse effects of the Flulaval Quadrivalent flu vaccine include: anaphylaxis, encephalopathy, syncope (fainting), Guillain-Barré Syndrome, arthritis, convulsions/seizures, life-threatening allergies, and influenza-like symptoms. In addition, the manufacturer states that the vaccine *"has not been evaluated for carcinogenic, mutagenic potential, or infertility."*[223]
- The National Vaccine Information Center reported:

As of July 31, 2020, there have been more than 176,294 reports of influenza vaccines reactions, hospitalizations, injuries and deaths following influenza vaccinations made to VAERS, including 1,748 related deaths, 14,062 hospitalizations, and 3,558 related disabilities.[224]

Measles, Mumps, Rubella (MMR)—The measles vaccine was introduced in the 1960s and combined with the mumps and rubella vaccines in the 1980s. MMR vaccine has been implicated in many adverse reactions, as noted by the vaccine manufacturer in the package insert, including atypical **measles,** vasculitis, pancreatitis, thrombocytopenia, anaphylaxis, arthritis, encephalitis, seizures, encephalopathy, GBS, transverse myelitis, febrile convulsions, ataxia, pneumonia, Stevens-Johnson syndrome, ocular neuritis, deafness, and death, to name a few.[225]

- In 1993, Japan banned the MMR vaccine *"after 1.8 million children had been given two types of MMR and a record number developed non-viral meningitis and other adverse reactions.*"[226]

- The MMR vaccine loses its immunity after a period of time, allowing the spread of the three diseases to others through shedding the live viruses.[227]

- There was a **5-fold increase** in the rate of febrile seizures following the MMR vaccine than from the measles infection based on a Danish study published in 2004. Seizures occurred in about 1 in 640 children within 2 weeks of vaccination and about 300 seizures lead to epilepsy each year as a result of the MMR vaccine.[228, 229]

- Dr. Yazbak, a pediatrician who is an authority in the area of autism and vaccines, published a study in August 2000, showing that a child may develop autism if the mother received the live virus MMR vaccine around conception, pregnancy, or delivery.[230]

- Studies show that these mild infectious diseases, when contracted as a child, strengthened the immune system while conferring lifelong immunity. Researchers have noted the benefits of contracting these common childhood diseases. For example, getting measles and mumps as a child has been shown to decrease the risk of cardiovascular disease later in adulthood.[231]

- Since the advent of the MMR vaccine, new atypical versions of the disease now occur later in life in a more serious form. People receiving the vaccine are still able to contract the disease and are able to spread it to others through shedding of the live virus induced by the fever from the measles vaccination.[232]

- A 2014 study in China showed that there have been more than 700 measles outbreaks between 2009 and 2012, in spite of mandatory vaccine compliance.

The reported coverage of the measles-rubella (MR) or measles-mumps-rubella (MMR) vaccine is greater

than 99% in Zhejiang province. However, the inci-
dence of measles, mumps, and rubella remains
high.[233]

- An international study by Deisher et al. looked at the
  impact of environmental factors on autism prevalence,
  which included the MMR vaccine that contains human
  fetal cells. They wrote:

  Thus, rising autistic disorder prevalence is directly
  related to vaccines manufactured utilizing human
  fetal cells. Increased paternal age and DSM revi-
  sions were not related to rising autistic disorder
  prevalence.[234]

  In other words, autism correlated with the use of human
  fetal cells in vaccines whereas older fathers and the change
  in diagnostic classification did not explain the rise in
  autistic cases.

- Dr. Peter Fletcher, former Chief Scientific Officer of the
  British Dept. of Health, stated:

  Clinical and scientific data is steadily accumulating
  that show that the live measles virus in MMR can
  cause brain, gut, and immune system damage in a
  subset of vulnerable children…It is entirely possible
  that the immune systems of a small minority simply
  cannot cope with the challenge of the three live viruses
  in the MMR jab, and the ever-increasing vaccine
  load in general.[235]

Measles (Rubeola)—a mild immune-building viral infectious disease
caused by the rubeola virus that can be contracted by being in close
contact with an infected individual. Disease symptoms include a

low-grade fever, head and back pain, sensitivity to light, and a severe rash over the whole body. Treatment involves bed rest, fluids to prevent dehydration, and efforts to reduce itchiness.

- The death rate from measles had declined by 97.7% between 1900 and 1955, 8 years before the vaccine was introduced in the United States. The death rate went from 13.3 to 0.03% per 100,000 population.[236] That is **3 deaths out of 10,000,000 people.**

- A study conducted by WHO in 1969 showed that vaccinated children were **15 times** more likely to contract measles than those who were unvaccinated.[237]

- Sencer et al., came to the premature conclusion that the *"Effective use of these vaccines during the coming winter and spring should ensure the eradication of measles from the United States in 1967."*[238] However, a study by Poland and Jacobson, based on a review of 18 separate reports, found that measles outbreaks occurred in highly immunized school populations in the U.S. and Canada. In their conclusion, they wrote, *"The apparent paradox is that as measles immunization rates rise to high levels in a population, measles becomes a disease of immunized persons."*[239]

- Prior to the measles vaccine, infants rarely contracted measles because mothers passed on protective maternal antibodies to their babies through the placenta in the womb, having contracted the natural virus when they were young. As mothers were increasingly vaccinated, it was no longer possible to pass natural immunity on to their babies, thereby making infants more susceptible to contracting measles. As a result, measles is now occurring more often in children younger than one year old and in adults when the temporary immunity wears off, making the disease much more severe and deadlier.[240]

- Since the measles vaccine contains the live virus, vaccinated children are able to transmit measles to other individuals, as also noted in the manufacturer's vaccine product insert.[241, 242] Live viral vaccines include: MMR, chickenpox, zoster, yellow fever, rotavirus, and influenza (intranasal).

- Measles outbreaks in vaccinated populations are common. For example, in 2011, there was a large measles outbreak in Quebec, Canada, in which the authors conclude that the elimination of measles may not be possible even with a 100% vaccination rate.[243]

- By contracting the measles virus naturally, the immune system is actually strengthened, reducing the risk of heart attacks, strokes, cancers, and Parkinson's disease.[244, 245]

- A study in Senegal showed that children who were infected by the measles virus had a lower death rate over the next 4 years than children who did not contract the natural virus, suggesting once again that contracting the natural virus strengthens one's immune system.[246]

- The *PDR* lists the following adverse reactions to the measles vaccine: encephalitis, febrile and afebrile convulsions, anaphylaxis, seizures, ataxia, subacute sclerosing panencephalitis, GBS, ocular palsies, angioneurotic edema, retinitis, deafness, dizziness, optic neuritis, headache, and death.[247]

- According to Dr. Anne Schuchat, the director of CDC's National Center for Immunization and Respiratory Diseases, there have been no deaths from measles between 2004 and 2015 in the United States, but there have been **108 deaths** caused by the MMR vaccine based on the VAERS database during this same 10-year period.[248] In other words, the measles vaccine may actually increase measles deaths instead of reducing them.

- Vitamin A deficiency is a risk factor for a severe measles reaction. High vitamin A supplementation has been shown to be effective in reducing mortality from measles and is an effective alternative to the MMR vaccine in treating the measles virus.

*Combined analyses showed that massive doses of
vitamin A given to patients hospitalized with measles
were associated with an approximately 60% reduction
in the risk of death overall, and with an approximate
90% reduction among infants.*[249]

Mumps—a mild infectious childhood disease caused by the mumps
virus that causes swelling of the salivary glands. Symptoms include
a fever between 100 and 104 degrees, loss of appetite, headache, and
back pain. After a few weeks, symptoms usually subside. No medical
treatment is required except to rest in bed, along with a soft diet and
lots of fluids, and icing to reduce swelling.

- The naturally occurring disease confers lifelong immunity
  while the mumps vaccine confers only short-term protection.[250] Once the vaccine's temporary immunity wears
  off, a more serious reaction can occur later in life as seen
  in the current mumps outbreak among high school and
  college students.[251, 252]
- Between 1967 and 1971, 75% of all mumps cases occurred
  in children age 14 and younger; by 2004, 79% of all mumps
  occurred in people between age 15 and 24, as a result of
  the vaccine itself.[253] Consequently, the widespread use of
  the mumps vaccine has shifted the incidence of the disease
  to adolescence and adults who are more susceptible to
  complications of testicular and ovarian infections, which
  can lead to sterility.
- In 1992, Albonico and Klein reported on 180 European
  doctors who indicated that the mumps vaccine can trigger
  diabetes, causing the medical community in Switzerland to
  resist the MMR immunization campaign.[254] In that same
  year, a study by the *New England Journal of Medicine* also
  confirmed that the vaccine can cause diabetes as well.[255]
- The *Physician's Desk Reference (PDR)* listed the following
  severe side effects from the vaccine: aseptic meningitis,
  encephalitis, orchitis, diabetes mellitus, parotitis (**mumps**),

anaphylaxis, and death.[256] The NVIC reported the following severe vaccine reactions: seizures, brain inflammation and encephalopathy; thrombocytopenia; joint, muscle and nerve pain; gastrointestinal disorders; measles like rash; conjunctivitis and other serious health problems.[257]

Rubella (German Measles)—"Rubella" comes from the Latin word, meaning "little red." It is a mild acute viral disease that causes fever and a rash that spreads from the face and scalp to the arms and body and then fades away after 2 or 3 days. Treatment includes rest and adequate fluids with rare complications reported. Rubella may cause congenital rubella syndrome (CRS), which damages the fetus, causing birth defects if a woman contracts the disease during the first trimester of her pregnancy.

- Before the rubella vaccine came onto the market in 1969, 85% of adults were immune to the disease from childhood by contracting the disease, which provided permanent protection.[258] However, after 5 years of receiving the rubella vaccine, 25% of those vaccinated showed no immunity.[259]
- Because the rubella vaccine now prevents girls from contracting the natural disease as a child, they become more susceptible to contracting CRS later on during the childbearing years.[260]
- Before the vaccine was licensed, 77% of rubella cases occurred in children younger than 15 years old, but by 1990, 81% of all cases were in children 15 years or older. The greatest increases were between the ages of 15 and 29 years when women are in their prime childbearing years. Consequently, CRS has become a greater risk for pregnant women as a result of the vaccine.[261]
- Adverse reactions from the vaccine noted by the pharmaceutical company included: arthritis, arthralgia, myalgia, GBS, polyneuritis, polyneuropathy, anaphylaxis, and death.[262] Other adverse reactions reported include: encephalitis, meningitis, GBS, and joint pain.[263]

Chickenpox (Varicella Virus)—a mild infectious disease of childhood caused by the *varicella-zoster* virus that confers lifelong immunity and helps to protect against heart disease, cancers, and allergic reactions.[264] Symptoms include a rash of red blisters, fever, headache, backache, and loss of appetite. Small red spots appear after a day or two, becoming blisters that form scabs that fall off within a week or two. Though complications are rare in children, adolescents and adults are at a much greater risk for a severe reaction.

- The vaccine was introduced in 1995. The vaccine product insert states that the virus from the vaccine causes "shedding" up to 6 weeks after vaccination and that close contact with others including pregnant women, newborns, premature infants, and immuno-compromised individuals should be avoided.[265]
- Although chickenpox declined after vaccination, cases of shingles at all age levels increased by 90%, and in ages 25–44, shingles increased by 161%.[266] In another study, children who receive the chickenpox vaccine are also getting shingles from the virus in the vaccine.[267]
- According to the findings of a CDC-funded study by Goldman & King:

> *Varicella vaccination is less effective than the natural immunity that existed in prevaccine communities. Universal varicella vaccination has not proven to be cost-effective, as increased HZ [herpes zoster] morbidity has disproportionately offset cost savings associated with reductions in varicella disease. Universal varicella vaccination has failed to provide long-term protection from VZV [varicella-zoster virus] disease.*[268]

- Serious vaccine reactions reported include: anaphylaxis, thrombocytopenia, encephalitis, transverse myelitis, GBS, Bell's palsy, seizures, aseptic meningitis, Stevens-Johnson syndrome, pneumonia, varicella, shingles, herpes zoster, pneumonia, arthralgia, Kawasaki syndrome, optic neuritis, blindness, MS, and death.[269, 270]

Shingles Vaccine—An increase in cases of shingles caused by the chickenpox vaccine has created the opportunity for Merck to develop the shingles vaccine (Zostavax). Unfortunately, this vaccine has had its problems as well, as summarized by the vaccine manufacturer in the clinical trials on safety and efficacy. Zostavax does not protect all vaccine recipients, and the duration of protection beyond 4 years after vaccination is unknown. Adults older than 80 who received the vaccine had more than twice as many cases of shingles than those who were not vaccinated. Four percent of the subjects died after taking the zostavax vaccine. The vaccine product insert listed adverse reactions, which included: **vaccine strain herpes zoster**, arthralgia, anaphylactic reactions, retinitis that can lead to permanent loss of vision, GBS, and facial paralysis.[271, 272]

NBC10 News in Philadelphia reported, as of June 2019, there have been 37,000 complaints from adverse reactions regarding Zostavax, with hundreds of lawsuits against Merck currently pending.

Human Papilloma Virus (HPV)—There are more than 200 HPV virus strains, a few of which have been theoretically linked with cervical cancer. It is estimated that the HPV virus is present in at least half of the normal population according to the CDC. "More than 90% of the infections are resolved within 2 years without treatment, often without signs, symptoms or health problems."[273] There is no evidence that cervical cancer appears more often in women with the virus than in those without the virus, indicating causality has never been proven. Yet this vaccine is pushed on young girls and even boys with dubious justification.

- In 2006, the Gardasil vaccine for HPV, developed by Merck, was approved by the FDA and recommended by the CDC for girls 9 to 15 years old, even though the clinical trials were on women 16 to 26 years old.[274]

- At the 4th International Public Conference on Vaccination, held in Virginia in October 2009, Dr. Diane Harper, lead researcher in the development of the HPV vaccines Gardasil and Cervarix, gave a surprise announcement. Instead of promoting these vaccines, she explained that *"the cervical cancer risk in the U.S. is already extremely low; vaccinations are unlikely to have any effect upon the rate of cervical cancer in the United States."*[275] This is hardly a glowing endorsement of the HPV vaccine from someone who helped design the safety studies in order to approve Gardasil.

- The efficacy of the HPV vaccine is quite limited according to Dr. Harper, who stated, *"There is no data showing that it remains effective beyond five years."*[276] If the average age for women getting cervical cancer is in their 50s, what is the rationale for girls as young as 9 years old getting this vaccine?

- In 2009, the CDC approved the HPV vaccine for males aged 9 to 26, to prevent the likelihood of acquiring genital warts or anal cancer, even though there is little evidence to claim its efficacy.[277]

- A 2011 report in the *Annals of Medicine* on the HPV vaccine questions Merck's claim that Gardasil is effective in preventing cervical cancer and in fact, the vaccine may actually enhance cervical disease in women with pre-existing HPV infections. They reported:

  While the world's leading medical authorities state that HPV vaccines are an important cervical cancer prevention tool, clinical trials show no evidence that HPV vaccination can protect against cervical cancer.[278]

- The National Vaccine Information Center lists numerous adverse events reported to VAERS, including anaphylaxis, lupus, transverse myelitis, ALS, central nervous system demyelination, MS, GBS, pancreatitis, inflammatory bowel syndrome, optic neuritis, autoimmune hepatitis, vasculitis, thrombocytopenic purpura, and CFS, to name a few.[279]

- HPV vaccine was responsible for **63.8%** of all deaths and **81.2%** of all permanent disabilities compared with all other vaccines in the United States reported to VAERS as of March 25, 2012. They informed the reader to keep in mind that:

> *the primary interest of a pharmaceutical company is developing and selling pharmaceutical products. One must ask whether rational vaccine policy decisions should be based on conclusions derived from an uncritical acceptance of flawed vaccine safety and efficacy estimates provided by the vaccine manufacturer.[280]*

- In a 2013 French health journal interview, Dr. Dalbergue, a former pharmaceutical industry physician with the Gardasil manufacturer, Merck, stated:

> *I predict that Gardasil will become the greatest medical scandal of all time because at some point in time, the evidence will add up to prove that this vaccine, technical and scientific feat that it may be, has absolutely no effect on cervical cancer and that all the very many adverse effects, which destroy lives and even kill, serve no other purpose than to generate profit for the manufacturer. Gardasil is useless and costs a fortune! In addition, decision-makers at all levels are aware of it! Cases of Guillain-Barré syndrome, paralysis of the lower limbs, vaccine-induced MS and vaccine-induced encephalitis can be found, whatever the vaccine.[281]*

- A report from the 2015–2016 National Health and Nutrition Examination Survey showed HPV vaccine increased the odds of asthma **8 times greater** in the vaccinated population than in the unvaccinated.[282]
- A 2016 Canadian study looked at 195,000 girls who were given the HPV vaccine. Within 42 days of vaccination more than 20,000 vaccine injuries were reported—19,351 emergency room visits and 958 hospitalizations. That means **approximately 10%** of the girls in this study ended up in the emergency room because of the adverse effects of the vaccine *itself.* Surprisingly, the investigators concluded, *"Rates of AEFI [adverse events following immunization] after HPV immunization in Alberta are low and consistent with types of events seen elsewhere."*[283] One has to wonder, What would be considered a significant concern regarding an adverse event? 25%?, 50%?, 100%?
- Annual deaths from cervical cancer in the United States are 2.3 deaths per 100,000, whereas the death rate reported in the Gardasil clinical trials was **85 deaths** per 100,000. This means that the chances of dying from the vaccine is **37 times greater** than dying from cervical cancer.[284]
- As of May 31, 2019, in the United States alone, there have been 62,393 adverse reactions from the HPV vaccine with **503 deaths,** 6,286 hospitalizations, and 3,018 disabling conditions, as reported to VAERS.[285]
- The Gardasil clinical trials had numerous exclusion criteria. Not allowed to participate in the trials were people with: severe allergies; prior abnormal Pap test results; more than four lifetime sex partners; a history of immunological disorders and other chronic illnesses; reactions to vaccine ingredients, including aluminum, yeast, and benzonase; or a history of drug or alcohol abuse—yet Merck administers Gardasil to the general public with few to no exclusions.[286]
- In the original Gardasil clinical trials, Merck used an aluminum adjuvant instead of a true placebo that was

supposed to be a nontoxic inert saline solution. In this way, Merck can falsely claim that the reaction between the "placebo" and the Gardasil vaccine were similar and that therefore the vaccine was safe. In 2014, Merck used the Gardasil vaccine as the placebo in the clinical trials for the new Gardasil 9 vaccine in order to obscure safety concerns, by comparing one toxic substance with another.[287]

- Merck monitored the adverse reaction to Gardasil for only 14 days and *then* attempted to refuse claims of injury stating that they "weren't related to the vaccine...Half (**49.6%**) of the clinical-trial subjects who received Gardasil reported serious medical conditions within seven months. To avoid classifying these injuries as adverse events, Merck dismissed them as new medical conditions."[288]

- *Children's Health Defense* reported that *"According to Gardasil's package insert, women are **100 times** more likely to suffer a severe event following vaccination with Gardasil than they are to get cervical cancer."*[289]

- In a 2020 study entitled *"Will HPV vaccination prevents cervical cancer?"* the authors noted numerous problems with the clinical trials on HPV, concluding:

> *It is uncertain whether HPV vaccination prevent cervical cancer. The trials were not designed to detect this outcome, which takes decades to develop. For most outcomes, follow-up data exist for an average of only four or five years.*[290]

Refer to Appendix E, ***How to Identify Vaccine Reactions,*** put out by the National Vaccine Information Center (NVIC); it provides a useful summary for evaluating adverse vaccine reactions that should be reported to VAERS.

Mouse Toxicity Test—The Division of Biologic Standards (DBS) of the Public Health Services (PHS) developed a toxicity test to determine a vaccine's safety in which "the vaccine is injected into the abdominal cavities of young mice to see if they continue to gain weight over a period of time. If the mice do not die and continue to gain a specific amount of weight, vaccine manufacturers and the FDA consider the vaccine safe for children." Unfortunately, *"the most troublesome aspect of the toxicity test was that some children had and still have serious and even fatal reactions from vaccines that have successfully passed this test."*[291] This is what the DBS apparently considers sufficient evidence for concluding that a vaccine is safe enough to inject into children.

Related Vaccine-Induced Conditions

Sudden Infant Death Syndrome (SIDS)—A sudden unexplained death of children younger than 1 year of age. It usually occurs during sleep and as a consequence is also referred to as "crib death." SIDS has become the catchall term that the medical community too often uses to evade responsibility for the deleterious effects of vaccines. 95% of SIDS deaths happen in the first 6 months of life with most occurring between 2 and 4 months of age. The vast majority of these babies die within hours or days of receiving multiple-dose vaccinations. In spite of the worrisome connection between vaccines and SIDS, the CDC website states:

> *The timing of the 2-month and 4-month shots and SIDS has led some people to question whether they might be related. However, studies have found that vaccines do not cause and are not linked to SIDS.*[292]

There is nevertheless a good deal of research that contradicts such a blank assertion. It's not as if these children got vaccinated and nothing happened. Typically, infants who have an adverse reaction shortly after vaccination can develop a skin rash and hives; a high fever, vomiting and diarrhea; cough, runny nose and ear infections; high-pitched screaming and persistent crying; collapse or shock-like episodes; seizure disorders: convulsions and epilepsy; loss of muscle control; blood disorders: thrombocytopenia and hemolytic anemia; diabetes and hypoglycemia; and death.[293, 294]

Neil Miller cites a study on SIDS by Dr. Viera Scheibner that measured episodes of apnea (cessation of breathing) and hypopnea (abnormal shallow breathing) following the pertussis vaccination in which an infant's breathing would become intermittent or stop completely. The study's author concluded *"vaccination is the single most prevalent and most preventable cause of infant deaths."*[295] In another study by Miller and Goldman, they found:

> *a high statistically significant correlation between increasing numbers of vaccine doses and increasing infant-mortality rates...Despite the United States spending more per capita on healthcare than any other country, 33 nations have better IMRs [Infant mortality rates].*[296]

Miller's Review of Critical Vaccine Studies lists 8 studies that *"provide strong evidence that hexavalent* injections significantly increase the risk of sudden and unexpected deaths in young children."* For example, Miller summarized the findings of one study showing that *"There was a **13-fold increase** in the risk of SIDS after the hexavalent vaccination compared to an earlier period when the multi-dose vaccine was unavailable."*[297] There is a curious lack of any acknowledgement in the standard medical literature that SIDS could in fact be associated with vaccines.

[*Hexavalent refers to a six-in-one vaccine for diphtheria, tetanus, pertussis, poliomyelitis, Haemophilus influenza type B and hepatitis B].

Peanut Allergies—Peanuts are a common cause of severe allergy attacks. In the early 1990s, the peanut allergy epidemic took off at the same time that there was a dramatic increase in vaccines using peanut oil, as an excipient to enhance and prolong the immune effect. Though it has been argued that peanut oil is no longer used in vaccines, it is impossible to know for sure because the FDA does not require manufacturers to make public every ingredient in a vaccine owing to the proprietary rights of confidentiality. There is also what is called "cross-reactivity," in which *a person allergic to peanut proteins may also react to nuts, even though they are from different plant families.*"[298]

Today, about 2% of U.S. children are allergic to peanuts, which is the number-one cause of deaths out of all food-allergy reactions. That's why food products in the grocery store have labels at the bottom of the packaging, saying something to the effect of, "This product was made in a factory where peanuts were handled." This is a relatively new development as a result of peanut allergies having become so deadly. In her 2011 book, *The Peanut Allergy Epidemic,* Heather Fraser blamed the dramatic increase in peanut allergies on the sudden proliferation of vaccines starting in the late 1980s and concluded, *"The peanut-allergy epidemic in children was precipitated by childhood injections."*[299]

Shaken Baby Syndrome (SBS)—The AAP defines SBS as "a serious and clearly definable form of child abuse." Violently shaking a baby causes serious brain injury. SBS is identified by a physician based on three conditions: 1) Subdural hematoma (bleeding on the protective layer of the brain), 2) cerebral edema (brain swelling), and 3) retinal hemorrhage (bleeding behind the back of the eye). This syndrome was initially advanced by three physicians from the AAP (Drs. David Chadwick, Robert Reece, and Carol Jenny) who were considered SBS authorities back in the 1980s. Based on these assumed medical symptoms, physicians have reported to legal authorities adults and child caregivers suspected of killing their babies. There have been estimates as high as 3000 people who have been incarcerated as a result of SBS diagnosis. In recent years, other investigators have come out criticizing the rush to judgment in claiming child abuse based on evidence that does not take into consideration other possible explanations for brain trauma.[300]

The movie *The Syndrome* (2016) chronicled the misdiagnosis of SBS in cases of people being imprisoned, many of whom have been given life sentences, accused of killing their babies. Unfortunately, the symptoms attributed to SBS can be caused by a number of different conditions described in the movie. Due to the growing controversy over SBS, the AAP now refers to this condition as abusive head trauma.

Vaccines have been implicated in these infant deaths that have been falsely blamed on SBS. For example, the DPT vaccine is able to create essentially the same condition as SBS: inflammation and swelling of the brain, causing bleeding. Instances of SBS proliferated in the late 1980s and early 1990s around the same time that vaccines were dramatically increased.[301] Though there are clearly instances of child abuse, many of these SBS cases were not the result of abusive behavior. Consequently, people have been falsely accused of murder when in fact adverse vaccines reactions may have been the cause of the problem.

Gulf War Syndrome (GWS)—Described as medically unexplained illnesses of the Gulf War veterans with symptoms that included: chronic fatigue, blackouts, joint pain, insomnia, lesions of the brain, heart, and lungs, inability to concentrate, skin rashes, vertigo, auto-immune disorders, allergies, liver damage, Tourettes syndrome, chronic headaches, neurological problems, respiratory disorders, memory problems, depression, post-traumatic stress disorders, and birth defects in children of Gulf War veterans. The anthrax vaccine, which contains the adjuvants aluminum hydroxide and squalene, is highly reactogenic, meaning that it is able to produce an adverse reaction. The anthrax vaccine has been implicated in GWS, according to *the Research Advisory Committee on Gulf War Veterans' Illnesses Government Report (RAC-GWVI)*. "Vaccine Syndrome," the 2017 film on GWS, reported, *"More than 35,000 soldiers have died due to* *the adverse effects from the anthrax vaccine."* In a 2009 VA Report, *"One out of three returning veterans, including those who had not seen combat, require treatment for depression and post-traumatic stress syndrome."*[302] According to the RAC-GWVI government report in 2011, *"More than 1 million U.S. soldiers suffer from Gulf War illnesses due to the anthrax vaccine."*[303]

The French who served in the Gulf War did not receive the anthrax vaccine and did not come down with GWS. The only ones who did contract GWS, regardless of whether they were deployed to the Gulf War or not, were among the American, British, and Australian soldiers who were vaccinated for anthrax. Even though the anthrax vaccine was never approved by the FDA, the government went ahead anyway and mandated that all soldiers receive the vaccine, with disastrous results. While government officials are always quick to praise *"the brave and courageous soldiers who defend our country,"* apparently that doesn't carry much weight when the financial interests of the pharmaceutical industry are a priority. So, despite the clear evidence that the anthrax vaccine has caused such irreparable damage to so many of our military men and women, the official decree is to get the shot, whether you like it or not.

Childhood and Adult Cancers—At the same time that the vaccine schedule has dramatically increased since the early 1990s, the rates of childhood cancers have soared. After accidents, cancer is the second leading cause of death in children between the ages of 1 and 14, according to the American Cancer Society. The vaccine ingredient formaldehyde has been associated with leukemia, which is the number-one cancer in children. Mercury, aluminum, and Polysorbate 80, have all been linked to various forms of cancer as well.[304]

The polio vaccine developed in the 1950s, was contaminated with the Simian Virus (SV40), known to cause various cancers including lymphomas, mesotheliomas, and brain cancers. Rosa FW et al. conducted a study of nearly 59,000 women and found that "children of mothers who received the polio vaccine (with SV40) between 1959 and 1965 had brain tumors at a rate 13 times greater than mothers who did not receive those polio shots." In other words, mothers who received the contaminated vaccine inadvertently passed on cancer to their offspring at a rate **13 times greater** than mothers who did not receive the polio vaccine with SV40.[305] In another study by Garcea & Imperiale, they wrote, *"the case of SV40 infecting humans and contributing to cancer has become more compelling, supported by both experimental and circumstantial evidence."*[306] It is important to note that none of the vaccines on the market have ever been evaluated by the pharmaceutical industry to determine if they are carcinogenic.

Regarding the many cancer charities that raise money through well-publicized funding campaigns, there is a sordid history that is not well known by the public. **Appendix F,** *Bogus Cancer Charities,* recounts the extent of corruption by these cancer charities that prey on the good intentions of an unsuspecting public, as highlighted in a 2014 CNN report. In that year, 8 of the top 15 worst charities listed in the United States were cancer organizations. The Cancer Fund of America, for example, spent about 97% of donations on themselves and fundraisers, while only 3% went to cancer patients. Similarly, the Kids Wish Network raised millions in donations in the name of dying children while spending less than 3% on actually helping kids.

Obsessive–Compulsive Disorder (OCD)—Obsessions are recurrent thoughts or feelings that one is unable to ignore that creates doubts and worries while compulsions are repetitive and ritualized actions in order to ward off fears and anxieties. Examples include compulsive hand washing and the need to retrace one's steps when negative thoughts occur. Together, they create stressful situations that interfere with daily living. Today, it is estimated that OCD affects between 1% and 2% of children and as much as 3% of teens and adults. In the later part of the 1980s, OCD increased dramatically, whereas prior to the 1980s, it was considered to be quite rare. This surge in OCD closely coincides with the uptick in vaccinations during this period. The possible link between vaccines and OCD is suggested by the negative impact of vaccinations on the immune system causing disruption of the immune function.

In 2017, research findings at the *Yale Child Study Center* were published that showed an association between vaccinations and increased incidences of several neuropsychiatric disorders, including OCD. The influenza vaccine in particular correlated with higher rates of OCD, anorexia nervosa (AN), and anxiety disorders. Vaccines for Hepatitis A and B and Meningitis were also associated with OCD, AN, and tic disorders.[307]

THE PHARMACEUTICAL INDUSTRY'S INFLUENCE ON GOVERNMENTAL AGENCIES, THE MEDICAL COMMUNITY, POLITICIANS, AND THE NEWS MEDIA

"If you tell a big enough lie and tell it frequently enough, it will be believed." —Adolf Hitler

"We now know that government by organized money is as dangerous as government by an organized mob." — Franklin D. Roosevelt

The influence of money in politics is nothing new. We have seen it with the tobacco industry, the military-industrial complex, the nuclear industry, the oil cartels, the biotech industry pushing genetically modified foods (GMOs), and now the attempt to push through the 5G technology in spite of dire warnings. Therefore, it should not come as any surprise that the pharmaceutical industry has done the same but even more skillfully. The efforts by the drug industry to use its financial wealth to influence the CDC, FDA, AMA, AAP, the medical community in general, the scientific studies, the politicians, and the news media can hardly be overstated. It is worth noting that the drug companies are the most profitable industry in the world. While most sectors of the economy make annual profits in the 5% range, the pharmaceutical industry can make gains approaching 20% a year. In 2015, the averaged annual gain of the Fortune 500 companies was 4.9%, while the drug companies averaged 18.6%.[308]

A 2019 Gallup poll ranked the pharmaceutical industry as the most poorly regarded industry in America, with a 58% negative rating, placing it last on a list of 25 industries.[309] Having stated that, let's look more closely at the corrupting influence of "Big Pharma."

As previously emphasized, vaccine companies do not have to advertise because vaccines are mandated by law, and, at the same time are exempt from any liability for injury to others, unlike with prescription drugs. The industry employs almost three times as many Washington lobbyists (1450+) than all the elected officials in both Houses of Congress (535). In 2020 alone, the pharmaceutical industry contributed approximately twice as much money lobbying politicians as the next highest lobbying interest. The numbers below are in millions of dollars, indicating that Big Pharma spent $306,000,000. Do you think this might have some impact on how politicians vote? (*Source: Center for Responsive Politics*)

Leading Lobby Industries in the United States in 2020, by Total Lobbying Spending
(in million U.S. dollars)

Pharmaceuticals/Health Products	306
Electronics Mfg & Equip	156.9
Insurance	151.85
Real Estate	131.84
Business Associations	119.53
Oil & Gas	110.69
Hospitals/Nursing Homes	108.83
Misc Manufacturing & Distributing	105.78
Air Transport	105.02
Telecom Services	104.82
Electric Utilities	104.74
Securities & Investment	102.65
Health Services/HMOs	99.76

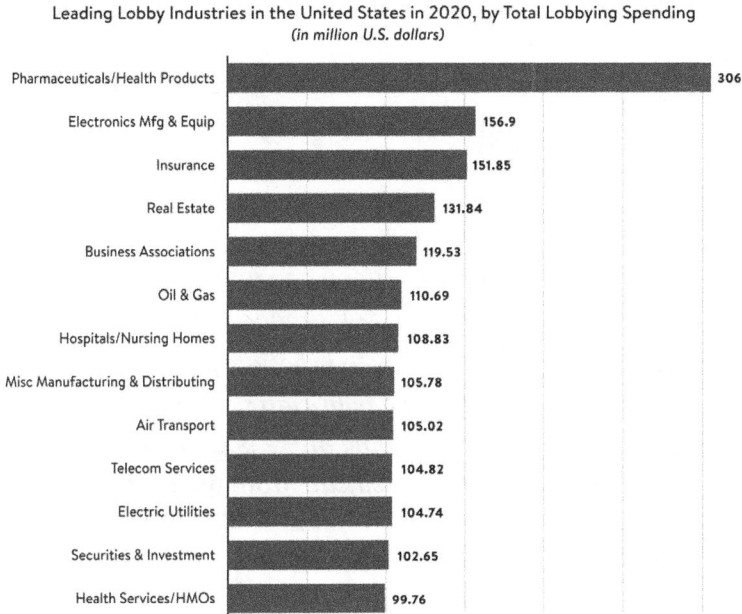

It is estimated that the pharmaceutical industry spends $20 billion each year in advertising to influence doctors to sell its drugs,

> *by sending sales representatives to doctor's offices for face-to-face visits, providing free drug samples and other swag, offering payments for speeches, food and beverages, travel, and hosting disease education.*

In addition, another $6 billion is spent on advertisement to influence the public through direct-to-consumer (DTC) marketing, mostly on TV and in magazine ads.[310] The inordinate influence of the pharmaceutical industry on the medical community is discussed in more detail in **Appendix G,** under the heading, *A Brief History of the Pharmaceutical Influence on the Medical Field.*

Medicare has been unable to negotiate drug costs with the pharmaceutical industry in spite of unanimous agreement that this could save billions of dollars in prescription costs for the public at large. The drug companies have spent enormous amounts of money keeping that from happening—that is the power that Big Pharma wields over politicians and the political system in spite of repeated pledges to rein in drug costs. By the way, the United States is the only developed country that does not regulate drug prices.[311] Wendell Potter, writing for *The Center for Public Integrity,* stated:

> *The Congressional Budget Office estimates that the government could save $112 billion ($112,000,000,000) over the coming decade if Congress reconsidered its 2006 gift to drug makers and gave Medicare the ability to negotiate prices. Remember that the next time you hear a politician say that the only way to keep the program from going broke is to cut benefits and raise the eligibility age for Medicare from 65 to 67.[312]*

The *British Medical Journal* wrote:

> *Growing evidence shows that extensive financial relationships between industry and healthcare decision makers distort scientific research, medical education, and the practice of medicine. The biggest problem is that industry-sponsored studies produce more favorable results, creating biased evidence that overplays benefits and downplays harms.[313]*

Today, the pharmaceutical industry funds many, if not most of the studies on vaccines and other drugs at universities and medical institutions. It often has the final say on what is reported to the public, and when unfavorable findings are discovered in these largely industry-sponsored studies, they are often minimized or even excluded while the positive results are exaggerated. A study by Dr. John Ioannidis who is considered "one of the foremost experts on the credibility of medical research" indicated that much of the published studies are *"misleading, exaggerated, and often flat-out wrong. He charged that as much as **90%** of the published medical information that doctors rely on is flawed.*[314] It should be emphasized that the actual vaccine research is not conducted by the FDA or the CDC, as the public might think, but instead is left to the pharmaceutical companies themselves, who may not be the most objective source of information given their financial stake in the outcome.

Doctor David Healy is an internationally recognized psychiatrist, scientist, and author of 20 books on the medical industry and of more than 150 peer-reviewed articles. In his 2012 book, *Pharmageddon*, Healy wrote about the corrupting influence of pharmaceutical companies on the healthcare industry. Healy discusses how studies are manipulated by drug companies in order to negate negative findings. The pharmaceutical industry will use ghostwriters to write up the results of the studies it funds. Dr. Healy has raised serious doubts on the legitimacy of such studies that the drug companies oversee. The following graphs, taken from *Vision Launch Media*, show the studies that have been done on these various drugs and what happens between the initial test findings and what actually ends up being presented in medical journals.

In each graph, below the red line are all the negative findings and above the red line are all the positive findings. The first graph is what the FDA looks at from the actual studies.

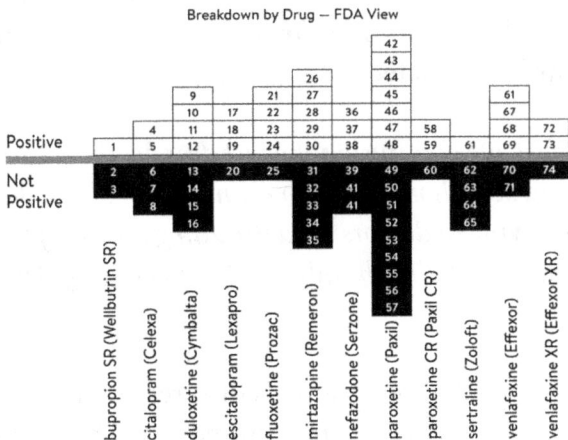

Breakdown by Drug — FDA View

	bupropion SR (Wellbutrin SR)	citalopram (Celexa)	duloxetine (Cymbalta)	escitalopram (Lexapro)	fluoxetine (Prozac)	mirtazapine (Remeron)	nefazodone (Serzone)	paroxetine (Paxil)	paroxetine CR (Paxil CR)	sertraline (Zoloft)	venlafaxine (Effexor)	venlafaxine XR (Effexor XR)
								42				
								43				
						26		44				
			9		21	27		45			61	
			10	17	22	28	36	46			67	
		4	11	18	23	29	37	47	58		68	72
Positive	1	5	12	19	24	30	38	48	59	61	69	73
Not Positive	2	6	13	20	25	31	39	49	60	62	70	74
	3	7	14			32	41	50		63	71	
		8	15			33	41	51		64		
			16			34		52		65		
						35		53				
								54				
								55				
								56				
								57				

(N Engl J Med 2008; 358: 252-260, DOI: 10. 1056/NEJMsa065779)

In the next graph, what we see is what actually gets put into the journals. In other words, the negative findings somehow disappear, and in some cases, the negative findings are moved into the positive column above the red line.

Breakdown by Drug — Journal View

```
                                          42
                                          43
                                          44
           9                              45                    66
           10          21   27            46                    67
     4     11    17    22   28    36      47    58              68
     5     12    18    23   29    37      48    59   61         69   72
     6     13    24    30   38            49    60   62         71   73
Positive 1 7  14 19    25   31    39
─────────────────────────────────────────────────────────────────────
Not                         32            50
Positive                                  56
```

| | bupropion SR (Wellbutrin SR) | citalopram (Celexa) | duloxetine (Cymbalta) | escitalopram (Lexapro) | fluoxetine (Prozac) | mirtazapine (Remeron) | nefazodone (Serzone) | paroxetine (Paxil) | paroxetine CR (Paxil CR) | sertraline (Zoloft) | venlafaxine (Effexor) | venlafaxine XR (Effexor XR) |

(N Engl J Med 2008; 358: 252-260, DOI: 10. 1056/NEJMsa065779)

In **Appendix H, *Pharmaceutical Settlements,*** ProPublica summarizes the fines levied against all the major drug companies for fraudulent marketing practices between 2009 and 2014, amounting to more than $13 billion. Now contrast that with the four vaccine makers in the United States alone (Merck, GSK, Pfizer, and Sanofi) who have been charged **more than 100 times** for criminal conduct. Robert F. Kennedy Jr. stated:

> *In the past 10 years, just in the last decade, those companies have paid 35 billion dollars in criminal penalties, damages, fines, for lying to doctors for defrauding science, for falsifying science, for killing hundreds of thousands of Americans knowingly.*[315]

In spite of this dubious track record, researchers who question the safety of vaccines end up being discredited and marginalized in a seemingly coordinated effort by government agencies, medical officials, and the news media. Grants funded by the pharmaceutical industry have been taken away from researchers who pursue findings that run contrary to the fiscal interests of the vaccine makers. Researchers have even been threatened with losing their medical licenses or their jobs for going against the vaccine orthodoxy. Joseph Mercola, DO, sums up the problem in this way:

> *Industry funded "science" has tainted our world and turned science-based evidence into science-biased propaganda. Universities are laundering money through foundations to intentionally hide relationships, while scientists secretly nurture their relationships with corporate executives...Negative outcomes go unpublished...Media is paid handsomely to ensure the public that "the science is settled," especially when corporate liability is a primary concern. Raw data is held captive, conflicts of interest are not fully disclosed, and studies are designed to specifically obtain a desired outcome.*[316]

The conflicts of interest among the drug manufacturers and those in authority at the CDC, FDA, WHO, AAP, and EPA raise serious concerns regarding the apparent collusion in which the dangers of vaccines are downplayed and dismissed. Those who have attempted to speak up have essentially been silenced by those in charge in order to avoid incrimination. What follows is a brief critique of these agencies.

The Centers for Disease Control and Prevention (CDC) operates under the DHHS, purporting to be a government health advocacy organization. Funding for the CDC's work is provided through the CDC Foundation, established by Congress as an independent, non-profit organization with its office in Atlanta, Georgia. The foundation works with the CDC and private-sector resources, including "Big Pharma," to raise money to support programs that essentially promote vaccinations, which is part of the CDC's mission statement. The CDC's close ties to the pharmaceutical industry, however, raises serious concerns regarding possible conflicts of interest, given that the Foundation takes money from the pharmaceutical industry in its efforts to promote vaccines. While it is commonly assumed that the CDC is an independent agency monitoring the vaccine-approval process, in fact, it owns *"56 vaccine patents pertaining to various aspects of vaccine development, manufacturing, delivery, and adjuvants"* that generate huge profits by promoting vaccines under the guise of childhood safety.[317]

The process for the approval of vaccines is determined by the Advisory Committee on Immunization Practices (ACIP), a committee made up of physicians and researchers handpicked by the CDC who determine which vaccines are to be mandated by law. In 2000, Rep. Dan Burton headed the Committee on Government Reform looking into the vaccine-approval process and the numerous "conflicts of interest" involving the members of the ACIP.[318] Those who were determining which vaccines were to be mandated simultaneously owned stocks and held patents on the same vaccines that they were authorized to approve. Others got research money from the drug companies to monitor vaccine testing or received funding for academic departments at universities. Members of the committee were routinely given conflict-of-interest wavers. For example, Paul Offit, an ACIP member, who has a patent on the Rotavirus vaccine, was allowed to approve his own vaccine on three separate occasions. The Children's Health Defense reported *"CDC or NIH employees whose names appear on vaccine patents can receive up to $150,000 in licensing fees per year (in perpetuity)."*[319] This suggests that there is a major incentive to turn out vaccines that can bring in big financial rewards.

The CDC has also worked in collaboration with and provided financial support to the Immunization Action Coalition (IAC) whose mission is:

> to increase immunization rates and prevent disease by creating and distributing educational materials for healthcare professionals and the public that enhance the delivery of safe and effective immunization services.[320]

IAC is essentially

> a leading vaccine front group that receives significant funding from both vaccine manufacturers and the CDC and lobbies for the removal of vaccine exemptions.[321]

In the book *Master Manipulator: The Explosive True Story of Fraud, Embezzlement, and Government Betrayal at the CDC* (2016), James Ottar Grundvig told how the CDC manipulated data in six vaccine safety studies starting around 2000 to hide the connection between vaccines and autism. Much of the story centered around Poul Thorsen, an opportunistic Danish scientist, who was essentially given "carte blanche" by the CDC to come up with skewed studies to prove that thimerosal (mercury) in vaccines was safe and had no connection to the autism epidemic. This was done with the covert support of the CDC's bosses that included Dr. Coleen Boyle, Director of the National Center on Birth Defects and Developmental Disabilities, who led the effort to stonewall any association between vaccines and autism.[322]

Thorsen was eventually *"indicted on 22 counts of wire fraud and money laundering"* in 2011, in which he diverted CDC grant money approaching $2 million to his personal account so that he could live a lavish lifestyle that included buying *"a home in Atlanta, a Harley-Davidson motorcycle, an Audi automobile, and a Honda SUV."*[323]

He ended up evading imprisonment by moving back to Denmark, where he works at Odense University Hospital. The CDC has had the opportunity to extradite him back to the United States to face trial for his offenses but CDC officials are apparently not too interested in drawing attention to his sordid history with their organization.

The Food and Drug Administration (FDA) is responsible for six major departments, including the Center for Biologics Evaluation and Research (CBER), whose mission is "to protect and enhance the public health through the regulation of biological and related products, including blood, **vaccines,** allergenics, tissues, and cellular and gene therapies."[324] The FDA is supposed to regulate the drug industry, along with vaccines, but once again its focus seems to be more aligned with the financial interests of the drug industry than the welfare of the general public. In fact, approximately 45% of the FDA's budget comes from user fees paid by the pharmaceutical companies when applying for approval of a medical device or drug. In essence, Big Pharma is paying for nearly half of the FDA's salary which creates a kind of symbiotic relationship that raises the question, "Who is really in charge?"

In 2000, the U.S. House Committee on Oversight and Government Reform discovered that many on the Advisory Board of the FDA who make the decisions regarding vaccine approval have conflicts of interest.[325] These include paid consultants to drug companies, grant recipients from the industry, vaccine developers who own patents, and shareholders in drug stocks. Based on the FDA's Vaccines and Related Biological Products Advisory Committee approval and licensing of new vaccines, the CDC's ACIP would then determine what vaccines were to be added to the childhood schedule.

A 2006 survey developed by the Union of Concerned Scientists (UCS), given to 5,918 FDA scientists to examine the state of science at the FDA, resulted in a troubling picture of an agency that has been compromised by outside-money interests. The survey described the environment within the agency as one of intimidation, censorship, and scientific fraud. Forty percent of FDA scientists feared "retaliation" for voicing safety concerns over prescription drugs. Only 47% of the scientists thought the *"FDA routinely provides complete and accurate information to the public."*[326] Once again, the evidence suggests that the FDA has been co-opted by the pharmaceutical industry's financial interests with secondary concern for the public's safety.

In an October 2013 article in the *Journal of Law, Medicine, and Ethics* (JLME), entitled, *"Institutional Corruption of Pharmaceuticals and the Myth of Safe and Effective Drugs,"* Donald W. Light et al. wrote:

> *The authorization of user fees in 1992 has turned drug companies into the FDA's prime clients, deepening the regulatory and cultural capture of the agency...Meeting the needs of the drug companies has taken priority over meeting the needs of patients. Unless this corruption of regulatory intent is reversed, the situation will continue to deteriorate.*[327]

In the book, *Altered Genes, Twisted Truth*, the author, Steven M. Druker, described in detail how the *"U.S. FDA enabled the commercialization of genetically engineered foods by covering up the warnings of its own scientists, repeatedly lying, and deliberately breaking the law."*[328] The FDA concluded, for example, that genetically modified organisms (GMOs) are safe based on testing done by Monsanto, the nation's largest manufacturer of GMOs, despite the fact that 60 countries have banned or severely regulated their use. This essentially parallels how the FDA pushes vaccinations, and at the same time, minimizes concerns, distorts facts, or withholds evidence of vaccine problems. Three experts from Harvard Medical School reviewed the FDA approval process for pharmaceuticals from 1983 to 2018, revealing "a troubling shift toward FDA use of 'less data' to approve drugs and biologics (vaccines)—alongside an escalating reliance on pharmaceutical industry payments to cover the salaries of the very FDA reviewers issuing the approvals."[329]

Robert F. Kennedy Jr. has reported:

> *In 1992, Congress passed the Prescription Drug User Fee Act, allowing pharmaceutical companies to make payments to the FDA (called 'user fees') in exchange for expedited approval of drugs and biologics, including vaccines... Moreover, in fiscal year 2017, **75% of FDA's annual budget increase came from user fees**, with the pharmaceutical industry in essence paying regulators' salaries.*[330]

This might help to explain the agency's apparent emphasis on protecting the interests of the drug industry as opposed to the general welfare of the public. An article in *Global Research* describes the FDA as:

> *one of the most dangerous government agencies in the United States. The sheer scope of people it affects with its corruption is staggering...the FDA's own webpage admits that the drugs it certifies as safe contribute to more than 100,000 deaths per year...It is a system built upon conflicts of interest that leaves consumers completely in the dark about the true consequences of taking Big Pharma products.*[331]

The American Academy of Pediatrics (AAP)—The AAP is a private-for-profit corporation headquartered in Elk Grove Village, Illinois. It has been described as a front group for the vaccine industry that receives funding from the four U.S. manufacturers of childhood vaccines, Merck, Pfizer, Sanofi, and GSK. A 2008 CBS news report stated, *"The vaccine industry gives millions to the AAP for conferences, grants, medical education classes and even helped build their headquarters."*[332] The bulk of the pediatricians' income can come from administering vaccines, which is tied to the additional rembursements from the medical insurance companies, for assuring high vaccination rates. For example, Blue Cross-Blue Shield has a rewards program in which

> *Providers receive $400 for each eligible two-year-old who has received all 24–25 vaccines by that age—but only if the provider manages to administer at least 63% of patients… therefore stand to make an additional $40,000 in bonus payments for every 100 fully vaccinated two-year-olds, creating a formidable incentive not to let any patients slip through the cracks, and a disincentive to continue serving families who decline one or more vaccines.*[333]

The AAP has also received more than $20 million in funding from the CDC in the past 10 years, reflecting their closely aligned agendas when it comes to advocating for vaccines. And according to the AAP, vaccines prevent cancer, the link between autism and vaccines has been disproven, and vaccines are safe when following the CDC vaccine schedule. Unfortunately, when asked to provide evidence of these assertions, none is forthcoming. Nevertheless, since vaccines are proven *"safe and effective,"* AAP sees no need to study vaccines any further. The science has been settled, according to the AAP. No problem with vaccines at all.[334] Richard Gale and Gary Null, writing about the myth of 'settled science,' stated:

> *A medical science that refuses to ask new questions and settles upon disputed beliefs to sustain an industry's financial*

portfolio is Scientism, a quasi-faith-based creed now insti-
tutionalized to promulgate repressive laws. These laws then
advance Scientism's authority. Unfortunately, today this
accurately represents the sad state of vaccine research and
vaccination policy.[335]

The AAP sees baby formulas as being beneficial just like breastfeeding, denying that there is significant differences between artificial genetically modified foods (GMOs) and organic foods, and pushes vaccines on infants and children without any concern for number of shots given, no matter how early, how often, and how much. One could hardly find a more pro-industry partner to promote artificial solutions over natural sources and remedies, but that is not all.

An article in the *Journal of Pediatrics,* by Chervenak, et al., suggests that refusing to vaccinate children may be viewed as child neglect since *"a child is exposed to some potential risk of harm by a parental act of omission."* The authors make a number of assumptions about *"herd immunity,"* the *"negligible risks"* of vaccines, and the *"overwhelming net clinical benefit of early childhood vaccinations."* These seem like reasonable assertions, unless you actually look at the research that puts all of these assumptions into question. The implication of the article is that pediatricians know what is best for children, due to their *"evidence-based clinical judgment"* and if parents don't come around, there should be consequences for their

misinformed or false beliefs...If parents remain unpersuaded,
their informed refusal becomes child neglect, because they
are refusing to authorize evidence-based, effective, and
safe preventive care required by the best interests of the
child standard as a norm. There is a strict legal obligation
to report child neglect to the local child health protective
services agency.[336]

Can you see where this is going?

Environmental Protection Agency (EPA)—The EPA was established in 1970 by President Nixon, and was initially seen as an agency to protect public health. Unfortunately, with time it became mired in controversy, devolving into an agency more attuned to maximizing corporate profits. The agency has increasingly come under the influence of corporate interests and money. The former coal lobbyist Andrew Wheeler was confirmed as head of the agency in 2018, after his predecessor, Scott Pruitt resigned due to numerous federal investigations for illegal practices.

A chemical safety law that was passed by Congress in 2016, under the Obama administration, was later overseen by Nancy Beck, a President Trump appointee. Beck, who was initially hired by Pruitt, was a former executive and lobbyist for the American Chemistry Council (ACC),[337] who reversed EPA positions on hazardous chemicals and environmental laws, exposing Americans to more toxic chemicals while supporting corporate interests.

The Trump administration ended up reversing many of the regulations under the Obama administration: turning back cleaner car standards; curtailing the Clean Air Act by allowing greater emissions of mercury and other toxins; reducing the Clean Water Act, allowing industries more latitude in dumping waste and chemicals into water supplies; reversing the Clean Power Plan that was supposed to cut dangerous factory emissions; withdrawing the U.S. from the Paris Agreement; and deleting references in government documents to such terms as, *"climate change"* and *"greenhouse gases."*

Now the EPA considers glyphosate (Round Up) to be safe, in spite of numerous studies to the contrary indicating that glyphosate-based herbicides cause or contribute to human cancer. Despite the public outcry, the EPA released the following statement on January 30, 2020:

> *The EPA thoroughly evaluated potential human health risk associated with exposure to glyphosate and determined that there are no risks to human health from the current registered uses of glyphosate and that glyphosate is not likely to be carcinogenic to humans.*[338]

Nevertheless, Bayer, who bought Monsanto in 2018, is involved in litigation with more than 100,000 plantiffs claiming that glyphosate has caused cancer. To date, Bayer has been ordered to pay more than $10 billion, with numerous lawsuits still pending.[339]

World Health Organization (WHO)—The organization states on its website that its primary role is *"to direct international health within the United Nations' system and to lead partners in global health responses."* Half of the WHO's funding comes from the 194 member states, while the other half is funded by the pharmaceutical interests, of which the Bill and Melinda Gates Foundation (BMGF) pays the lion's share, being the single largest donor to the WHO. As a result, Gates has an undue financial influence over WHO's operations, in which the corporate interests of his pharmaceutical partners seemingly supersede other concerns. Gates, who has no medical background, nevertheless plays a major role in the development and distribution of vaccinations worldwide, which has become a big and profitable business with little oversight. The partnership between BMGF and WHO has been criticized for pushing vaccines on third-world countries without doing the proper testing to determine their safety and effectiveness.

Dr. Soren Mogensen and Dr. Peter Aaby were commissioned by the Danish government and Novo Nordisk Foundation in 2017 to study the results of the vaccine program in the West African nation of Guinea Bissau. Much to their surprise, they found that girls vaccinated with DTP died at a rate **10 times greater** than those girls who were not vaccinated. Though the children were protected from DTP, they ended up being more susceptible to other deadly diseases because of the DTP shots' adverse effect on the immune system. In their conclusion, they wrote that the *"DTP was associated with 5-fold higher mortality than being unvaccinated,"* when combining the mortality-hazard rate (HR) results from both infant girls (9.98) and boys (3.93).[340]

In a March 1, 2020 article in the *Foreign Policy Journal*, Jeremy Hammond discussed a controversial malaria vaccine (Mosquirix), sponsored by the WHO and GSK. Intended to stop malaria, the vaccine actually increased its risk because the vaccine's effect waned over a 4-year period. In addition, there was a **10-fold** increased risk of meningitis and twice the death rate among female children. He also mentioned a dengue-vaccine program implemented by the Philippine government, the WHO, and the Sanofi Pasteur drug company that "was shown to increase the risk of serious dengue infection among children who had not already experienced a prior infection...WHO had ignored early warnings from clinical trials that the vaccine might cause precisely that outcome." Hammond concluded his article by asserting:

> *The WHO's experimentation on African children without informed consent is but the latest illustration of how our children's health and our fundamental human rights are being threatened by powerful people acting not in the public's interests but in service to the pharmaceutical industry.*[341]

Another example of WHO's willful misconduct is covered in the documentary, *Infertility: A Diabolical Agenda*, produced by Dr. Andrew Wakefield and Children's Health Defense. It details the WHO's intentions to produce an anti-fertility vaccine "under the guise of a neonatal tetanus prevention program" that had been deliberately sterilizing women [in Kenya]—either using a vaccine to abort existing pregnancies or to prevent future pregnancies." These measures by the WHO were taken in order to reduce the population in third world countries without people's knowledge or consent going back to the mid-1990s. In 1995, the Catholic Women's League of the Philippines took the WHO to court in order to stop the UNICEF tetanus program after it was discovered that the anti-fertility-laced vaccine was used to effectively end or prevent pregnancy.[342]

In an article in *The National Review* entitled, "*Stop Funding WHO Until It Cleans Up Its Act*" (June 14, 2017), Jeff Stier stated, "WHO is plagued by persistent wasteful spending, utter disregard for transparency, pervasive incompetence, and failure to adhere to even basic democratic standards." He went on to question the new head of the organization, writing:

Dr. Tedros, as he likes to be called (he has a Ph.D. in community health), is a leader of Ethiopia's brutal minority party, the Tigray People's Liberation Front, a wing of the ruling Marxist-rooted Ethiopian People's Revolutionary Democratic Front. He served the violently repressive regime as minister of foreign affairs from 2012 to 2016, after a stint as health minister.[343]

In October 2017, Tedros was roundly criticized for recommending Zimbabwe President Robert Mugabe as a WHO goodwill ambassador. Tedros had to quickly withdraw his controversial appointment based on Mugabe's history of human-rights abuses being cited by both the United States and the European Union.[344]

Critics of the Pharmaceutical Industry

Marcia Angell, MD, worked at *the New England Journal of Medicine* for more than 2 decades and became the first female editor-in-chief of the journal. In 1997, *TIME* magazine listed her as one of the 25 most influential people in America. She left the journal in 2000 over her criticism of the kinds of articles that were being accepted by the journal, as with other medical publications that were being systematically influenced and neutralized by the pharmaceutical interests. In a 2004 book, *The Truth About the Drug Companies*, published in the *New York Review of Books*, Angell wrote:

Over the past two decades, the pharmaceutical industry has moved very far from its original high purpose of discovering and producing useful new drugs. Now primarily a marketing machine to sell drugs of dubious benefit, this industry uses its wealth and power to co-opt every institution that might stand in its way, including the U.S. Congress, the FDA, academic medical centers, and the medical profession itself.[345]

In March of the same year, **Richard Horton,** editor of the *Lancet,* reiterated Angell's view, stating, *"Journals have devolved into information-laundering operations for the pharmaceutical industry."*[346]

Meryl Nass, MD, board member of the Alliance for Human Research Protection, gave a talk in 2019, in which she stated:

> *The pharmaceutical industry exerts enormous influence on government regulators, their advisors, professional medical organizations, key opinion leaders, and medical journals as well as the mass media and lawmakers. This is not debatable—there are dozens of studies proving it. Merck has a list on this website of more than 1,000 candidates for state and federal offices to whom they gave money in 2018. Merck also lists payments to hundreds of professional medical organizations, patient organizations, Pharma lobbying groups and scores of Republican and Democratic PACs and committees.*[347]

David Lewis, PhD, a former U.S. EPA Research Microbiologist, wrote:

> *After buying out the news media, pharmaceutical companies are focused on controlling scientific journals and lobbying Congress to lower standards for data used by the FDA and CDC to approve and recommend their products. Congress has shielded pharmaceutical companies from lawsuits over vaccine-related injuries, and it's moving toward mandating all CDC-recommended vaccines.*[348]

Pharmaceutical companies spend an enormous amount of money on advertising in comparison to research and development. *The British Medical Journal* noted that drug companies spent **19 times** more money on marketing their drugs than on research and development.[349]

Richard Smith was the editor of the *British Medical Journal* until 2004 and received the Health Watch Award for 2004 from the

Medical Society of London. His talk at that event was summarized in an article entitled, *"Medical Journals: An Extension of the Marketing Arm of Pharmaceutical Companies?"*[350] The following is a summary of Smith's list of examples of shady methods that pharmaceutical companies use to get the results they want from clinical trials:

- Conduct a trial of your drug against a treatment known to be inferior.
- Trial your drugs against too low a dose of a competitor drug.
- Conduct a trial of your drug against too high a dose of a competitor's, making your drug seem less toxic.
- Use multiple endpoints in the trial, and select for publication those that give favorable results.
- If there is no subgroup that does well, do not publish that study at all.
- Do multicenter trials, and select for publication results from centers that are favorable.
- Conduct subgroup analyses, selecting those publications that are favorable.
- Present results that are most likely to impress—for example, reduction in relative rather than absolute risk.

Peter Gotzsche is a Danish physician, medical researcher, and former head of the Nordic Cochrane Center in Copenhagen, Denmark, and the cofounder of the center in 1993. He was expelled from the Governing Board in 2018, over his criticism of the pharmaceutical industry's influence on medicine, which threatened the transparency and legitimacy of research. Gotzsche ultimately wrote a book, *Deadly Medicines and Organized Crime (2013),* in which he equated the drug industry with the mafia or mob. He wrote:

> *The main reason we take so many drugs is that drug companies don't sell drugs, they sell lies about drugs...Virtually everything we know about drugs is what the companies have chosen to tell us and our doctors.*[351]

In 2010, two virologists, **Stephen Krahling and Joan Wlochowski,** who worked for Merck, filed a lawsuit alleging that the drug company had defrauded the United States going back to 1990 by exaggerating the MMR vaccine's effectiveness. They claimed in the lawsuit that they had witnessed firsthand the improper testing and data falsification by which Merck artificially inflated the vaccine's efficacy findings. This court case is still pending in spite of the vaccine company's attempt to have it thrown out.[352]

Andrew Wakefield, a gastrointestinal surgeon with a specialty in inflammatory bowel disease, has been ostracized for his research into the measles vaccine. He has published more than 140 original scientific articles and written a 250-page manuscript reviewing the literature on the safety of the measles vaccine. Wakefield was contacted by parents of children with autism and severe gastrointestinal symptoms because of his research on the measles vaccine. He worked with one of the world's leading pediatric gastroenterologists, Prof. Walker-Smith, doing clinical workups on these autistic children. In 1998, Wakefield and 12 other scientists published a *Lancet* article indicating that the findings were preliminary and that further studies were recommended regarding a possible association between the MMR vaccine and autism. This created a media firestorm among the medical community, although his study has since been replicated **28 times** by scientists in the States and other countries.[353] However, in 2004, the editor of *The Lancet* declared that the 1998 article was "fatally flawed" because Wakefield had failed to disclose financial conflicts of interest. The British General Medical Council (GMC) ultimately took away his license in May 2010 and retracted the 1998 article. He was accused of scientific fraud, undisclosed financial conflicts of interest, and ethical breaches in performing tests on sick children. There were no complaints from the families involved in the study and the parents were prevented from testifying on his behalf. Wakefield received no private compensation for his work, and he was not a patent holder for a separate measles vaccine, as was claimed by GMC.

The Center for Personal Rights, a non-profit public-interest law firm in the United States, found no evidence of scientific fraud on the part of Wakefield and Prof. Walker-Smith. The British High Court overturned the findings of the GMC, stating that it had made *"fundamental errors, distorted evidence, and based its findings on an inadequate analysis of the facts."* Nevertheless, Andrew Wakefield has continued to be vilified in the news media to date. In January 2011, Wakefield was interviewed by Anderson Cooper on CNN that ended up being more like an interrogation than an actual interview. Cooper repeatedly cut off Wakefield, at one point, stating, *"But sir, if you're lying, then your book is also a lie. If your study is a lie, your book is a lie."*[354] Apparently, this is what passes for objective news media coverage when one dares to question the vaccine orthodoxy.

Judy Mikovits, PhD, is a biochemist and molecular biologist who specializes in neuroimmunology and has researched cancer, HIV, Chronic Fatigue Syndrome (CFS), autism, and other diseases. In 2011, she discovered that 30% or more of the vaccines at that time were contaminated with gammaretroviruses from mice used in their development. These retroviruses introduced via vaccinations are then incorporated into the DNA of humans—children and adults alike—and will then stay there and be passed on to future generations. Dr. Mikovits contended that these new retroviruses can contribute to conditions such as CFS, autism, cancers, leukemia, lymphoma, Alzheimer's, and Parkinson's disease.

When Dr. Mikovits released her findings, it created such a backlash that she was told to destroy her data. When she refused, she was fired and subsequently arrested under the pretext of stealing data from the workplace. A gag order from the court was placed on her work over a 4-year period in which she could not talk about her research. Since that time, she has written two books, *Plague, One Scientist's Intrepid Search for the Truth About Human Retroviruses and Chronic Fatigue Syndrome, Autism, and Other Diseases*, and *Plague of Corruption: Restoring Faith in the Promise of Science,* in which she chronicles her work and the attempt by the U.S. government to silence her, and to hide the truth regarding chronic diseases caused by vaccines.[355]

Brandy Vaughan was a former Merck pharmaceutical sales executive who left the company because of the *"pharmaceutical industry's agenda to make and keep people sick for profit—and take away our right to decline medical procedures, treatment, and pharmaceutical drugs."*[356] In December 2020, Ms. Vaughan, the founder of the educational non-profit organization, *LearnTheRisk.com* (previously *Council for Vaccine Safety*), died unexpectedly at the age of 45. Because of her outspoken criticism of the pharmaceutical industry and numerous anonymous threats on her life, Ms. Vaughan wrote in a Dec. 2019 post:

> *If something were to happen to me, it's foul play, and you know exactly who and why—given my work and mission in this life. I'm also NOT accident prone. And I got the highest health rating possible when I went through a battery of medical tests...*[357]

In 2014, **Dr. Brian Hooker,** a scientist and father of an autistic child, had a series of four phone conversations with **William Thompson,** a senior CDC epidemiologist, as recounted in the book *Vaccine Whistleblower: Exposing Autism Research Fraud at the CDC* (2015) by Kevin Barry, an attorney specializing in autism who is also a father of an autistic child. In these conversations, William Thompson regretfully acknowledged that he and his coauthors had destroyed research data establishing a causal connection between the MMR vaccine and autism, most notably in African-American males before the age of 36 months. This corrupt action, back in 2004, was at the direction of senior CDC officials including branch chief and lead author, Frank DeStefano.[358]

Here we have a situation where a drug company, Merck, conspired with CDC officials at the highest level to engage in criminal behavior, when in fact, the CDC should have been providing oversight. Thompson, realizing the seriousness of this decision, ultimately kept records that were eventually turned over to Congressman Posey in 2014. He was seeking federal whistleblower protection and stated that he was willing to testify under oath before the House Committee on Oversight and

Government Reform (OGR). However, the CDC officials and OGR chairman, Jason Chaffetz blocked him from appearing, and the House has since conveniently avoided any attempt to look into this matter.

Dr. Lucija Tomljenovic, through the FOIA, was able to uncover more than 30 years of government documents that deliberately hid information regarding the dangers of vaccines in which

> *the British Joint Committee on Vaccination and Immunization (JVCI) made continuous efforts to withhold critical data on severe adverse reactions and contraindications to vaccinations to both parents and health practitioners.*

While ignoring questions of safety, they also actively censored unfavorable data on vaccines to perpetuate the notion that they were safe and effective.[359]

A study by Public Citizen, a nonprofit consumer-advocacy organization, reported on **412 legal settlements** against pharmaceutical companies between 1991 and 2017. In spite of these numerous illegal activities, they concluded:

> *Financial penalties continued to pale in comparison to company profits, with the $38.6 billion in penalties from 1991 through 2017 amounting to only 5% of the $711 billion in net profits made by the 11 largest global drug companies during just 10 of those 27 years (2003–2012).*[360]

The president of a network news division informed Robert F. Kennedy Jr. that the mainstream media receives as much as **70%** of its advertising revenues from pharmaceutical ads. The CEO went on to say that, *"He would fire a host who brought onto his station a guest who lost him a pharmaceutical account."*[361] This would suggest that what is approved for public consumption in the mainstream news media depends on who is paying the bills. As the saying goes, *"Don't bite the hand that feeds you."*

And what about the news media, especially on T.V., where the public is bombarded by one drug commercial after another in which we are told all the awful things that can happen as a result of taking their pills while at the same time showing images of smiling people blissfully prancing around without a care in the world. This continual onslaught of drug commericials, one after another, stating all the negative contraindications, over time has had the effect of desensitizing the public.

For example, Humira, prescribed for rheumatoid arthritis, one of the most advertised drugs on the market, warns:

> *Humira can lower your ability to fight infections, including tuberculosis. Serious, sometimes **fatal** infections and cancers, including lymphoma, have happened, as have blood and nervous system problems, serious allergic reactions, and new or worsening **heart failure**...*[362]

Under normal circumstances, one would be shocked at such an array of potentially negative outcomes, but when repeated over and over, it becomes less objectionable as the potential benefits are emphasized while concerns are subtly minimized by portraying positive imagery that suggests it is an acceptable risk.

In the book *Selling Sickness: How Drug Companies Are Turning Us All Into Patients (2005)*, **Ray Moynihan and Alan Cassels** explained how drug companies widen the definition of illness to include the healthy in order to increase the need for medicines. In this way, mild health issues are labeled as serious; common complaints become medical conditions requiring the need for medicines (e.g., erectile dysfunction, restless leg syndrome, social anxiety disorder, in other words, shyness). One only has to turn on the TV to see the impact of the pharmaceutical industry pushing drugs on the public. Regarding the influence of money, they wrote:

> *The doctors, the drug reps, the medical education, the ads, the patient groups, the guidelines, the celebrities, the*

conferences, the public awareness campaigns, the thought leaders, even the regulators, and advisors at every level, there is money from the drug companies.[363]

The United States and New Zealand are the only countries in the world that are allowed to advertise prescription drugs and vaccines directly to the public on TV. While the U. S. makes up roughly **4%** of the world population, Americans consume **50%** of the drugs produced in the world and **80%** of the world's opioids. I guess that answers the question, "Do pharmaceutical advertisements work?" The current opioid epidemic in the U.S. has largely been driven by the financial interests of the pharmaceutical industry. According to the CDC, between 1999 and 2018, more than 232,000 deaths from drug overdoses have occurred in the U.S., in large part due to the over-prescription of opioids, in particular OxyContin, with nearly 50,000 opioid deaths in 2018 alone.

Defenders of the Pharmaceutical Industry

Dr. Anthony Fauci, "America's doctor," is at the top of the list of those siding with the pharmaceutical industry, in his capacity as Director of the National Institute of Allergy and Infectious Diseases (NIAID) since 1984. In the seminal book, *The Real Anthony Fauci* (2021), Robert F. Kennedy Jr. painstakingly chronicles Fauci's long history at NIAID, detailing how he has repeatedly served the interests of the pharmaceutical industry and his own, to the detriment of public health. He wields enormous power in his position, controlling billions of dollars, in which he is able to dictate what scientific research gets funded and to whom. Fauci has pushed the use of the toxic chemical, AZT, to the exclusion of more effective drugs, causing the needless deaths of thousands of AIDS patients; reduced the NIAID standards for drug approval, allowing poorly tested products to come to market; backed the pharmaceutical industry's atrocious experiments on vulnerable subjects, including minority orphan and foster children; unloaded harmful drugs and vaccines on third world countries that were banned in the U.S.; and promoted the toxic and costly drug, remdesivir, on COVID patients.

Working in concert with Bill Gates and Big Pharma, and coupled with his coercive financial influence over mainstream news, and social media, Fauci has been able to push drug and vaccines mandates with little resistance. This is especially apparent in the rapid introduction of the current experimental COVID vaccines that have never been properly evaluated for safety or efficacy. Fauci has portrayed vaccines as the only viable solution to this current crisis, while simultaneously, denying successful and cost-effective treatments for COVID that are being intentionally suppressed. The real medical experts on the frontline, attempting to sound the alarm as to what is actually going on, have been vilified and censored, leaving the public largely manipulated and misinformed.

Kennedy asserts that the U.S. response to COVID-19, under Fauci's leadership, has been abysmal; pointing out that while Americans make up 4.2% of the world population, the U.S. is responsible for 20% of the COVID deaths worldwide. When compared to China, which has a 3 per million death rate from COVID, the U.S. death rate is 2,107 per million—the worst in the world. Whereas, China was able to get the virus under control in 2 months by using chloroquine on a national level, the U.S. banned hydroxychloroquine, ivermectin and other effective treatments, in favor of the COVID vaccines that have only prolonged the virus and increased the death rate.

Bill Frist, the Senate Majority Leader and the White House, back in 2005, conspired with drug industry lobbyists to pass "*a sweeping liability provision that shields the industry from lawsuits over products used to treat pandemic illnesses, even in cases of gross negligence or gross recklessness.*" This shield provision was attached to a

> *defense appropriations bill in the dead of night, with the aid of House Majority Leader, Dennis Hastert...The industry deployed at least 158 lobbyists to influence policies relating to vaccines and pandemic preparedness in 2004 and 2005, including 84 who were previously employed by the federal government.*[364]

In 2009, **Dr. Scott Reuben,** an anesthesiologist from Tufts University in Boston, was sentenced to prison and had his medical license revoked for **falsifying data on 21 studies** sponsored by the Pfizer pharmaceutical company on the pain medications, Celebrex, Bextra, and Vioxx. No patients were ever enrolled in any of his studies, and the medical journals had to retract more than 30 bogus articles that Reuben had simply made up.

Paul Offit MD, the Director of the Vaccine Education Center at the Children's Hospital of Philadelphia, is the pro-vaccine advocate brought before the news media whenever the issue of vaccinations arises. You can count on Offit to extol the virtues of vaccines while readily dismissing concerns regarding vaccine safety. In 2010, Dr. Paul Offit was voted "Denialist of the Decade" by the *Age of Autism,* for his dismissive attitude toward vaccine injuries in spite of voluminous evidence to the contrary.[365]

Offit was a consultant for Merck when he developed the Rotavirus vaccine, receiving millions of dollars for the development of the vaccine in addition to a $1.5-million research chairmanship at Children's Hospital of Philadelphia paid for by Merck. The hospital also benefited financially as co-owner of the rotavirus vaccine patent along with Offit. At the same time, Offit sat on the ACIP, where he approved on three separate occasions his own vaccine, pointing to an obvious conflict of interest. In addition, Merck purchased 20,000 copies of Offit's book, *Vaccines: What Every Parent Should Know,* to distribute to doctors' offices throughout the United States exhorting the virtues of vaccination. Let's look at some of Offit's most fallacious quotes:

- Offit has suggested, *"Each infant would have the theoretical capacity to respond to about 10,000 vaccines at any one time."*[366] He initially stated that infants could tolerate 100,000 vaccines but then modified this number, realizing that was a bit too much even for him.
- He has also made the unsubstantiated claim that there are 20,000 studies proving that vaccines are safe. However, when it comes to acknowledging any legitimate studies

showing vaccines to be unsafe, Offit is quick to minimize any concerns.

- Offit has repeatedly stated that there is no connection between vaccines and autism, contrary to numerous studies showing a link. In an interview, Offit asserted that the number of autistic children has not increased in the past 30–40 years.[367] Really? And this is the pediatrician who is touted as a medical authority on the subject of vaccines and autism.

- In 2013, on Offit's vaccine-education center website, it stated, *"Aluminum is considered to be an essential metal… It is found in all tissues and is also believed to play an important role in the development of a healthy fetus."*[368] No, it is not. It is a heavy metal neurotoxin that, when injected into a body can cause numerous adverse reactions, as noted in numerous scientific studies. For example, a 2011 paper by Dr. Kawahara, stated:

> *Whilst being environmentally abundant, aluminum is not essential for life. On the contrary, aluminum is a widely recognized neurotoxin that inhibits more than 200 biologically important functions and causes various adverse effects in plants, animals, and humans.*[369]

Julie Gerberding served as the Director of the CDC from 2002 to 2009. After she took over as head of the agency, many of the scientists and leaders left the CDC, and she replaced them with people who had close ties to the vaccine industry. While heading the CDC, Gerberding was quite reluctant to acknowledge that autism was on the rise, while maintaining that there was no evidence of a link between vaccines and autism. As CDC director, she helped Merck in promoting Gardasil while ignoring negative findings; prevented the disclosure of Merck's chickenpox vaccine that was causing shingles; and silenced Dr. Thompson when he confessed that the CDC, in coordination with Merck, were destroying documents showing a connection between Merck's MMR vaccine and autism. Then in 2009, she left the CDC to take over as the president of Merck's vaccine division, where she received a $2.5 million salary, in addition to stock options. In January 2020, Gerberding sold more than half of her Merck stock shares worth $9.1 million, according to the Childrens Health Defense Chairman, Robert F. Kennedy, Jr.[370] Gerberding is a perfect example of how government officials who establish close ties with private industry, end up cashing in when they leave their government positions to take up lucrative jobs in the private sector. As a matter of fact, 59% of the pharmaceutical/health product lobbyists in the U.S. were previous government employees, according to an article, "Which Industry Spends the Most on Lobbying?" by Jake Frankenfield in *Investopedia.com* (Nov 1, 2021).

Congressman Billy Tauzin, a republican from Louisiana, is another example of how the revolving door between government and the private sector works. Tauzin retired from Congress in 2005 and became a lobbyist for the Pharmaceutical Research and Manufacturers of America (PhRMA), a lobbying association for drug companies. Between 2006 and 2010, he made $19,359,927 working as a lobbyist who was instrumental in blocking a proposal to allow Medicare to negotiate drug prices. In his final year working for PhRMA, he was paid $11 million. There are others in Congress highlighted in Lee Fang's article, *When a Congressman Becomes a Lobbyist, He Gets a 1,452% Raise (On Average)* simply by going to the private sector.[371]

Congressman Adam Schiff (D), in his attempt to silence critics of the vaccination program, directed Facebook and Google in 2019 to remove any online content that expresses *"anti-vaccination informa- tion."*[372] Accepting the vaccine orthodoxy on faith, Schiff has unknowingly bought into the media propaganda that "antivaxxers" are deluded, uninformed, and dangerous. As previously noted, "antivaxxers" more often than not are "exvaxxers" who learned the hard way that vaccines aren't always as safe as advertised. This forced censorship by politicians in coordination with social media and reinforced by the medical establishment further erodes the First Amendment rights that protect freedom of speech and effectively shuts down any legitimate discussion.

This is the kind of suppression of information that one expects to see in a totalitarian state, as opposed to a democratic society where open debate and differences of opinion are allowed to be freely expressed.

At the international level, unethical conduct on the part of the pharmaceutical industry is commonplace. When a vaccine is taken off the U.S. market because of its deleterious effects, the pharmaceutical company will just ship it off to another country instead. A perfect example is the Bayer pharmaceutical company back in the 1980s that produced the hemophiliac drug, Factor VIII, that was contaminated with the AIDS virus and ended up being responsible for thousands of deaths. As a result, Bayer took it off the U.S. market and unloaded the drug on 22 other countries in Europe, Asia, and Latin America. There ended up being a multi-million-dollar settlement against Bayer, which was kept from the public as part of a gag order, that became effective in 2010 involving thousands of hemophiliacs.[373]

The WHO and the Bill Gates-funded organization, the **Global Alliance for Vaccines and Immunization (GAVI)** are another example in which the DTP vaccine was given to African babies, after it was discontinued in the United States and other developed countries due to its severe adverse reactions.

And when it comes to drug trials using unsuspecting people in poor countries, where regulatory oversight is essentially absent, it is a great way to test potentially harmful vaccines and drugs on those who are most vulnerable and least capable of having anything to say about it. Often in these trials, informed consent is not obtained, and participants are not given accurate information regarding the purpose of these vaccine and drug studies. The **Bill and Melinda Gates Foundation (BMGF)** and the Gates-funded organization, GAVI, have been investigated by the India Supreme Court pending a lawsuit over deaths and injuries occurring during the HPV vaccine trials in 2014. In most of the cases, the girls and their parents were pressured into the vaccine trials without knowing what was involved. The researchers were also cited for other ethical violations that included forging consent forms and refusing to provide medical assistance for those who were injured. Out of the 23,000 girls between the age of 10 and 14 who were vaccinated, *"Approximately 1200 girls suffered severe side effects, including autoimmune and fertility disorders. Seven died."* No follow-up medical care was offered to the victims. A report funded by BMGF dismissed these adverse reactions, contending that the injuries were unrelated to the Gardasil vaccine.[374]

The BMGF has also been involved in an effort to eradicate polio in India by mandating the repeated use of the oral polio vaccine for children younger than 5. Though the wild poliovirus has declined, the related nonpolio acute flaccid paralysis (NPAFP) exploded between 2000 and 2017, with **490,000 cases** of paralyzed children above the expected numbers reported.[375] Indian doctors blamed the Gates campaign to eliminate polio for only exacerbating the crisis through the overuse of the oral vaccine that has induced more polio cases with symptoms that are more severe. In 2017, the Indian government reversed course in the vaccine program and told Gates to leave India. As a result, the *"NPAFP rates dropped precipitously."* Even the WHO in 2017 acknowledged reluctantly that the global explosion in polio was largely the result of the oral polio vaccine campaign. Similar epidemics have been noted in the Congo, Afghanistan, and the Philippines, with **70%** of the global polio cases being related to the vaccine itself.[376]

Another devastating example of abuse occurred in a small village in Chad, Africa, in December 2012. Five hundred children

> *were locked into their school, threatened that if they did not agree to being force-vaccinated with a meningitis A vaccine, they would receive no further education. These children were vaccinated without their parents' knowledge ...Within hours, one hundred and six children began to suffer from headaches, vomiting, severe, uncontrollable convulsions, and paralysis.*

The government financially compensated the families for the injured children but then told the parents that the injuries were not related to the vaccine. *"During investigations, it was discovered that the whole project was being run by the Bill and Melinda Gates Foundation."*[377]

Indian authorities have noted that BMGF has close ties to Big Pharma, as exemplified by the GAVI, funded by BMGF that promotes vaccinations globally. The board members included drug-company reps with *"conflicts of interest,"* pushing vaccines that have caused adverse reactions while at the same time, denying any culpability for vaccine injuries and deaths.[378]

Edward Bernays and Propaganda—The modern-day origins of manipulating public opinion are, in large part, attributed to Edward Bernays (1891–1995), known as the "father of public relations." In his famous work, *Propaganda*, he explored ways of exploiting emotions for commercial gain. Joseph Goebbels, Hitler's minister of propaganda, admired Bernays' techniques for manipulating the public and as a result, developed five principles used in Nazi propaganda summarized in an article from Children's Health Defense, entitled *Vaccine Coverage in Mainstream Media—Variations on a Theme of Propaganda*:

1. Avoid abstract ideas—appeal to the emotions.
2. Constantly repeat just a few ideas. Use stereotyped phrases.
3. Give only one side of the argument.
4. Continuously criticize your opponents.
5. Pick out one special "enemy" for special vilification.

The article asserts that "Big Pharma" uses propaganda in a similar manner when it comes to vaccines:

> *Today we are witnessing the layers of deceit, propaganda machinations, and engineered consent, all rolled up into a series of big lies: that vaccines are safe and effective, that the science is settled, that measles will kill us if we do not vaccinate, that there is no link between vaccines and autism, and that people that question are to be deemed misinformed, misinforming, and irresponsible, or worse yet, criminal.*[379]

Nathan Shasho, in his book, *Perspective: Making Sense of It All,* he wrote:

> *Indoctrination and propaganda, coupled with an uninformed public, are powerful tools that have been used throughout history by those who would make us their pawns. Critical thinking, along with a well-informed public, is the only way to combat this indoctrination.*[380]

In **Appendix I, *How to Win the Vaccine Credibility War,*** by Ted Kuntz, he shows how the pharmaceutical industry uses propaganda to effectively "brainwash" the public by following 10 devious methods in an attempt to convince people that vaccines are safe and effective.[381]

Astroturf and Other Fictions—Astroturf is a fake, grassroots, citizen's group or coalition, created and funded by corporations and political interests as a PR tactic used for political gain in which actors pretend to represent spontaneous grassroots support for a particular agenda.

The Astroturf movement was best exposed by Sharyl Attkisson in a TED Talk that noted such Astroturf websites as Left Brain-Right Brain, ScienceBlogs, skeptics.com, Neuroskeptic, Skeptical Raptor, Science-Based Medicine, HealthNewsReview, and the government-corporate-funded, American Council on Science and Health.[382]

In her presentation, she talked about how Astroturf blogs portray credible scientists and researchers as incompetent, quacks, frauds, and so on, while referring to legitimate scientific research as controversial, weak, flawed, and junk science.

This propaganda operates with the moral support of the vaccine industry and its government partners, reinforcing one another's faulty critiques. Reporters who do not do their own research will rely on this disinformation from Astroturf blogs and other pharmaceutical-influenced sources. The news media presents articles and stories that promote the pro-vaccine position to the exclusion of research that is contradictory. Authors that are pro-vaccine get special treatment in the media. Two recent books are a case in point:

- *Neurotribes* by Steve Silberman (2015).
- *In a Different Key: The Story of Autism* by Donvan and Zucker (2016).

Both books are written by news journalists who make assertions based largely on speculation, such as, autism as we see it now has always been with us and the changes in diagnostic classification explains why we are identifying so many autistic children today. Unfortunately, in these books, there is a notable absence of any discussion of the numerous scientific studies that support the proposition that vaccines are associated with autism and other neurodevelopmental disorders. Both books talk about the **neurodiversity** that emphasizes the acceptance of autistic children for who they are. While this is an appropriate response in addressing the needs of autistic children, it shouldn't negate the search for a greater understanding of what factors contribute to autism. But **Steve Silberman** nevertheless believes that the cause of autism is apparently unknowable, like schizophrenia. Therefore, the focus should be on the acceptance of autism while providing support services, instead of trying to pursue causation. Silberman wrote, *"Whatever autism is, it is not a unique product of modern civilization. It is a strange gift from our deep past, passed down through millions of years of evolution."*[383] This rather romantic interpretation of the origins of autism negates the fact that autism has reached epidemic levels today, since its dramatic growth starting around 1990. The proof of the sudden rise in autism and other neurodevelopmental disorders are to be found in the schools, where special-needs services are being severely impacted today.

Similar to Silberman, **Donvan and Zucker** stated that one cannot do anything to prevent autism, so we just need to accept it. They asserted that the autism-vaccine link has been *"thoroughly debunked by the scientific community."* According to them, *"Autism is not a disease to be cured but a genetically rooted identity with its own distinctive qualities to be respected and celebrated."*[384] Well, tell that to the parents of normally developing children who regress into an autistic state in which they become unresponsive, losing their ability to relate with family members, regress in language, speech, and cognitive functioning, develop seizure disorders and other physical anomalies, engage in ritualistic behaviors of hand flapping, rocking back and forth, head banging, and acting out uncontrollably and often aggressively, reflecting the palpable physical and emotional pain they are experiencing.

More than 80% of autistic children will need some degree of care for the rest of their lives, with the most severe cases requiring constant 24-hour supervision. Close to 50% are intellectually disabled and 40% are unable to speak, more than 25% exhibit self-injurious behaviors; roughly 90% of adult autistics are jobless; and health conditions range from asthma, skin and food allergies, ear infections, diarrhea, constipation, convulsions, and colitis. They also tend to have significant issues with ADD/ADHD, obesity, OCD, and Tourette's syndrome. It would seem that this description of autism would be closer to a nightmare for autistic children and their parents than *qualities to be respected and celebrated.*"

Refer to **Appendix J** for examples of *Censorship in Science,* when scientific evidence does not go along with the conventional wisdom of the medical establishment and the financial interests of the corporate world.

Vaccine Safety Science Is Flawed as summarized below:
- U.S. government studies refuse to compare the effects of vaccinated children versus unvaccinated children, for fear that the results would show that vaccines are not so safe after all, as a number of independent studies have already shown. Instead, the vaccine promoters assert that the science on vaccines is already "settled," when in fact, science is a process that is forever engaged in challenging current assumptions.
- Drug companies compare the efficacy of a new vaccine with a previous vaccine that contains similar ingredients, thereby negating an attempt to compare the vaccine against an inert saline solution that is supposed to be non-toxic. For example, in the clinical trials on Gardasil 9,

the original version of Gardasil was used as the placebo making it impossible to assess the vaccine's safety, if, in fact, one vaccine is being compared to essentially another questionable vaccine.

- Vaccines are **not,** and never were, tested in a double-blind placebo-controlled study, wherein neither the subject nor the researcher know in advance which treatment is being used, so that conclusions can be based on unbiased observation.

- The rapid approval of vaccines without adequate study makes it impossible to determine their long-term effects. The pharmaceutical-sponsored studies on vaccine reactions may follow the effects of a vaccine over only a **48-hour period.** This can exclude the majority of vaccine reactions that may occur weeks, months, or even years before there is any evidence of an adverse effect, as in the case of rheumatoid arthritis, cancers, diabetes, and so on. For example, the Salk vaccine was approved in **only 2 hours.** As mentioned previously, this led to the infamous "Cutter Incident" in 1955 in which the laboratory mistakenly released the live virus polio vaccine to the public resulting in *"40,000 cases of polio leaving 200 children with varying degrees of paralysis and killing 10 children."*[385]

- Testing is done only on individual vaccines with no researcher ever considering the effects of multiple vaccines given at one time. Current research has repeatedly shown a direct correlation between the number of vaccines given to children and the increased chances of injury caused by the synergistic effect of combining toxic ingredients from multiple vaccines.

- The CDC recommends the use of vaccines on populations with no safety data to support their use (e.g., pregnant women, newborns, premature births and immunocompromised individuals), in spite of the fact that the vaccine manufacturers specifically list these contraindications on the vaccine product inserts that come with each vaccine. In addition, the manufacturers acknowledge that the vaccines have not been tested for carcinogenic properties, the possibility of mutations, or their effect on fertility.

- It is assumed that vaccine efficacy is synonymous with the ability to induce antibody production artificially through a combination of chemical ingredients, many of which are toxic. However, the ability of the vaccine to create antibodies does not have the same effect as when contracting the natural disease. That is why vaccines provide only temporary immunity—because long-term protection comes only from acquiring the natural disease.

- Children used in vaccine studies are carefully screened to make sure they are in excellent health with no medical history of problems, whereas vaccinations are routinely given out to children without any serious consideration for their medical history or current state of health, increasing the possibility of an adverse reaction in those most vulnerable.

- The FDA does not conduct its own research on proposed vaccines but instead relies on the pharmaceutical companies to test, evaluate, and endorse its own product. This would seem to raise concerns regarding the legitimacy of the test results, especially given the past sordid history of the drug industry. This is analogous to the fox being put in charge of the hen house.

- Adverse reactions from vaccines are often negated or seen as coincidental instead of contributory. The medical authorities are notoriously unwilling to pursue a finding that could be damaging to "pro-vaccine interests." For example, they ignore the fact that children vaccinated with the live virus can shed the disease to others. Instead, the medical establishment and the news media focus exclusively on the unvaccinated as the source of the problem in spreading disease.

Ethical Behavior and the Pharmaceutical Industry

The public's attitude regarding prescription drugs versus vaccines is quite different, though both are produced by the same pharmaceutical companies. For example, people have no trouble understanding the corrupt practices of "Big Pharma" when it comes to their involvement in creating the opioid crisis, and the hundreds of thousands of deaths, or when they hide the adverse effects of drugs like Vioxx, which has caused tens of thousands of heart attacks and deaths or Johnson & Johnson who knew that baby powder contained asbestos for decades and kept that information from regulators and the public. Yet when it comes to questioning the efficacy of vaccinations, there is a notable lack of concern, as if it would be inconceivable to imagine that these same drug companies would put an injurious vaccine product into our children for the sheer purpose of profit. Well, in fact, there are a multitude of examples in which "Big Pharma" has committed fraud, censored unfavorable data, falsified scientific studies, and continued using drugs and vaccines when it was quite clear that they were causing injuries, chronic illnesses, and deaths. Take for example, the customary practice in which the pharmaceutical industry will take a vaccine that has been banned from the U.S. market because of its ill-effects and then turn around and pedal it off on other countries. This would suggest that the drug industry is more concerned with their profits than ensuring the safety of the public. After all, the bottom line is about protecting corporate profits, and to jeopardize that would seemingly amount to "bad business practices."

PART VII

MANUFACTURING HYSTERIA

"The gods are innocent of man's suffering. Our diseases and physical pains are the product of excess." —Pythagoras (570–510 B.C.)

As the medical community, backed by the pharmaceutical industry and the media, hypes up the next great pandemic on the horizon, invariably, there are calls to create a new drug or vaccine to combat the latest feared disease. In this way, the pharmaceutical industry benefits financially even though these diseases often do not materialize as predicted. Hysteria is fermented over diseases such as AIDS, anthrax, the reemergence of smallpox, swine flu, avian flu, mad cow disease, SARS, Zika virus, measles virus, and most recently COVID-19.

The book *Virus Mania,* by Torsten Englebrecht, journalist, Claus Kohnlein, MD, Samantha Bailey, MD, and microbiologist Stefano Scoglio, PhD, presented evidence that contagious viruses are falsely claimed to be the source of many diseases. They wrote:

> *These alleged contagious viruses may be, in fact, alternatively seen as particles produced by the cells themselves as a consequence of certain stress factors such as drugs and toxins…and wrongly interpreted as epidemic-causing viruses by doctors who have been indoctrinated for more than 100 years by the theory that microbes are deadly and that only modern medications and vaccines will protect us from virus pandemics.*[386]

The authors looked at the use of pharmaceuticals, illegal drugs, pesticides, heavy metals, pollution, stress, and processed foods, including GMOs, as possible explanations for these so-called viral epidemics. They included such diseases as: HIV/AIDS, Mad Cow disease (Bovine Spongiform Encephalopathy or BSE), Severe Acute Respiratory Syndrome (SARS), Avian flu (H5N1), Swine flu, and the current coronavirus (SARS-CoV-2), referred to as COVID-19. What follows is a very brief summary of these diseases covered in *Virus Mania,* which questions many of the scientific assumptions that these apparent epidemics are the result of viruses.

Virus Mania

Swine Flu (1976)—The medical establishment and the CDC urged Americans back in 1976 to get vaccinated in order to avert a deadly swine flu epidemic. More than 40 million people were inoculated, and anywhere between 20 and 40 percent experienced adverse reactions, including some cases of paralysis and death. The vaccine was taken off the market, and the CDC director, David J. Sencer, was subsequently fired over the swine-flu fiasco, and damage claims due to the vaccine totalled $2.7 billion. Ironically, in the end, there was no swine flu outbreak, and even Dr. Sencer later acknowledged in a CBS *60 Minutes* interview that there were no confirmed cases of the swine flu in the world, outside of one soldier at Fort Dix, New Jersey, who was identified as having the swine flu. However, more than 500 people developed Guillain-Barré syndrome (GBS), a severe paralytic condition as a direct result of the swine-flu vaccine.

Human Immunodeficiency Virus /Acquired Immunodeficiency Syndrome (HIV/AIDS)—AIDS is a loosely defined syndrome that may include:

> *anyone suffering from a few common and non-specific symptoms like weight loss plus diarrhea and itching...people are declared to have AIDS if they have a 'positive' antibody test,*

and simultaneously suffer from at least one of 26 likewise,
well-known diseases.[387]

HIV is described as a retrovirus that was first discovered by Luc
Montagnier and was considered to be the cause of AIDS, though even
Montagnier admitted that *"there is no scientific proof that HIV causes
AIDS."* The authors stated that the tests used for identifying HIV: the
HIV antibody tests, the PCR (polymerase chain reaction) test, and the
helper cell count, are unlikely to distinguish between HIV and other
possible conditions. For example, the HIV test may react to others
who survived tuberculosis, as well as other symptoms, which could
include pregnancy or a simple flu.

They presented evidence that AIDS could be explained by the use
of illegal drugs and medications like antiviral and antibiotics and by
malnutrition. AIDS victims have a history of consuming drugs such
as poppers (nitric oxide), cocaine, heroin, LSD, crystal meth, barbitu-
rates, and amphetamines. In the gay community, poppers were widely
used as a sexual stimulant. This abuse of drugs has had a detrimental
effect on the immune system, causing the kinds of symptoms that
are seen in AIDS patients. Unlike viruses and homosexuality, which
have been around throughout history, AIDS is a recent phenomenon
*"triggered by environmental factors like drugs, medications, and insuf-
ficient nutrition."*[388] For example, a standard AIDS treatment, AZT,
that was actively promoted by Dr. Fauci, who falsely claimed that it
was safe and effective, turned out to be a highly toxic antiretroviral
medication that destroyed bone marrow and caused innumerable
deaths that were then deceptively attributed to the AIDS virus.

**Mad Cow Disease (Bovine Spongiform Encephalopathy or
BSE)**—The human version is referred to as Creutzfeldt-Jakob disease. They wrote that no one actually succumbed to this supposed
epidemic, though it was predicted that as many as 10 million people
might die. The assumption that BSE was an infectious disease
found in meat that could be passed on to humans has never been

verified. On Oct. 13, 2001, the *British Medical Journal* called the *"Creutzfeldt-Jakob disease: the epidemic that never was."*[389] More likely, BSE was precipitated by poisoning with insecticides, heavy metals, copper deficiency, or autoimmune reactions. For example, phosmet, a highly toxic insecticide, used on cows to keep warble flies away, can penetrate through the skin, causing severe neurological damage commonly associated with BSE.

Severe Acute Respiratory Syndrome (SARS)—In 2003, SARS was feared to be the next epidemic on the rise. The WHO hyped up the estimated 800 SARS fatalities that occurred in China out of a population of more than 1 billion people. It was portrayed as a highly contagious virus by the medical authorities and in the media, though no epidemic ever took place. The medical solution was to administer antiviral and antibiotic medications, such as Zovirax, Relenza, and Tamiflu, to address the lung infections. Unfortunately, the drugs prescribed, which could also include cortisone and other steroids, only served to further weaken the immune system by damaging bone marrow, causing breathing difficulties, and reducing kidney and liver function, as noted on the pharmaceutical package inserts. In addition, they pointed out that the area in China where SARS broke out happened to be where all forms of electronic equipment were shipped from all over the world and then disassembled under hazardous conditions, causing toxic fumes that adversely affected the unprotected workers.

Avian Flu (H5N1)—In 2005, a new pandemic was predicted, triggered by the avian flu virus named, "H5N1." The United Nations chief coordinator, David Nabarro, stated in September 2005, *"A new flu pandemic can break out any moment—and it can kill up to 150 million people."*[390] The H5N1 hysteria was hyped up in the media and even Anthony Fauci, director of the National Institute of Allergy and Infectious Diseases (NIAID), warned that the H5N1 is *"a time bomb waiting to go off."*[391] In spite of these dire warnings, only 153 deaths were attributed to the bird flu spreading to humans and even that number was considered suspect. Nevertheless, doctors prescribed medications, like Tamiflu, which proved to be useless. They reported on a 2011 study that concluded, *"Taking Tamiflu can lead to a sudden deterioration in health and subsequent death."*[392]

Swine Flu (2009)—In the summer of 2009, the so-called swine flu caused fears of another epidemic, hyped up by the mainstream media that simply parroted the medical authorities that were closely linked to the pharmaceutical interests. The authors stated that the dreaded swine flu ended up being milder than other flu seasons, with only 258 deaths being counted. The swine flu vaccine itself was regarded as similar to other flu vaccines and therefore considered as safe, though it had been tested for only a few weeks. The vaccine contained a number of toxic ingredients, including thimerosal, aluminum, formaldehyde, Polysorbate 80, and squalene, causing severe side-effects, resulting in cases of narcolepsy, paralysis, and death.

Zika Virus

The Zika virus, not covered in *Virus Mania*, is yet another example of a disease hyped up by the media. Agencies like the CDC, the NIH, and the WHO, push for drastic measures to combat this supposedly fearful epidemic that is responsible for causing microcephaly. Microcephaly is a medical condition in which a newborn's head circumference is smaller than normal because of the lack of brain development, causing mental retardation.

The Zika virus, spread by mosquitoes, was first discovered in Uganda's Zika forest in 1947. Symptoms are exhibited roughly 20% of the time and are described as generally mild and of short duration, typically including a rash, pink eye (conjunctivitis), muscle aches, and a fever. That is the extent of the Zika virus. Prior to the current hysteria regarding the claim that the virus causes microcephaly, Zika had been around for over half a century without any previous association with microcephaly, in spite of a number of outbreaks. Based on insufficient evidence and skewed statistics, presumed to be correct, without considering other factors, the CDC, NIH, and WHO were quick to conclude that the Zika virus was the cause of microcephaly. In a paper published in the *New England Journal of Medicine*, four CDC employees stated, "*This study marks a turning point in the Zika outbreak. It is now clear that the virus causes microcephaly.*"[393]

Alternative theories regarding the cause of microcephaly were dismissed by the CDC without any further investigation, including the possible connection between microcephaly and toxic chemicals. The doctor's group, the Brazilian Association for Collective Health, stated its belief that the widespread use of chemicals in Brazil was contaminating the environment as well as people. They blamed the international chemical industry and its close financial connections with Latin American ministries of health, the WHO, and the Pan American Health Organization.[394]

A report published by physicians from the crop-sprayed villages of Argentina suggested that the chemical, pyriproxyfen, was the likely cause. The authors stated, "Malformations detected in thousands of children from pregnant women living in areas where the Brazilian state added pyriproxyfen to drinking water are not a coincidence..." The Brazilian Health Ministry placed pyriproxyfen into the water reservoirs in the state of Pernambuco, 18 months before the jump in birth defects. This region was where 35% of Brazil's microcephaly cases were reported. Sumitomo Chemical, a subsidiary of Monsanto, produces pyriproxyfen which is:

> *a growth inhibitor of mosquito larvae which alters the development process from larva to pupa to adult, thus generating malformations in developing mosquitoes and killing or disabling them.*"[395]

So, pyriproxyfen is "*a growth inhibitor*" of developing organisms, which sounds like the kind of chemical that might prevent a child's brain from developing normally. But never mind this apparent connection between pyriproxyfen and microcephaly. The CDC and the NIH have decreed that Zika is the culprit. So, now they can muster all their resources for attacking the Zika virus by killing off all the mosquitoes using more toxic chemicals that can cause more microcephaly, which will then justify more spraying and the rationale for developing a vaccine.

This is the kind of faulty circular reasoning that justifies spending billions of dollars on research and development of a vaccine to prevent a problem created by the toxic chemicals that are the cause of the problem to begin with. At the same time, these agencies are able to dismiss pesticides as being responsible for these birth defects and thereby avoiding liability. After all, who is going to go up against the authority of the CDC, the NIH, the WHO, and the mainstream news media that perpetuate the myth that the mosquitoes carrying the Zika virus are what causes children to contract microcephaly?

Severe Acute Respiratory Syndrome Coronavirus 2 (SARS-Co-2)

The ongoing fears regarding the coronavirus portrayed in the news media have been a motivating force in driving the push to create a vaccine, held up by the government, medical authorities, and media as the only viable solution to defeating this virus. The rapid roll-out of these new vaccines, as a result of Operation Warp Speed through Emergency Use Authorization (EUA), without the benefit of long-term studies, raises questions about their potential to cause unforeseen adverse events. The FDA sanctions manufacturers in the private sector to develop medical countermeasures through EUA in order to advance experimental treatments, including vaccines, during a public health crisis, as in the case of the current COVID-19 outbreak. [COVID-19 is an acronym: 'CO' stands for corona,'VI' for virus, 'D' for disease, and '19' for 2019].

> *Under an EUA, FDA may allow the use of unapproved medical products…in an emergency to diagnose, treat, or prevent serious or life-threatening diseases or conditions when certain statutory criteria have been met, including that there are **no** adequate, approved, and available alternatives.*[396]

In fact, there are alternative treatments as noted in numerous studies from the U.S. and other countries that have proven to be extremely effective in combatting SARS-CoV-2 without the adverse effects of the current COVID vaccines being used. The medical establishment has turned a blind eye, even censoring these alternative treatments that have been very effective, as in the case of ivermectin, in favor of the more lucrative vaccine measures taken. Though a multitude of vaccine injuries and deaths have occurred as a result of the rapid roll-out of mass vaccinations, this information has been largely kept out of mainstream media coverage.

Vaccines authorized under the EUA are, by definition, experimental, and the FDA cannot mandate these new vaccines until formally approved. Therefore, individuals have the right to refuse vaccinations since it is illegal to force participation in a medical experiment under EUA guidelines without one's consent. Introducing these experimental vaccines on such a large scale so quickly, poses a risk, especially when considering the growing number of physicians, scientists, and others who are witnessing the unprecedented injuries and deaths as a result of these vaccinations. In spite of this, the government has attempted to coax, bribe, shame, and now threaten those who refuse vaccination, essentially blaming the unvaccinated for impeding society's recovery from COVID-19. The government has increasingly resorted to gimmicks (eg. donuts, beer, baseball tickets, million-dollar lotteries) in order to entice the public to get jabbed, along with fear tactics to pressure people into getting vaccinated with absolutely no long-term evidence of safety and mounting evidence of harm. Under normal circumstances, vaccine development takes years in order to go through the proper safety testing, as opposed to a few months. In this rushed process fueled by fear, it seems that safety concerns have taken a backseat to the optimistic assertion that these vaccines are the solution, while at the same time, conveniently providing a highly profitable incentive to rush vaccines to the market. This short-sighted and dangerous approach in which professional voices are being openly censored for expressing grave concerns with the direction that things are headed, point to dire consequences down the road.

Dr. Mike Yeadon, Pfizer's former Vice President and Chief Scientist for the company, has "spent over 30 years leading new [allergy and respiratory] medicines research in some of the world's largest pharmaceutical companies." He wrote:

> *There is absolutely no need for vaccines to extinguish the pandemic. I've never heard such nonsense talked about vaccines. You do not vaccinate people who aren't at risk from a disease. You also don't set about planning to vaccinate millions of fit and healthy people with a vaccine that hasn't been extensively tested on human subjects…Any such proposals of universal inoculation are not only completely unnecessary but if done using any kind of coercion at all, illegal.*[397]

In a July 7, 2020 article by Robert F. Kennedy Jr., he cited documents by Axios and Public Citizen, indicating that the NIH partnered with Moderna to develop the COVID vaccine, in spite of the fact that Moderna has never been engaged in vaccine development previously. Nevertheless, Dr. Fauci approved a $483 million grant to Moderna through the Biomedical Advanced Research and Development Authority (BARDA), which made *"Moderna CEO Steve Bancel a billionaire and further enriched Fauci's mentor and co-investor Bill Gates."* According to these documents, the NIH apparently owns half of the patent and therefore half of the royalties for Moderna's COVID vaccine. *"In addition, four NIH scientists have filed their own provisional patent application as co-inventors"* who can then *"collect up to $150,000 annually in royalties,"* raising concerns about the potential for regulatory corruption.[398]

This is especially troublesome given that the 2020 Public Readiness and Emergency Preparedness Act (PREP Act), authorized by the DHHS, which declared that entities and individuals who are *"involved in the development, manufacture, testing, distribution, administration, and use of countermeasures,"*[399] are immune from any and all liability. Once again, the pharmaceutical industry and the medical community won't be held accountable for any adverse vaccine reactions that could cause serious injuries or deaths, regardless of their culpability. Instead, that will fall on the families who will be left to deal with the consequences of any adverse vaccine reactions.

One of the most disturbing aspects of the push to mandate vaccinations is the attempt by government to order children in school, as young as 5 years old, to be inoculated with experimental vaccines without sufficient evidence of safety. This is especially alarming, given the extremely rare occurrences of injury and death in children from the virus itself, compared to the abundance of data that show the COVID-19-vaccine-related disabilities and fatalities, as is currently observed in the unprecedented numbers of myocarditis seen in the 12–17 age group. How did school districts so willingly follow the dictates of the federal government in lockstep, in spite of parental pleas to abandon the vaccine requirement? In order to understand these marching orders, to mindlessly adhere to school mandates, one has to simply "follow the money," as the expression goes. Since the beginning of the COVID-19 crisis, Congress has passed trillions of dollars in stimulus funds, with billions going to schools, with the proviso that school boards adopt policies consistent with federal guidelines. In other words, do what the government says or lose your funding. Even though the science for the efficacy of these measures was lacking, the Department of Education (DOE), in coordination with the CDC's recommendations, initially enforced lock downs, and then required masking, social distancing, contact tracing, screening tests, and ultimately, aggressively pushing vaccinations as a condition for school attendance.[400]

The Impact of Worldwide Lockdowns—While so much fear and hysteria over COVID-19 has been provoked by the medical community, government leaders, and the media, little attention has been devoted to the impact of the worldwide lockdown itself. The delay in providing critical early medical care, the censorship of effective alternative treatments, and the adverse effects of the vaccines themselves, has increased the number of COVID-19 cases being admitted to the hospital. As a result of the primary emphasis on treating COVID-19 patients to the exclusion of other patients needing life-saving medical procedures, deaths from tuberculosis, HIV, malaria, cancers, heart attacks, have skyrocketed. Starvation and famine due to lockdowns in 2021 has been catastrophic with more than 2 million *children predicted to die in the coming year.* Domestic and sexual abuse has soared, with teen pregnancies up, along with suicide and drug problems. Cases of depression in the U.S. has increased 3-fold and substance abuse has led to overdoses and deaths at the highest point ever in a 12-month period. Perhaps most visible, has been the enormous negative impact on the economy and poverty: 150 million people have been forced into extreme poverty; over 110,000 U.S. restaurants permanently closed with unemployment tripling among young Americans, 52% now living with their parents; a disproportionate number of evictions for Black and Latino tenants, *exacerbating a homeless crisis;* and worldwide, an estimated 225 million full-time jobs lost in just 2020 alone.[401]

In another study from the Brownstone Institute, Paul Elias Alexander, summarized more than 400 studies on the failure of compulsory COVID-19 interventions, that include: lockdowns, shelter-in-place policies, school closures, and mask mandates. He reported that governments that have attempted compulsory measures to control the virus,

> *[H]ave failed in their purpose of curbing transmission or reducing deaths. These restrictive policies were ineffective and devastating failures, causing immense harm especially to the poorer and vulnerable within societies.*[402]

Vaccine Effectiveness—As with all vaccines, immunity is temporary, raising the question, "How long will this protection last and what does one do afterwards?" Since the initial COVID-19 vaccines provide protection that may last only 6 months, the obvious solution put forth are booster shots to prolong immunity. However, as noted previously, with each additional booster, the vaccine's effectiveness wanes even more rapidly, as viruses tend to become increasingly resistant to repeated vaccinations. This is what has happened with the overuse of antibiotics that breed bacterial resistance, causing bacteria to mutate while at the same time, making antibiotics increasingly ineffective. As acknowledged by vaccine makers, the COVID-19 vaccines were not designed to block the infection or prevent transmission to others, but only to lessen the disease. This, in fact, is the primary concern with the COVID shots, since they are not able to prevent the infection,

SARS-Co-2 is allowed to persist and adapt through mutation, as in the case of the Delta and Omicron variants.

Regrettably, the role of one's immune system has been ignored, as if naturally acquired immunity plays no part in one's response to the virus, when in fact, it is the only real solution, given that the natural immunity to the SARS-CoV-2 virus is superior to vaccine-induced immunity. It offers broader and longer-lasting protection, helps in reducing the spread of the virus to others and also protects against reinfection. By acquiring the natural infection, the body develops a more diverse array of antibodies and T cells that target all of the components of the virus, whereas the COVID shots focus on only one portion of the virus, namely, the spike protein. This then prompts the need for a booster shot to address what was supposedly not covered in the previous inoculation. This sets in motion the push for repeated boosters, dictated by the increasingly less effective vaccine response, as seen being played out in Israel, to be discussed shortly in further detail.

The independent virologist and vaccine expert, Dr. Geert Vanden Bosche, wrote an open letter to the World Health Organization on March 6, 2021, warning that the global mass vaccination effort is causing the emergence of new and deadly mutations. He stated:

> *Vaccinologists, scientists, and clinicians are blinded by the positive short-term effects in individual patients, but don't seem to bother about the disastrous consequences for health. Unless I am scientifically proven wrong, it is difficult to understand how current human interventions will prevent circulating variants from turning into a wild monster... From all of the above, it's becoming increasingly difficult to imagine how the consequences of the extensive and erroneous human intervention in this pandemic are not going to wipe out large parts of our human population. One could only think of very few other strategies to achieve the same level of efficiency in turning a relatively harmless virus into a bioweapon of mass destruction.*[403]

What is repeatedly reinforced in the mainstream news media is that the COVID-19 pandemic is a crisis of the unvaccinated. However, as more people are getting vaccinated, COVID-19 infections are increasingly seen in the fully vaccinated, as a result of this waning effect of vaccines. What started out providing immunity for 6 months, may now only last as long as one month, due to the repeated use of booster shots that further suppresses the immune system. Instead of providing greater protection from viruses, vaccines are making people more susceptible to future variants, as a result of weakened immunity. Today, the rising cases of COVID-19 infections observed in the vaccinated are politely referred to as "breakthrough infections," when, in fact, they clearly reflect vaccine failures.

Relative Risk Versus Absolute Risk

Mark Twain said that there were three kinds of lies: lies, damn lies, and statistics. Well, in regards to COVID-19, the use of statistics usually falls into the category of damn statistical lies. In order to understand how statistics can be manipulated, it is critical to make a distinction between "relative risk" versus "absolute risk." Relative risk compares the risk in two different groups, however it doesn't say anything about the actual odds of something happening within a total populace, whereas absolute risk does that. While relative risk is often used to show the benefits of a treatment, it tends to exaggerate the effect of an intervention. Whereas, the absolute risk gives a better representation by measuring the difference between the number of people experiencing an event in relation to the total population being studied.

If a study shows that out of 10,000 subjects in the experimental group, only 1 person contracts a disease and in the control group of 10,000 subjects, 2 people contract the same disease, the relative risk of getting the disease in the placebo group would be 100% greater, since 2 people would be 100% greater than 1 person. In this way, it would seem that the experimental group benefited greatly from the drug or vaccine used in the trial. However, using absolute risk (also referred to as risk difference), we would see that the risk between the treatment group and the control group is only between 1 and 2 people out of 10,000 subjects. So, the question becomes, "Is the treatment worth it?", if in fact, 10,000 people would have to be treated in order for 1 person to benefit. This is why it is essential to understand the reduction in absolute risk vs. relative risk, if you want to do an accurate cost-benefit analysis. The drug companies are notorious for only using relative risk reduction that purposely distorts the findings in order to accentuate the positive effects of a treatment. In this case, by listing the relative risk without understanding the absolute risk, it renders the information essentially nonsensical.

Adverse Reactions—From the beginning, severe reactions have been reported in all of the COVID-19 trials by Moderna, Pfizer, Johnson & Johnson, and Astra-Zeneca, yet we are told, based on limited information presented to the public by the developers, that these vaccines are up to 95% safe and effective. In spite of questionable claims of vaccine efficacy, VAERS data, maintained by the CDC and FDA, released on July 8, 2022, showed "a total of 1,329,135 reports of adverse events from all age groups following COVID vaccines, including 29,273 deaths and 241,910 serious injuries between Dec.14, 2020 and July 1, 2022." These vaccines have been associated with cases of blood clotting disorders (14,171), GBS (895), miscarriage or premature birth (1,761), anaphylaxis (2,285), myocarditis and pericarditis (4,251), and Bells Palsy (3,623). It also reported, "32,543 adverse events, including 1,843 rated as serious and 44 reported deaths" among 12- to 17-year-olds.[404]

In the United Kingdom, just within the first 6 months that the COVID vaccines were introduced, there were 30,305 deaths reported within the first 21 days of the COVID shot. The number of deaths in the U.S. following the COVID vaccinations in just 9 months outstripped the deaths from all other vaccines combined that have been reported over the past 30 years.[405] But, this is only the tip of the iceberg based on the July 19, 2021 sworn testimony by a whistleblower, who goes by *Jane Doe*. In order to preserve confidentiality, she wished to remain nameless out of concern for her personal safety and that of her family. She is a computer programmer with expertise in healthcare data analytics who disclosed evidence contained in her Declaration that VAERS under-reported deaths caused by the COVID-19 vaccines. In the written testimony it stated:

> *Jane Doe queried data from CMS [Centers for Medicare and Medicaid Services] medical claims, and has determined that the number of deaths occurring within 3 days of injection with the Vaccines exceeds those reported by VAERS by a factor of at least 5, indicating that the true number of deaths caused by the vaccines is at least 45,000.*[406]

Earlier attempts to develop a coronavirus vaccine, going back more than 2 decades, have triggered what is referred to as antibody-dependent enhancement (ADE). ADE is a condition in which a vaccine is able to create the opposite effect, actually enhancing the virus' ability to infect the cells and then replicate, causing a more severe disease, as in the case of previous coronaviruses (CoVs).[407] In the medical field, ADE is euphemistically referred to as *"immune enhancement"* when, in fact, it reflects *"disease enhancement,"* whereby the body's exposure to pathogens can precipitate an autoimmune reaction, referred to as *"pathogenic priming."* An April 2020 study in the *Journal of Translational Autoimmunity* asserted that pathogenic priming likely contributes to serious illnesses and mortality due to the vaccinations causing autoimmunity and warned that animal studies *"should be undertaken before use of any vaccine against SARS-CoV-2 is used in humans.*"[408] Going ahead with human trials without first doing the customary animal studies is especially troublesome, given the experimental nature of the new mRNA (messenger ribonucleic acid) gene therapy technology. The long-term consequences of the mRNA vaccines have presented *"unique and unknown risks"* involving an inflammatory response that could trigger an autoimmune condition.[409]

The mRNA vaccines, developed by Pfizer and Moderna, do not really qualify as a vaccine in the true sense of the word since the manufacturers never claimed that the mRNA vaccine created immunity or prevented transmission, which meets the criteria for a vaccine. Instead, the manufacturer and the FDA describe the mRNA as a form of gene therapy that serves only to reduce the symptoms of the person being vaccinated.[410] The mRNA vaccines are designed to instruct the cells to manufacture spike proteins that will trigger an immune response, producing antibodies that will presumably protect the vaccinee from getting infected with COVID-19. However, mRNA injection contains a synthetic and nondegradable chemical called Polyethylene glycol (PEG), which has been associated with adverse immune reactions, including anaphylaxis. Documents from Moderna showed that the company is *"well aware of the risks associated with PEG and other aspects of its mRNA technology but is more concerned with its bottom line."*[411]

The SARS-Co-2 spike protein found in the coronavirus is what has caused the most severe symptoms of COVID-19. However, the genetically modified spike protein found in the mRNA vaccines is materially much worse than the spike protein in the coronavirus itself. The COVID-19 shot utilizes lipid nanoparticle technology to facilitates the transfer of the modified spike proteins into the cells that are then programmed to reproduce additional modified spike proteins. The problem with the spike protein is that it can attach to the walls of the small blood vessels, imped-ing the flow of blood due to the spike protein's rough surface. Clotting results when the blood cell platelets encounter these rough spots in the capillary network. Sensing that the blood vessel is damaged, the platelets will accumulate at the spot of the spike protein forming an abnormal blood clot. And given that the spike protein can spread throughout the body via blood circulation, it can end up in the lungs, heart, brain, bone marrow, liver, spleen, adrenal glands, lymph nodes, and ovaries. In addition, it is not known how long the spike protein will be able to continue replicating within the cells with the potential to cause ongoing havoc.

The COVID-19 vaccine has also been shown to cause damage by *"dysregulating your innate and adaptive immune systems and activating latent viruses,"*[412] and with each successive shot, the damage to the immune system is accumulative. The harmful effects of the modified spike protein can exacerbate preexisting health conditions, such as leukemia and lymphomas, and can reactivate latent viruses, such as herpes zoster. Autoimmune disorders also caused by the spike protein may not develop until months or years afterwards, which begs the question as to why there has been such a rush to vaccinate without the proper time to study the long-term impact, especially when there were other treatments that were proven more effective against COVID-19.

Regarding the use of the COVID-19 vaccines on pregnant women, the CDC's claim that they are safe has been challenged by evidence to the contrary. Even the CDC-sponsored study by Shimabukuro et al. (2021) has been criticized for its shoddy statistics which suggested that *"there were no obvious safety signals precluding mRNA vaccine use in pregnancy."* The study claimed that spontaneous abortions occurred in only 12.6% of cases, however, re-analysis by Brock and Thornley indicated that there was

> a cumulative incidence of spontaneous abortions ranging from 82% (104/127) to 91% (104/114), 7–8 times higher than the original authors' results."

> In conclusion, they suggested, "The immediate withdrawal of mRNA vaccine use in pregnancy and those breastfeeding, alongside the withdrawal of mRNA vaccines to children or those of child-bearing age in the general population.[413]

Another study published in 2022 and funded by the NIH in the journal *Science Advances*, noted unexpected menstrual bleeding after SARS-Co-2 inoculations. The study surveyed approximately 40,000 women and found that 42% of those who were menstruating reported unexpected heavy bleeding after getting the COVID shot and 66% of postmenopausal women reported a reoccurrence of bleeding. Similar results were reported in other studies outside the United States.[414]

A study presented at the American Heart Association (AHA) Scientific Conference in November 2021, indicated that there is an increased risk of developing acute coronary syndrome (ACS), a sudden reduction of blood flow to the heart, after receiving the mRNA COVID-19 vaccines. The study author concluded that mRNA vaccines:

> *dramatically increase inflammation on the endothelium [interior surface of blood vessels] and T cell infiltration of cardiac muscle and may account for the observations of increased thrombosis [blood clots], cardiomyopathy [heart muscle weakness], and other vascular events following vaccination.*[415]

A recent phenomenon in the sports world has seen a surge in the sudden deaths of athletes starting around the latter part of 2021 that has not been covered in the mainstream media. The United Kingdom soccer legend and sports commentator, Matt Le Tissier has been outspoken in his attempt to draw attention to the large number of athletes who have been collapsing and even dying on the field of play and as a result of his efforts, he was fired from his job. In his 17 years playing soccer, Le Tissier has never seen anything like what is happening and can't understand why there has been no investigation into these events, over a 6-month-period, involving more than 400 'supposedly' healthy athletes. This has closely coincided with COVID, and could be a consequence of the illness, or it could be the result of the vaccine but the health authorities are simply ignoring the problem. There are numerous reports from the athletes themselves who have noted the ill-effects of the vaccine after being inoculated.[416]

Similar issues regarding vaccine safety have been raised by airline pilots who have suffered the adverse effects of vaccinations. Josh Yoder is an airline pilot who cofounded the U.S. Freedom Flyers (USFF), an organization against vaccine mandates for pilots. Yoder stated that "USFF has documented cases of blood clots, strokes, cardiac arrest, unconsciousness and sudden death among airline professionals which have been medically linked to the COVID-19 vaccinations." The *Advocates for Citizens' Rights,* committed to safeguarding human rights, has also cited numerous cases of pilots being injured or dying after vaccination. They have communicated these concerns to the Federal Aviation Administration (FAA), U.S. Dept. of Transportation, U.S. Dept. of Justice (DOJ), and all U.S. major air carriers about the increased risks to pilots flying with potentially abnormal health conditions that could lead to a catastrophic event.[417]

One of the most frightening discoveries have been reports, first noticed in 2021, by embalmers who are witnessing strange new blood clots never-before-seen post-mortem in vaccinees. The National Funeral Directors Association has cited numerous embalmers who are seeing odd long string-like clots that tend to stay intact when removed from the body. Richard Hirschman, a funeral director who has been embalming people for over 20 years, contends that the current vaccines are the likely cause in the deaths of around 65% of his cases. He is not aware of any unvaccinated people that displayed these unusual blood clots. Cary Watkins, another embalmer who has worked for over 50 years, relays the same concerns regarding these strange clots that only started happening after the COVID vaccines came out. Attempts to get the CDC to investigate this anomaly has been curiously met with silence.[418]

The National Health Federation, a non-profit health freedom organization, has compiled and summarized 559 recent scientific studies on COVID-19, referencing research that contradicts the prevalent view that vaccines are efficacious and essential to ending the pandemic. It covered various issues including adverse reactions from the COVID-19 inoculations. Specific examples of detrimental side-effects included: venous thromboembolism (blood clotting), myocarditis (inflammation of the heart muscle), irregular menstruation, spontaneous abortions, and other adverse reactions, as a result of a weakened immune system. This increased susceptibility has caused a drop in T cells which are supposed to keep viruses in check. Consequently, there has been an increase in shingles, HPV virus, uterine cancers, melanomas, Parkinson's disease, anaphylaxis, and hypertension, particularly in the elderly.[419]

In Oct 2021, Steve Kirsch, Executive Director of the COVID-19 Early Treatment Fund, put together a 181-page slide presentation entitled, *All you need to know about COVID vaccine safety*. He did an extensive review of vaccine studies, stating:

> *The vaccines kill more people than they can be expected to save for all groups, especially young adults. So far, more than 150,000 Americans have been killed by the vaccines... The FDA and CDC have deliberately ignored the safety signals, ignoring clear fraud in Phase 3 trials...The vaccines should be immediately HALTED. Instead, we are doing the opposite by mandating deadly, experimental vaccines that were never properly tested.[420]*

Kirsch is so confident in his research findings that he has even offered one million dolllars to anyone who can prove his calculations are incorrect. He has directly challenged the CDC and FDA to debate the efficacy of these vaccines, but they have avoided all attempts to respond to his allegations. Kirsch has emphasized that the early treatment of COVID using alternative approaches *"are far superior to vaccination in virtually every aspect."* Refer to Appendix K: *How to Report an Injury from COVID-19 Vaccine for Reimbursement.* The injury needs to be reported within one year of vaccination.

Falsifying Data—The standard PCR (polymerase chain reaction) test that is used to identify SARS-CoV-2 infections has been manipulated to give the impression that there are more cases of COVID-19 than actually exist. Dr. Kary Mullis, who won the Nobel Prize in Chemistry for inventing PCR, warned back in 1996 that his invention was exaggerating the numbers of AIDS cases.[421] Likewise, the current PCR test is being used inappropriately to amplify the

number of COVID cases. So, as more cases are being falsely identified in the media, it engenders a greater level of fear that one is more
susceptable to contracting the disease, and therefore, creating a greater
sense of urgency to get vaccinated. The procedure for determining
the PCR test results usually involves swabbing the nose of patients in
order to collect an RNA sample that is then amplified in cycles, called
cycle thresholds (CT). The higher the cycle threshold, the greater the
sensitivity of the test and the greater likelihood that healthy people
will be labeled as having COVID due to false positive readings. For
example, with a CT of 35 cycles or higher, the PCR test accuracy falls
below 3%, meaning that more than 97% of the test results end up being
false positives, based on a September 2020 study in *Clinical Infectious
Diseases.* Nevertheless, the WHO recommends setting CT at 45 and
the CDC and FDA suggest setting the CT at 40 cycles, rendering
the test results as useless in accurately identifying actual COVID-19
cases. In effect, many more people are being inaccurately labeled as
having Covid-19, as a result of more people being tested, even those
who are asymptomatic, meaning they have no symptoms yet are still
classified as having Covid because of the false positive test results.[422]

Another way in which the CDC has manipulated data is by
using two different criteria for determining whether patients have
contracted COVID-19. Those who have been vaccinated and are suspected of having COVID-19 are tested using a CT of 28 or less, while
the unvaccinated are tested with a CT of 40. In this way, the CDC can
falsely claim that the vaccinated are better protected, since they will
more likely test negative for COVID while the unvaccinated will test
positively more often, due to the inaccurate false positive readings.[423]

On August 23, 2020, the CDC released data indicating that
only 6% of COVID-19 deaths were attributed solely to the coronavirus, whereas the remaining 94% of deaths listed on average 2.6
comorbidities, in addition to COVID-19.[424] Therefore, out of 600,000
deaths attributed to COVID-19, hypothetically, only 36,000 deaths
would be attributed to COVID alone, when excluding other health
conditions. This is why it is especially critical to draw a distinction
between those who die **from** COVID as opposed to those who die

with COVID. It should be noted that the CDC abruptly changed the criteria that existed for the previous 17 years regarding the way pre-existing/comorbidity conditions are reported. This significantly alters death-certificate reporting, listing COVID-19 mortality cases as primary, when, in fact, other comorbidity conditions are the real cause of death. It is estimated that 80% of COVID deaths that occur in those 65 years and older, especially those in nursing homes, are largely due to pre-existing chronic diseases or medical conditions. Factors such as obesity, diabetes, cancers, high blood pressure, poor diet adversely impacting gut flora, and low vitamin D levels, have all been shown to contribute to a weakened immune system, making one more susceptible to the coronavirus.

An investigation by the Emmy Award-winning journalist, Sharyl Attkisson, of *Full Measure,* on the Sinclair Broadcasting Network, pointed out that numerous deaths throughout the country were being falsely reported as COVID–related, when in fact, people were actually dying from totally unrelated events, such as car and motorcycle accidents, homicide-suicide murders, terminal cancers and other chronic life-threatening conditions.[425]

The organization, Global Frontline Nurses was started by nurses who have witnessed the corruption and censorship within the medical system that has been the cause of so many injures and death due to the COVID-19 vaccines and procedures instituted by the hospitals and care facilities that blindly follow government mandates. These dedicated whistleblowers are being threatened for reporting patient abuses and in many cases losing their employment for exposing the truth about the shoddy conditions and lack of proper medical care. Nursing homes can collect $10,000 per COVID death, so that patient care may become a lower priority as a result.[426] In addition, hospitals are financially incentivized to count patient deaths as due to COVID-19 even when other comorbidity factors are the cause of death. In an August 1, 2020 Washington Examiner article, the CDC Director, Robert Redfield, confirmed that hospitals have a monetary incentive to overcount coronavirus deaths.[427] For example, if a Medicare patient has pneumonia and is also listed as having COVID-19, the federal government reimburses the hospital $13,000 and if that patient ends up on a ventilator, that amount increases to $39,000.[428] This would seemingly create a strong incentive for hospitals to list patients as having COVID whenever possible, regardless of other factors.

The issue of vaccine transmissibility has been widely debated, especially as it relates to asymptomatic cases, in which individuals test positive for COVID-19 but show no symptoms. The Chinese government ended up conducting a mass screening program of nearly 10 million residents of Wuhan between April and May 2020, to determine the current status of the COVID-19 epidemic. The study found that there was no indication that asymptomatic persons passed on the virus to others.

> *A total of 1174 close contacts of the asymptomatic positive cases were traced, and they all tested negative for the COVID-19…In summary, the detection rate of asymptomatic positive cases in the post-lockdown Wuhan was very low (0.303/10,000) and there was no evidence that the identified asymptomatic positive cases were infectious.*[429]

Dr. Robert Malone, the world-renowned virologist and immunologist who was instrumental in the development of the mRNA vaccine technology, has come out criticizing the notion that the vaccinated are protected from transmitting the COVID virus to others. He has described the fully vaccinated as being *"super-spreaders,"* adding that *"The idea that if you have a workplace where everybody's vaccinated, you're not going to have virus spread is totally false. A total lie."*[430] If this is the case, it raises the question, "Why are the vaccinated allowed privileges that the unvaccinated are denied, if, in fact, both are equally able to transmit the virus to others?

Treatment Options—Numerous studies have confirmed that there are alternative treatments to vaccination that have proven to be safe, effective, and inexpensive, especially in regards to the elderly population. These treatment options are able to guard against the COVID-19 virus while strengthening the immune system.[431] Simone

Gold, MD, founder of America's Frontline Doctors, reported on the use of **hydroxychloroquine** (HCQ) as an effective treatment for COVID-19, stating that HCQ has been an FDA-approved drug safely used for more than 65 years throughout the world. Despite numerous studies that have *"shown remarkable efficacy against SARS-CoV-2,"*[432] HCQ has been largely discredited by medical authorities as being ineffective and even dangerous. This was initially based on a flawed *Lancet* study that was later discredited and retracted from the journal. However, HCQ continued to be dismissed by the mainstream media in spite of evidence to the contrary showing that it has had a beneficial effect in treating COVID-19 when given in the correct dosage. Dr. Vladimir Zelenko recommended using **quercetin** as an alternative to hydroxychloroquine since it is a more readily available over-the-counter supplement. Quercetin is described as having "antiviral, anti-blood clotting, anti-inflammatory and antioxidant properties, all of which are important in the treatment of SARS-CoV-2 infection."[433]

Another remedy proposed by Dr. Joseph Mercola involved the use of **nebulized hydrogen peroxide** *"to combat infections and can be used both prophylactically after known exposure to Covid-19 and as a treatment for mild, moderate, and even severe illness."*[434]

The Front Line COVID-19 Critical Care Alliance (FLCCC), formed in March 2020, led by the founder and Co-Chief Medical Officer, Dr. Paul Marik, along with his colleagues, pioneered a treatment protocol known as MATH+ which stands for **M**ethylprednisolone, **A**scorbic Acid, **T**hiamine, **H**eparin, plus Ivermectin (IVM), Nitazoxanide, Dual Anti-Androgen therapy, Vitamin D, and Melatonin.

This protocol incorporates the use of **Ivermectin** (IVM), an anti-parasitic medicine that has *"anti-viral and anti-inflammatory properties against SARS-CoV-2 and COVID-19."* In the summary, FLCCC suggested:

> *The widespread use of this safe, inexpensive, and effective intervention could lead to a drastic reduction in transmission rates as well as the morbidity and mortality in mild, moderate, and even severe disease phases.*[435]

In January 2021, even the NIH approved Ivermectin as an effective option in the treatment of Covid-19. Yet, the CDC has continued to discourage and even threatened to expel doctors who attempt to use ivermectin and other treatment methods that have proven safer and less invasive than the current COVID-19 vaccines. In a related story, three researchers were awarded the Nobel Prize in Medicine in 2015 for discovering ivermectin as an extremely effective treatment against human infections caused by parasites as well as reducing deaths due to malaria.[436] Nevertheless, the mainstream media has repeatedly mocked ivermectin as "horse medicine" that is dangerous for use in humans. Monoclonal antibody therapy has also been used in the early treatment of mild to moderate COVID-19 cases but is administered in the hospital or a nursing home setting since it is given by IV (intravenously), with some restrictions based on age, health history, and the limited time period from the onset of symptoms. They are laboratory-made proteins that are designed to mimic the immune system's ability to fight off the virus, preventing it from entering the cells.

Dr. Peter McCullough, the vice chief of internal medicine at Baylor University Medical Center and leading authority on COVID-19, discussed the basis and rationale for early outpatient intervention in the treatment of SARS-CoV-2 infection. He emphasized the importance of treating patients at home within the first 5 days of contracting the virus, utilizing a combination of anti-viral medicines such as HCQ or IVM, along with antibiotic drugs like Azithromycin, and non-prescription treatments that include vitamin D3, zinc sulfate, vitamin C, and oxygen, in order to avoid hospitalization and the greater risk of death.[437] Unfortunately, the standard medical treatment for COVID-19 is generally not initiated until the patient becomes severely ill and then has to be admitted to the hospital, where the prognosis for recovery is diminished, especially when relying on ventilators as a last resort, which can cause lung damage and death. McCullough sees the emphasis on vaccines to the exclusion of early alternative treatments prior to hospitalization as the primary reason there have been so many unnecessary deaths and blames the profitability of vaccinations as the force behind the intentional suppression of effective treatments. The pharmaceutical industry has corrupted government agencies, the medical establishishment, the political system, and the mainstream media, to such a degree, that few are willing to risk their livelihood, to go up against the "official" sanctioned narrative.

The FDA's primary solution for treating COVID-19 patients in the hospital, was to approve Gilead Science's expensive drug, remdesivir, though there was little evidence that it did any good. WHO's Solidarity study, released in October 2020, *"conducted in 405 hospitals in 30 countries"* was the largest controlled study on remdesivir. It indicated that remdesivir *"does not reduce mortality or the time COVID-19 patients take to recover,"* and did not recommend its use because of its potential to do harm. WHO noted, *"a disproportionately high number of reports of liver and kidney problems in patients receiving remdesivir."*[438] Nevertheless, the FDA went ahead and authorized its in-hospital use with COVID-19 patients, while censoring safer, less costly, and more effective alternative medications.

The Association of American Physicians and Surgeons (AAPS) puts out, *A Guide to Home-Based COVID Treatment,* providing an overview of the SARS-CoV-2 coronavirus and symptoms related to COVID-19. The focus is on early home treatment that is especially critical for high-risk patients. The physician or licensed medical professional is provided with a format for initiating a home-based treatment plan. This informative guide presents a summary of prescription medicines, supplements, and other therapies that can be used to treat COVID-19. A free PDF copy of this e-booklet is available at *AAPSonline.org.*

The Origin of Covid-19—The question as to where the COVID-19 virus came from has been mired in controversy. Though Dr. Fauci and the CDC claimed that the virus originated in a Chinese market, there is overwhelming evidence to indicate that the virus was created in the Wuhan lab in China as a result of gain of function (GOF) research.[439] Luc Montagnier, the French virologist and recipient of the 2008 Nobel Prize in Medicine for his discovery of the human immunodeficiency virus (HIV), stated in a French interview in May

2020 that the COVID-19 virus was developed in the Wuhan lab. He speculated that the virus, derived from bats, was manipulated by researchers, in which components of HIV had been inserted into the coronavirus in an apparent attempt to develop an AIDS vaccine.[440] Even Dr. Redfield believed that the coronavirus came from the lab in Wuhan. In a CNN interview on March 26, 2021, contradicting Dr. Fauci, he stated: *"I am of the point of view that the most likely etiology of this pathogen in Wuhan was from a laboratory, you know, escaped...I do not believe this somehow came from a bat to a human."*[441]

GOF research is an experimental procedure in which scientists from the U.S. and China have taken viruses from nature and studied how they can be modified to become deadlier and more transmissible, supposedly to determine which viruses might threaten the public so they can design countermeasures. On May 15, 2020, Fred Guterl, the executive editor of *Scientific American*, wrote an article entitled, *"Dr. Fauci Backed Controversial Wuhan Lab with Millions of U.S. Dollars for Risky Coronavirus Research."*[442] Dr. Anthony Fauci, who heads the National Institute of Allergy and Infectious Diseases (NIAID), funded millions of dollars for these studies at the Wuhan Institute of Virology and other laboratories to research the bat coronaviruses. This GOF research was considered so controversial that it was halted under the Obama administration back in 2014 but then reinstated during the Trump presidency in 2017. In a senate hearing on May 11, 2021, Dr Fauci stated, *"The NIH has not ever, and does not now, fund gain-of-function research in the Wuhan Institute,"* in spite of clear evidence to the contrary based on documentation in which he authorized grants to Eco-Health Alliance and others to conduct GOF research on coronaviruses.[443] The manipulation of viruses in the lab, with the potential for infecting humans, was criticized by scientists, such as Richard Ebright, an infectious disease expert at Rutgers University, because of the risk of creating a pandemic from the accidental release of a new and virulent form of the virus. Fred Guterl indicated that, *"More than 200 scientists called for the work to be halted. The problem, they said, is that it increased the likelihood that a pandemic would occur through a laboratory accident."* Tom Inglesby of Johns Hopkins University and Marc Lipsitch of Harvard, added:

> *We have serious doubts about whether these experiments should be conducted at all...With deliberations kept behind closed doors, none of us will have the opportunity to understand how the government arrived at these decisions or to judge the rigor and integrity of that process.*[444]

There has been considerable pressure by the CDC, governmental officials, and the mainstream media to promote the idea that the coronavirus naturally evolved from bats and then spread to humans. At the same time, government squelched any suggestion that this was the result of GOF research that set off a catastrophic global crisis. Obviously, the admission of such a blunder, implicating both the United States and China, would have profound implications.

Yet, the most damning evidence exposing the corruption and fraud in regards to the origin of the COVID-19 pandemic came from Li-Meng Yan, MD, PhD, a Chinese researcher with specific training in coronaviruses and the research being conducted at the Wuhan lab. She stated that SARS-CoV-2 was developed in a Chinese military lab with the support of U.S. funding from Dr. Fauci's NIAID. She also implicated WHO as being involved in the cover-up along with the Chinese Communist Party (CCP). Yan claims that the military scientists from the CCP and coronavirus experts engaged in developing a bioweapon with the intent of ultimately undermining America's economic and social order.

At one point, the Chinese government became suspicious of Yan, who questioned what was going on, prompting her supervisor, Dr. Leo Poon, to warn her to keep silent or she will be "disappeared," which is how the government typically deals with dissenters. Out of fear for her safety, Yan escaped to the U.S. from Hong Kong in April 2020. She was subsequently interviewed on Fox News, on June 30, 2021, where she disclosed the experimentation that was conducted at the Wuhan lab.

According to Yan, hydroxychloroquine (HCQ) is being widely used in China for the treatment of COVID-19, which is sold over the counter throughout the country. She believes that the high death rates in the U.S. are due to the suppression and censorship of HCQ, in order to push the more lucrative vaccine option. Yan noted that China has profited greatly by being heavily invested in stocks from Pfizer, Moderna, and other pharmaceutical companies. Ultimately, she sees the COVID shots and the vaccine passports as part of the CCP's agenda to create an advanced 24/7 digital surveillance system, like in China, that can then closely monitor and control the actions of every person. Yan uses the example of what happened to Hong Kong, over a 2-year period starting in 2019, in which China was able to destroy democracy thereby enacting national security laws that took away personal freedoms and the right to privacy. Yan warns that China's ultimate goal is to achieve world dominance by 2035.[445]

Vaccine Passports are based on technology that uses Quick Response Code (QR Code), a type of barcode that can be read easily by a digital device, which stores information as a series of pixels in a square-shaped grid. It is a machine-scannable image like a barcode used at the supermarket. Since the emergence of COVID-19, vaccine passports have gained increased popularity, due to its suitability in quickly verifying one's vaccination status using the QR code. Using this technology to track those who are or are not vaccinated, has an Orwellian quality to it. Governments will increasingly have the unprecedented power to monitor citizens with this new technology, and by extension, the ability to enforce vaccine mandates that have the potential of endangering one's right to privacy and the freedom of choice.

In regards to those concerns, the proposed Immunization Infrastructure Modernization Act (H.R. 550), would create a federal vaccine database allowing the CDC to track one's immunization records. In this way, the federal government can condition federal money based on compliance with federal policy, as in mandating vaccinations. Though the bill denies that it would force federal vaccine mandates or digital health passports, as president-elect Biden initially stated, once in office he reversed his position and pushed for vaccine mandates.[446] On September 10, 2021, President Biden spoke in front of the American people stating,

> *Many of us are still frustrated with the nearly 80 million Americans who are still not vaccinated even though the vaccine is safe, effective, and free... this is a pandemic of the unvaccinated...We have been patient but our patience is wearing thin.*[447]

This implicit threat on those who refuse to get vaccinated, raises the question, "What happens if you don't?" To what ends will the government go, in order to force vaccine mandates on the public, effectively negating an individual's right to make personal medical decisions. Never mind that Biden's speech made false statements, such as, the COVID-19 vaccines are proven safe and effective, and that the pandemic persists due to the unvaccinated.

Currently, vaccine passports are being used in many countries, including the U.S., as a way of monitoring people's actions beyond the verification of one's vaccination status. They are seen as a precursor to digital ID's that will be able to collect and consolidate additional information on one's bank account, health records, and social credit system.

> *The plan is to collect and link as much personal information as possible, and there's no reason to think this data won't be shared for control, social engineering and profit—that's what Google, Facebook, and other platforms have done for years.*[448]

The Israeli Experiment—Israel entered into an exclusive agreement to administer **only** the COVID vaccine developed by Pfizer. It was one of the first countries to implement this vaccine mandate in spite of the fact that these shots were still in the experimental stage. The safety trials for the Pfizer vaccine were not set to be completed until 2023. Nevertheless, by February 2021, 70% of Israelis had received two doses of the Pfizer vaccine and while there was an initial reduction in the number of COVID cases, by summer, there was a dramatic uptick in hospitalizations. What initially appeared to be an effective treatment for COVID, after a few short months, the vaccine quickly waned. As a consequence, Israel went ahead with a booster shot due to the ineffectiveness of the original two shots, and now Israel is even initiating a fourth vaccine since the third shot appears to provide even less protection than the first two. In spite of the miserable results from this vaccine experiment, the Israeli Ministry of Health concluded that giving more booster shots was warranted. This brings to mind the definition of insanity, "Doing the same thing over and over and expecting a different result." In spite of Israel having one of the highest vaccinated rates in the world, it ends up having one of the highest daily infection rates as well.[449]

A large Israeli study by Gazit et al., involving more than 750,000 individuals, looked at the relationship between those who were fully vaccinated and the unvaccinated who'd recovered from the COVID disease. As it turned out, the vaccinated had a 27-fold increased risk of a symptomatic infection than the unvaccinated COVID-recovered cases and were 9 times more likely to be hospitalized for COVID.[450] In their conclusion, they stated:

> This study demonstrated that natural immunity confers longer-lasting and stronger protection against infection, symptomatic disease, and hospitalization caused by the Delta variant of SARS-CoV-2, compared to the BNT162b2 [Pfizer] two-dose vaccine-induced immunity.[451]

In an August 5, 2021 news interview, Dr. Kobi Haviv, director of the Herzog Hospital in Jerusalem, *"reported that 95% of severely ill COVID-19 patients were fully vaccinated, and that they made up 85% to 90% of COVID-related hospitalizations overall."*[452] It was not long ago that the U.S. public were assured that herd immunity would be achieved when 70% receive the COVID vaccines. But now there are more cases of COVID-19 occurring in the fully vaccinated, even when countries are above 75% vaccine compliance. As a matter of fact, a Sept 2021 study of 68 countries and 2947 counties in the United States, showed that the higher the rate of the fully vaccinated, the higher the percentage of COVID-19 cases per 1 million.[453] This suggests that the COVID vaccines may not be as safe and effective as portrayed and that maybe the benefits don't outweigh the risks.

On top of the previous concerns raised, the FDA wanted to give Pfizer **75 years** to completely release documents on their COVID vaccine. *"At the agency's proposed rate of 500 documents per month, the last documents would be released in 2096."* The nonprofit group, Public Health and Medical Professionals for Transparency (PHMPT), decided to sue the FDA, stating that the agency could release all this information within *"only 12 weeks with 19 reviewers working full-time to review and produce the documents."* The PHMPT is *"seeking safety and effectiveness data, adverse reaction reports and a list of active and inactive vaccine ingredients."*[454] One has to wonder the motives behind the FDA's proposed plan to withhold critical vaccine findings from the public for three quarters of a century. How useful will it be for people today, to not have access to all that data until the year 2096? Fortunately, U.S. District Judge Mark Pittman on January 6, 2022, ordered the FDA to release all of Pfizer's safety data in just over 8 months, instead of 75 years, stating that it was of "paramount public importance" to make this data available to the public as fast as possible.[455]

Japan's COVID-19 Vaccination Policy—In sharp contrast to Israel, the United States and most other countries in the world, Japan has taken a more cautious and reasoned approach to COVID-19 inoculations.[456]

- First, Japan provides information that warns the public about serious side-effects associated with COVID-19 injections, such as, the risk of myocarditis.
- Japan takes strict measures to monitor and report all side-effects from the vaccinations, including hospitals, that are

required to report, in detail, any adverse reactions that occur within 28 days of receiving COVID-19 vaccines.

- Japan is against compulsory vaccination and the Ministry of Health on its website includes a section on vaccines, stating that mandatory vaccination and discrimination against those who choose not to be vaccinated are not advised; this includes those in the workplace, where forced vaccination is not allowed.
- Japan supports the rights of individuals to receive informed consent and the freedom to decide whether to be vaccinated or not.

In Japan, responsibility for healthcare decisions is left to the individual or family; whereas the U.S. mandates vaccinations through a bureaucratic system that forces a medical procedure on an entire population indiscriminately without any liability for the outcome. So how does Japan's approach compare to the U.S.? Well, as of January 1, 2022, the U.S. population was approximately 334 million and in Japan, 126 million; that makes the U.S. population 2.65 times larger than Japan. But when looking at the death totals from COVID-19, as of January 3, 2022, the U.S. reported 847,408 deaths, while Japan had only 18,395 deaths. Whereas, the U.S. has close to **3 times** the population of Japan, the U.S. has roughly **46 times** as many deaths from COVID than Japan.[457]

The Great Barrington Declaration—In October 2020, this declaration was authored by Dr. Kullforff, professor of medicine at Harvard University; Dr. Sunetra Gupta, professor at Oxford University; and Dr. Jay Bhattacharya, professor at Stanford University Medical School. Approximately 60,000 medical and public health scientists and medical practitioners, and more than 850,000 concerned citizens from around the world, to date, have co-signed this declaration. The declaration recommends:

A more compassionate approach that balances the risks and benefits of reaching herd immunity" and allowing "those who are at minimal risk of death to live their lives normally to build up immunity to the virus through natural infection, while protecting those who are at highest risk.

They refer to this as *"focused protection… adopting measures to protect the vulnerable,"* especially the elderly. In conclusion, they wrote:

Those who are not vulnerable should be allowed to resume life as normal. Simple hygiene measures, such as hand washing and staying home when sick should be practiced by everyone to reduce the herd immunity threshold. Schools and universities should be open for in-person teaching. Extracurricular activities, such as sports, should be resumed. Young low-risk adults should work normally, rather than from home. Restaurants and other businesses should open. Arts, music, sport and other cultural activities should resume. People who are more at risk may participate if they wish, while society as a whole enjoys the protection conferred upon the vulnerable by those who have built up herd immunity.[458]

The Rome Declaration—In September 2021, the International Alliance of Physicians and Medical Scientists initiated the Rome Declaration at the International Global Covid Summit held in Rome, Italy. The event was attended by physicians, scientists, lawyers, and other professionals from around the world, protesting

the deadly consequences of Covid-19 policy makers' and medical authorities' unprecedented behavior: behavior such as denying patient access to lifesaving early treatments, disrupting the sacred physician-patient relationship and suppressing open scientific discussion for profits and power… These professionals, many of whom are on the front lines of pandemic treatment, have experienced career threats, character assassination, censorship of scientific papers and research, social media accounts blocked, online search results manipulated, clinical trials and patient observations banned, and their professional history and accomplishments minimized in academic and mainstream media.[459]

As of October 7, 2021, more than 11,000 physicians and medical scientists have signed the declaration, realizing that they are at risk of losing their medical licenses as a result. Nevertheless, the signatories have taken a strong stance, making it quite clear that they are no longer willing to go along with the manipulation and censorship of those in leadership who are abusing their authority.

Refer to **Appendix K:** *Physicians Declaration: Global COVID Summit–Rome, Italy,* to read the entire text of the Rome Declaration.

Refer to **Appendix L:** *How to Report an Injury from COVID-19 Vaccine for Reimbursement.* The injury needs to be reported within one year of vaccination.

Misinformation, Censorship, and Coercion

Misinformation, censorship, and coercion have been tactics used by governments throughout history in order to exert control over the public by suppression of free speech, spreading propaganda, and censoring any information that conflicts with the politically sanctioned narrative of those in power. This is one of the hallmarks of repressive totalitarian regimes, the very antithesis of a democratic society that allows for the open expression of differing points of view. Unfortunately, the current crisis over COVID-19 has created a politicized environment which has engendered a level of fear and stress stoked by the incessant state of alarm fomented by medical officials, the news media, and politicians. As a result, many people have been frightened to such a degree that they have unwittingly gone along with these draconian government measures that have curtailed individual freedoms.

The blatant censorship and suppression of information regarding any negative findings about COVID vaccines has been unparalleled in modern times. False and misleading information, with the intent to deliberately deceive the public at large, has been perpetuated by the pharmaceutical industry's undue influence over the medical establishment, political officials, and the mainstream news media. Those who resist being vaccinated are being shamed and vilified. World-renowned experts in the field of COVID research have been uniformly ignored, discredited, mocked, attacked, and accused of endangering the public by daring to question the efficacy of these experimental vaccines. By dismissing alternative treatments, people are left thinking that vaccines are the only real solution. One of the best examples of how information has been systematically distorted relates to the use of "Ivermectin," an antiparasitic medicine that the media has unfairly characterized as a "horse dewormer" only used by veterinarians, when in fact, it has been effective in a number of human treatment protocols, as previously noted. Even the WHO has placed ivermectin on their "List of Essential Medicines."

Since when does shutting down scientific inquiry make any sense, as if all the questions regarding COVID have been settled to everyone's satisfaction. This is hardly the case. There is substantial evidence of harm and even deaths that are occurring as a result of this rapid dissemination of these so-called "safe and effective" vaccines, though this information has been largely concealed from the public. One has to wonder why there has been such resistance to open debate. What is the unspoken agenda here? Is the U.S. government's primary concern with the welfare of the general public or rather, with the interests of Big Pharma, the medical establishment, High Tech, the mainstream media, and other entities that have benefited financially from this crisis?

The government's coercive intrusion into the lives of Americans is affecting society on many levels. The unvaccinated are being discriminately banned from public venues, losing their jobs, being fined for noncompliance, barred from travel, denied medical services, and even refused life-saving surgeries for refusing to be vaccinated. Children are being withheld from public school, and in some cases, removed from their homes because parents refuse to have them vaccinated. Government officials have even determined that 11-year-olds can now decide for themselves to be vaccinated without parental approval. What's next? Can individuals lose social security and Medicare benefits, not be allowed to renew one's driver's license or obtain a passport, or be blocked from filing taxes? This escalating encroachment on individual freedoms doesn't seem to reflect a society based on democratic principles but rather an oppressive system controlled by those in power who will unilaterally decide what is in the best interests of the public.

PART VIII

MEDICAL TREATMENT AND THE BIOMEDICAL APPROACH

"There is no need to poison our children's bloodstreams with toxins in the name of "prevention" when the real prevention to illness is a healthy immune system." —Dr. Letitia Dick-Kronenberg

Theories postulated back in the 1800s have had an enormous impact on opinions held today regarding the causes of diseases and subsequent treatments. A major controversy during that time evolved around germ theory vs. host theory that is summarized here.

Pasteur vs. Béchamp—During the 19th century, Louis Pasteur, a French chemist, credited himself with having developed the "germ theory" though it had been proposed by others, well before his time. Pasteur's germ theory claimed that diseases came from outside the body and that microorganisms, such as bacteria and viruses, were the main cause of disease and ill health. Therefore, Pasteur reasoned that the job of the physician was to identify the germ causing the illness and kill it through the use of drugs and other antimicrobials. In 1860, Florence Nightingale, the world-famous British nurse, more than 17 years before Pasteur advocated the germ theory, attacked the idea, stating that "There are no specific diseases; there are specific disease conditions."[460]

Dr. Antoine Béchamp, a French scientist and critic of Pasteur's germ theory, held an opposing view that emphasized the body's terrain, referred to as the "host theory" of disease. He was able to demonstrate in his lab experiments that diseases developed within the body and that disease-causing germs were the result of a weakened body owing to malnutrition, exposure to toxins, and the like. Béchamp realized that there was considerable variation in the ability of many pathogenic organisms to cause diseases with some pathogens being more virulent than others. In addition, there were also significant disparities among individuals in the immune system's ability to combat diseases with some people being more susceptible to illness as a result of a compromised host body. Béchamp focused on understanding and addressing the underlying conditions that allowed diseases to thrive. His work emphasized the body's natural ability to heal itself by cultivating a healthy lifestyle through diet, hygiene, exercise, detoxification, and so on. Consequently, his views were more in keeping with alternative medical approaches that, for example, view healthy foods as medicines that are able to strengthen the body's response to disease.

During this period, Pasteur often contradicted Bechamp's research findings, yet medical historians have pointed out that many of Pasteur's theories were appropriated from Bechamp's own work. Pasteur proved to be adept at self-promotion, giving him an unearned reputation as an authority, when in fact, he stole many of his ideas from others, as discussed in Ethel D. Hume's book, *Béchamp or Pasteur? A Lost Chapter in the History of Biology (1923).* Unfortunately, the importance of Béchamp's research was largely discredited and ultimately suppressed by Pasteur and the French Academy of Sciences. As a result, Pasteur's germ theory became the accepted standard for Western medicine and the foundation for understanding all diseases.

Unfortunately, with the advent of pharmaceutical drugs, the medical establishment and governmental agencies usurped traditional therapies in favor of the more convenient and profitable allopathic model. Access to alternative medicine was systematically excluded from mainstream medicine and stigmatized as "quackery" by those in power holding the "purse strings." Medical schools indoctrinated interns in the belief that the allopathic approach was the only legitimate medical model, and, at the same time, discredited alternative approaches, such as homeopathic and chiropractic disciplines.

Hippocrates, the Greek physician, who lived about 2,400 years ago, is considered the "Father of Modern Medicine." He is famous for the Hippocratic Oath, which has been summarized in the quote, *"First, do no harm."* It calls upon physicians to uphold specific ethical standards, such as caring for the sick to the best of one's ability. Hippocrates emphasized the innate healing capacity of people, writing that the *"natural forces within us are the true healers of disease."*[461]

Conventional Medicine—Conventional or allopathic medicine is practiced by a medical doctor (MD) involved in the treatment of diseases primarily through the use of pharmaceutical remedies and vaccines, along with medical interventions to address acute trauma or chronic degenerative conditions that require surgery, radiation, chemotherapy, and the like.

- The focus is disease-oriented, meaning that the emphasis is on disease intervention and the treatment of symptoms with less emphasis on addressing the underlying causes.
- The traditional medical model sees the physician as the authority who diagnoses the problem and prescribes a treatment, while the patient is seen as essentially a compliant participant following doctor's orders.
- Physicians are trained in pharmaceutical interventions but receive no formal training in the nutritional and supplemental remedies of alternative approaches.
- Doctors may prescribe new drugs on the basis of recommendations by drug representatives who rely on the pharmaceutical company's own studies. In a similar fashion, vaccines are dispensed based on the CDC's recommendation without much forethought or investigation on the part of physicians.

In *The Biology of Belief* (2008), Bruce H. Lipton, Ph.D., a recognized authority in the field of cell biology, wrote:

> *Medical doctors are caught between an intellectual rock and a corporate hard place; they are pawns in the huge medical-industrial complex ... In their postgraduate years, those same doctors receive their continuing education about pharmaceutical products from drug reps, the errand boys of the corporate healthcare industry. Essentially, these nonprofessionals, whose primary goal is to sell product, provide doctors with "information" about the efficacy of new drugs. Drug companies freely offer this "education" so that they can persuade doctors to "push" their products. It is evident that the massive quantities of drugs prescribed in this country violate the Hippocratic Oath taken by all doctors to, First do no harm.*[462]

Functional Medicine is also practiced by medical doctors, like orthopedic physicians, as well as other health practitioners, including chiropractors, naturopaths, homeopaths, and acupuncturists, with an emphasis on a holistic approach that is patient-centered, focusing on environment, lifestyle, diet, psycho-social factors, and stress.

- It is a health-oriented model associated with alternative approaches that emphasize strengthening the immune system in order to fight diseases from within. It views the body as having an innate ability to heal itself when making the right lifestyle choices.
- There is a greater focus on the underlying causality of diseases as opposed to addressing symptoms by asking how and why illnesses occur and attempts to restore health by addressing the root cause of disease for each individual.
- A treatment plan is developed with disease prevention and health promotion in mind, emphasizing the patient's involvement in the healing process.

- Functional medicine views diet and nutrition as critical to fostering optimal health, with more emphasis on the use of vitamins and other supplements and less reliance on pharmaceutical drugs whenever possible.

The popularity of conventional medicine and why it is so readily accepted by the general public is that it provides the hope of "a quick fix" to health problems—a magic pill, so to speak. There is less emphasis on the underlying cause, which requires a greater investment in one's overall health as emphasized in the functional medical model. In spite of these differences, a more comprehensive view of medicine would view allopathic and alternative medical approaches as being complementary rather than contradictory. Alternative therapies emphasize the **prevention** of illnesses by the promotion of health through lifestyle changes that include a healthy diet, regular exercise, fostering one's social and emotional well-being, and the like, all with the purpose of strengthening one's immune system as the primary defense against diseases. Meanwhile, the allopathic approach emphasizes **intervention** when preventive measures are insufficient. This is especially relevant in emergency situations that deal with acute injuries requiring immediate attention in order to stabilize patients and save lives. In general, the least invasive medical procedures should be considered first before taking a more intrusive course of action, such as surgery, which may be the only viable option left.

Biomedical Treatment Options for Autism—Biomedical in the field of autism refers to a treatment approach that looks at the biological basis of autistic behavior and attempts to address the myriad medical conditions seen in autism. The biomedical treatment of children with autism addresses numerous and varying conditions associated with metabolic dysfunction, gastrointestinal disorders, nutritional deficiencies, allergic reactions, sleep disorders, hyperactivity, obsessive behaviors, mood swings, aggressiveness, speech and language difficulties, avoidance of others, and so on.

Based on each child's unique physiological makeup, an individualized treatment plan is developed, taking into consideration nutrition, immune function, genetic and environmental factors, and other health-related issues. By incorporating a gluten- and casein-free diet, using supplements to bolster the immune system, detoxifying the body through methylation and chelation, and so on, the biomedical approach attempts to address the underlying factors that hinder the child's functional health. The fact that some children do recover from autism points to the environmental factors that can make a difference as demonstrated by the biomedical-intervention approach. Unfortunately, not all children are able to completely recover, but, clearly, improvements are possible through the various treatments that address issues around diet, nutrition, supplementation, and detoxification.

Homeopathic and naturopathic doctors as well as chiropractors and other naturalistic practitioners are generally more aware of biomedical treatments that focus on the underlying factors affecting autistic children. There are also MDs who are strong advocates of this integrative approach, such as Robert W. Sears, who authored *The Autism Book* (2010), detailing the biomedical method. Though Dr. Sears acknowledged that the link between vaccines and autism is still being debated, he cautioned against vaccinating children who have been diagnosed with autism, given the thousands of anecdotal reports by parents who believe vaccines contributed to their children's autism. He emphasized that there have been no placebo-controlled studies comparing the rate of autism between the vaccinated versus unvaccinated children, so that the link has not been disproven.

Regarding autism, there are significant differences between the mainstream medical beliefs regarding treatment options and that of the biomedical approach advocated by those working closely with families of autistic children. For example, Jay L. Hoecker, MD, in an article for the Mayo Clinic, wrote:

> *There is no cure for autism…As a result, many unproven alternative therapies are often suggested. However, these*

alternative therapies are usually found to be ineffective and sometimes harmful.[463]

This is the standard response from the medical establishment, which has little background or understanding of these alternative approaches. But those in the autistic community, out of necessity, tend to be well-versed in these alternative therapies and have benefitted from these procedures based on first-hand experiences. Behavioral interventions such as Applied Behavior Analysis, speech therapy, and occupational therapy play a necessary role, though limited in their impact, without first looking at the underlying biological and medical issues with autistic children. A multi-layered approach that addresses detoxification, nutritional factors, and cellular function that supports the mitochondria and optimal methylation is essential in understanding and dealing with the many underlying conditions affecting autistic children.

Jeff Bradstreet, MD, summarized the complex factors that contribute to an autistic diagnosis:

ASDs [Autism spectrum disorders] are associated with: oxidative stress; decreased methylation capacity; limited production of glutathione; mitochondrial dysfunction; intestinal dysbiosis; increased toxic metal burden; immune dysregulation; characterized by a unique inflammatory bowel disease and immune activation of neuroglial cells; and ongoing brain hypoperfusion [reduced blood flow].[464]

The following is a brief summary of some of the biomedical treatments and procedures used in combination to address the common concerns of ill health among autistic and other neurodevelopmentally injured children.

Detoxify the Body
- **Heavy metal chelation**—removing heavy metals from the body by intravenous injections of a chelating agent, such as EDTA and DMPS or an oral chelating agent, such as

DMSA. This is an important first step in addressing the toxic overload so commonly seen in autistic children.

- **Methylation**—injecting methyl B12 to restore myelin and glutathione that is depleted in autistic children, as a result of vaccinations. A stronger synergistic effect has been reported when methyl B12 is coupled with the hyperbaric oxygen treatment.

- **Hyperbaric oxygen treatment**—a medical treatment in which the child inhales 100% pure oxygen to enhance the body's natural healing process. It reduces inflammation, increases the flow of oxygen-rich blood to affected areas of the body, and decreases oxidative stress that can lead to cell and tissue damage.

- **Ozone therapy**—an anti-inflammatory therapy that stimulates the body to activate antioxidants while decreasing free radicals in order to fight infections. It can assist with medical problems, behavioral issues, immune system, GI tract, and dental-decay issues. It is usually administered with a stethoscope into the ear or rectally, though IVs can also be used if tolerated.

- **Infrared saunas**—heat from the sauna penetrates deep into the joints, muscles, and tissues of the body restoring and calming the nervous system and increasing oxygen flow, circulation, and detoxification.

- **Low dose immunotherapy (LDI)**—helps to reduce the inflammatory responses in the body and restore balance to the immune system in autistic children. It blends immunotherapy with the general principles of homeopathy that combines an extremely diluted mixture of allergens in order to desensitize the body to develop immune tolerance. It is in liquid form and administered in drops sublingually.

Improving the Microbiome—The human microbiome is a complex ecosystem composed of trillions of microbes, including bacteria, viruses, and fungi, most of which live in the gut. It is instrumental in determining our level of health by affecting metabolic functions, protecting against pathogens, balancing hormones, supporting the immune system, detoxifiying the gut, and so on. The foods we eat to a large extent will determine the quality of our microbiome. Examples of some of the healthy foods that nurture the microbiome follow:

- Eating diverse and unprocessed fruits and vegetables that are organic and locally grown, such as leafy greens, broccoli, beets, kale, cauliflower, arugula, radish, asparagus, and carrots; citrus fruits; various berries, including blueberries, raspberries, and cranberries.
- Organic and locally farmed eggs that are free range; meat without antibiotics, such as grass-fed chicken, beef, and lamb; organ meat; bone broth; fish caught in the wild like salmon. Avoid animal meat injected with growth hormones and farmed fish with chemical additives.
- Organic herbs such as garlic, onion, leeks, chives, cinnamon, thyme, turmeric, green tea, parsley, cilantro, oregano, rosemary, ginger, and basil.
- Organic nuts and seeds like walnuts, pistachios, almonds, and macadamia, flax seed, and Brazil nuts.
- Organic olive oil, coconut oil, and avocado oil. Avoid all vegetable oils, like canola, peanut, corn, safflower, and palm oil.
- Fermented foods like sauerkraut, kombucha, miso, and probiotic yogurt.

Allergen Free Diet—Identifying allergens that are causing havoc in the body.

- **Gluten-Free Diet**—Autistic children are often allergic to gluten found in wheat, rye, barley, oats, and bread products such as cookies, cakes, muffins, pasta, pizza, and breaded items, such as chicken nuggets and fish sticks.
- **Casein-Free Diet**—Many of these children are also allergic to dairy products that need to be eliminated, including

milk, cheese, butter, low-fat yogurt, ice cream, and products containing whey.

Bolster the Immune System with Vitamin and Mineral Supplementation

- **Digestive enzymes**—supplements that help with digestion,
  especially those enzymes that digest casein and gluten
  proteins.
- **Targeted vitamins and essential minerals**—such as,
  vitamins A, B complex, C, D, E, selenium, magnesium,
  zinc, calcium, iodine, chromium, N-acetyl-cysteine (NAC),
  taurine, folinic acid, glycine, and dimethylglycine (DMG).
- **Probiotics**—supplements that contain good bacteria to help
  keep the gut healthy; they counter the effects of antibiotics and other medicine that can destroy healthy gut flora.
- **Fish oil or Cod liver oil**—supplements rich in omega-3
  fatty acids that support the gut, reduce inflammation, and
  strengthen the immune system.
- **Methyl B12 shots**—a form of vitamin B12 that helps the
  body make red blood cells. In autistic children, it has
  been associated with improved attending skills, increased
  language and social skills.
- **Antioxidants**—foods rich in antioxidants (fruits, vegetables, nuts) help to limit the damage caused by free radicals
  that can make cells vulnerable to pathogens. Glutathione
  is a critical antioxidant produced in the cells that can be
  given intravenously, topically, as an inhalant or as an oral
  supplement. It is instrumental in reducing oxidative damage in children with autism.
- **Chlorine dioxide (MMS)** is a controversial drug promoted
  by Kerri Rivera that has been highly censored in the mainstream media. In her book *Healing the Symptoms Known
  as Autism,* she contends that the drug is safe when used
  correctly and has been extremely effective in addressing
  autistic symptoms.

Obviously, pursuing a biomedical treatment plan requires a good deal of investigation on one's part requiring time and effort, well beyond what is briefly outlined here. The books noted below provide a possible starting point for those families dealing with the needs of vaccine-injured children.

The Autism Book: What Every Parent Needs to Know About Early Detection, Treatment, Recovery, and Prevention by Robert W. Sears, MD (2010). He details the biomedical approach to working with autistic children from diagnosis to multiple treatment modalities.

Healing and Preventing Autism (2009) by Jenny McCarthy and Jerry Kartzinel, MD, is especially geared toward families raising an autistic child. It provides highly specific information on the biomedical approach focusing on the need for early intervention, diet, supplements, detoxification, and food sensitivities. It covers numerous concerns associated with autism, along with related issues dealing with asthma, allergies, seizures, attention deficit disorders (ADD/ADHD), Tourette's syndrome, and obsessive-compulsive disorders (OCD).

The Unvaccinated Child: A Treatment Guide for Parents and Caregivers (2017) by Judith Thompson, ND and Eli Camp, ND, focuses on alternative treatments to vaccination that emphasize preventing illness by fostering a healthy immune system. In keeping with the aforementioned biomedical approach, naturopath doctors stress the importance of nutrition, diet, herbal medicine, breastfeeding, exercise, exposure to microorganisms, and homeopathy. A chapter is devoted to each of the major childhood diseases; the book provides a number of specific recommendations for alternative treatments in lieu of vaccinations.

Steven R. Gundry, MD, in his book, *The Longevity Paradox: How to Die Young at a Ripe Old Age* (2019), emphasizes the importance of the foods we eat and how one's diet is crucial to the overall health of each of us. The microbes or bacteria in our gut make up the microbiome that helps to determine the quality of our health. Foods that are detrimental to the microbiome over time, such as sugars and starches, have the effect of causing "leaky gut syndrome" which can lead to a multitude of problems throughout the body, affecting the brain, joints, skin, thyroid, colon, sinuses, and adrenals. Finding a doctor, well-versed in the biomedical approach who has extensive experience in working with special needs children is a critical first step in guiding and supporting families dealing with a multitude of complex issues. There are a number of resources listed in the bibliography, such as Generation Rescue, the National Vaccine Information Center, the Children's Health Defense, The Highwire, A Voice for Choice, Autism Action Network, the National Health Federation, the American Frontline Doctors, and AutismOne, that are invaluable sources of information. Many of these organizations create a network of support for special needs families, provide needed resources, and hold conferences and other events that present the most up-to-date research on autism and other neurodevelopmental disorders.

Refer to **Appendix J: How to Report an Adverse Event to VAERS** (Vaccine Adverse Event Reporting System). The injury must be reported within three years of the vaccination.

PART IX

SUMMARY AND RECOMMENDATIONS

"The media is the most powerful entity on Earth. They have the power to make the innocent guilty and to make the guilty innocent because they control the minds of the masses." —Malcolm X

Highlighting Major Points

Since grade school, we have been taught to believe that vaccines have been responsible for saving millions of lives from deadly infectious diseases. This widely accepted belief is the reason that most people don't question the science behind vaccines today. Stories of the eradication of diseases like smallpox and polio are so ingrained in our thinking that it is hard to imagine it not being so. An accurate reading of history, however, shows that diseases have declined steadily as living conditions in the world have improved. Vaccines came into play after most childhood diseases were on the decline due to better sanitation, nutrition, and medical care. However, the medical community, backed by the pharmaceutical industry, has falsely credited vaccinations as the reason for the dramatic reduction in deaths from childhood diseases, such as smallpox, measles, diphtheria, whooping cough, and poliomyelitis.

By stepping in and mandating vaccines for the "greater good," government has taken the position that it knows what is best when it comes to medical decisions, and as a result, the rights of the individual to choose has been effectively negated. The question then becomes, "What other medical decisions can the state decide for us in the name of the common good?" This is especially worrisome given the questionable assumptions regarding vaccine safety that are perpetuated by the medical establishment and mainstream news media, on behalf of the pharmaceutical interests.

Using disease statistics from third-world countries to justify the need for vaccinations in the United States and other developed countries is a common tactic used to push vaccines by instilling fear that these diseases are the same everywhere regardless of environmental conditions. The kinds of diseases seen in impoverished areas of the world today are the same diseases that were prevalent in the United States and Europe back in the 19th century, when living conditions were abysmal, especially in crowded inner cities with a lack of sanitation, poor hygiene, contaminated water supply, and essentially no access to medical treatment.

Man has evolved and adapted over millions of years without the benefit of vaccines and managed to survive in spite of diseases. As a matter of fact, man's ability to survive is in large part a result of the very illnesses that are so maligned.

Common childhood diseases in the past, such as measles, mumps, and chickenpox, were considered unpleasant but not catastrophic, whereas now they are portrayed as dangerous and deadly diseases. Children growing up in the 1950s were much healthier than kids today in spite of contracting these common diseases. Autism, childhood cancers, peanut allergies, seizure disorders, and autoimmune problems were not perceived concerns back then like they are today. In spite of the obvious increases in childhood disorders, the medical community continues to assert that adverse reactions from vaccines are minuscule, "one in a million," which obscures the fact that children are sicker today than ever before. The proof of this is not to be found in doctor's offices but in the classrooms, where schools are struggling to keep up with the increasing demands to provide special-education services. This dramatic surge in services started around the same time that the CDC expanded the number of vaccines required for school attendance. By some estimates, special-needs children make up as much as 25% of the student population today as noted in some areas of the country.

Children are now being exposed to toxins in the environment like never before, starting on day one of life, in large part due to vaccinations. That is not to say that there are not other environmental exposures to toxins, but one would be hard pressed to find a more ubiquitous collection of toxins than what is found in vaccines: aluminum, mercury, formaldehyde, antibiotics, lead, Polysorbate 80, foreign proteins derived from animals and aborted fetal tissue injected into infants starting shortly after they come out of the womb.

The most insidious aspect of the controversy around vaccine safety has been the medical community's dismissive attitude toward the tens of thousands of parents who have witnessed their children regress after being vaccinated. Those in the medical field are reluctant to acknowledge that vaccines could be the cause of serious problems, and doctors have been trained in the belief that vaccines are safe and effective. Doctors rarely research the data behind vaccines, instead relying on what they have been told as part of their training, namely that vaccinations are essential to the well-being of children. Often information on drugs and vaccines is relayed to practicing doctors by drug reps from the pharmaceutical companies who push for the sale of these drugs and vaccines. But for those parents who have witnessed their children injured or died as a result of vaccinations, they have a far different perspective that is personal and traumatic. Many of these parents end up doing the research that doctors don't do, and consequently, have become better informed and justified in their own beliefs regarding the undeniable dangers of vaccines.

Legitimate scientific research points to the unintended consequences of injecting children with toxins found in vaccines at levels never used before. This reliance on and overuse of vaccines prevents children from contracting the natural diseases, as in the past, that essentially provided lifelong immunity. The artificial immune response from vaccinations was supposed to be equivalent to immunity from the naturally acquired disease, but, when that turned out to be false, booster shots were introduced. The original term, "herd immunity," was used in reference to immunity as a result of a majority of people contracting the natural disease. The medical community has usurped the term to mean immunity due to vaccinations. Unfortunately, herd immunity through vaccination has proven to be ineffective even in situations where children have been vaccinated essentially 100% of the time. Due to the waning effects of vaccines, individuals can become susceptible to more serious reactions later on, as demonstrated in the recent cases of mumps outbreaks on college campuses. In addition, vaccinated children are able to spread the disease through "shedding" the live virus to others, particularly those who are vulnerable: pregnant women, premature infants, and immunocompromised individuals.

Today, in addition to the reemergence of common diseases like measles, mumps, and whooping cough, which were thought to be behind us, we are now seeing new and divergent mutated forms of these diseases that are resistant to many of the current vaccines, not unlike the crisis we are seeing with the overuse of antibiotics. Increasingly, we are tampering with a complex and not totally understood immune system as though there are no limits to our intrusion. Basically, this is an experiment in which mostly children are being used as "guinea pigs" without clearly understanding how the long-term implications of disrupting the immune system will play out. This is especially crucial when considering the vaccines that incorporate foreign DNA injected into newborns and infants without really knowing what genetic effects this will have on future generations. The current rush to eliminate COVID-19 by administering experimental mRNA vaccines never used before on humans is but another example of how we toss caution to the wind out of fear. This is not the first time that society has been convinced to follow the edicts of the medical establishment that have turned out to be deleterious to one's health.

The pharmaceutical industry is big business and its impact on the news media, politicians, and the medical establishment cannot be overstated owing to the corrupting influence of money. Officials in the CDC, FDA, AMA, and AAP, as well as other agencies, have been coopted by "Big Pharma," rendering unbiased oversight largely unattainable. Instead, what we are left with is the reiteration of the "vaccine orthodoxy" that vaccines are safe and effective and that the benefits outweigh the risks. How can medical science support the notion of the "one-size-fits-all" vaccination policy when taking into consideration the unique individual differences of each person? Here-in lies one of the major problems: the assumption that all vaccines for all children will work equally well without a hitch. It is no coincidence that the high infant-mortality rate in the United States today directly correlates with the high rate of vaccines given.

The medical establishment and the news media routinely repeat that there is no connection between vaccines, autism, and other neurodevelopmental disorders, making false assertions, as on the CDC website that, "vaccines don't cause autism." The manufacturer's own vaccine product inserts have stated that there are numerous adverse reactions, including autism, that have occurred as a result of vaccinations. Unbiased scientific research, independent from those sources that have something to gain by being less than truthful, has shown a convincing correlation between autism and vaccines. In the span of 4 decades, we have seen autism go from roughly 1 in 10,000 to less than 1 in 36. At the same time that there has been a 7-fold increase in the number of vaccines given, there has been a dramatic increase in vaccine injuries. In addition, the drug companys' vaccine inserts state that these vaccines have not been tested to determine whether they might be carcinogenic, injurious to pregnant women or fetuses, cause infertility, or lead to genetic mutations. Most egregious is the fact that vaccines have never been tested in combination, yet infants are routinely given 6, 8, 10 or more vaccines at one time when they are ill equipped to withstand the onslaught of toxic ingredients at such an immature and vulnerable age.

The enormous increase in the rate of autism and other neuro-developmental disorders has never been addressed by governmental agencies or the medical authorities in any serious way. All they can say is that they are not sure what's going on: it must be genetics or changes in classification, or maybe it has to do with older male fathers or nerdy silicon types who are socially inept, and so on. One gets the impression that the medical authorities are not that keen on finding out what is really going on because that would create a dilemma of having to confront the elephant in the room that is being overlooked, by the name of "Vax."

To be clear, there has been a chorus of critics going back to the beginning of vaccinations when Jenner came up with the smallpox vaccine supposedly derived from cowpox. Unfortunately, these critics have been mostly ignored, dismissed, and vilified for daring to dissent. The intentional distortion of facts for fear of what the truth might show is best exemplified by the flawed vaccine-safety science that is presented to the public by those in authority. If it were widely understood that vaccines are the cause of serious injuries and deaths in children today, there would be a lot of people called to account for their actions. If it was determined, for example, that the autism epidemic is largely the result of the overuse of vaccines and that the pharmaceutical industry, along with government officials and medical authorities, were engaged in a cover-up, the financial implications would be staggering. So, there is a very strong incentive to defend the pro-vaccine agenda by whatever means necessary by denying, deflecting, and distorting the facts, whatever the cost.

The influence of money on politics largely dictates what gets communicated to the American people. To the degree that the mainstream news media is silenced by special interests, then we can expect the worst. No longer will we get the truth; instead, we will get the propaganda that is so cleverly presented to the public through the mainstream news outlets, social media, Astroturf websites, and other sources that squelch the critics and negate legitimate scientific inquiry. Hearing the "vaccine orthodoxy" lie repeated over and over, it ends up becoming the "truth" for an unsuspecting populace who can't envision the degree to which governmental agencies and others have been co-opted by those pulling the strings behind the screen, like in *The Wizard of Oz*.

The unfortunate truth about vaccines is that we have started down a path that is going to be difficult to undo, given what has been set in motion. The financial interests of the pharmaceutical industry have infiltrated and neutralized the mainstream news media, and now they have convinced the politicians to shut down the internet regarding any conversation that is critical of vaccinations, regardless of the facts. The censorship of information is unprecedented. Scientific studies showing the ill effects of the current COVID vaccines are being kept from the public, and the scientists and medical physicians attempting to sound the alarm are being silenced. The pharmaceutical industry's influence over the medical establishment, government officials, and the mainstream news media is chilling. It makes a mockery of the entire vaccination program, which is manipulated by the money interests of Big Pharma and other entities that greatly profit from this clever deception.

We need to take a break from this incessant rush to vaccinate and stop to look at the devastation that is being created. This is going to be a difficult task, given how the odds have been stacked against a largely misinformed public. What is left are the citizenry, the families and individuals who know the truth based on their personal experiences. The need for a "grass-roots" movement is more critical than ever before if we are going to have any hope of shifting public opinion. It will not come from the "top" alone, given those in authority who hold the "purse strings" and the media-driven consensus that vaccines are safe and effective. It must first take root at the local level, if we are to convince pro-vaccine parents and the largely compliant medical community that the unvaccinated are not the problem and that the solution is not more vaccines. There are those who may feel this view is too extreme and may still opt for some or all vaccines, and it is within their right to make those decisions. Likewise, the ability to refuse vaccination should also be honored because whenever there is a risk of injury or death, individuals must have the ultimate choice to decide for themselves. All medical procedures should be based on free and informed consent without exception. Otherwise, there will be no edict by government decree that cannot be enforced under the guise of public safety. Given the history of medical malfeasance, as exemplified by past inhumane medical experimentations, performed on unsuspecting individuals, endorsed by the medical establishment, authorized by the government and propelled by financial interests, one should be cautious, if not highly suspicious, when the state asserts it is acting in the "best interests" of everyone. Mandating any medical procedure against the will of an individual amounts to medical tyranny by an authoritarian system that does not respect human rights. The time to take a stand is NOW, otherwise, it may be too late to reverse course down the road.

What follows are suggestions for what individuals can do in the local community as well as what changes are needed at the state and federal levels in order to protect personal freedoms while exposing the "vaccine orthodoxy."

Personal Actions
- Become informed—learn by reading many of the excellent resources, such as those listed in the bibliography, watch videos, and attend talks on the subject.
- Know your rights and what choices you have, especially as it relates to vaccine exemptions, particularly at the local and state levels.
- Get involved—let your views be heard. Share with others who are willing to listen to what you have learned.
- Join a support group in your local community. Become part of an organization or website supporting vaccination choice (e.g., *National Vaccine Information Center, Children's Health Defense, A Voice for Choice, Generation Rescue, Informed Consent Action Network, Mercola.com, Andy Wakefield Podcast*).
- Work with others to put together a presentation that may include videos, referenced in the **Bibliography,** like "Vaxxed" or "Vaxxed II" to be shown to a group of concerned parents from school, daycare, your local church, or another community organization.
- Attend meetings of the School Board or Board of Supervisors to discuss your concerns regarding vaccine

legislation, providing a short, concise summary of major points you wish to convey.

- Write a letter to the editor of the local newspaper or other news sources expressing your concerns on specific issues regarding vaccine safety, pointing out the contradictions highlighted in this book and other resources.
- Contact your state and federal legislators, sharing your concerns, especially if you have a child who has been adversely affected by vaccinations. Setting up face to face meetings with representatives are more impactful than corresponding by email or phone, especially if you communicate in a respectful manner and come organized with keys points that you wish to emphasize.
- "Think outside the box" when trying to see what else is possible that can make a difference in shifting the "vaccine orthodoxy."

Recommendations at the national and state level in order to reverse the undue influence of money by drug corporations on the medical establishment, the mainstream news media, and the politicians who pass laws based on faulty information.

- Current laws, like the one in California, mandating vaccinations should be reversed. At both the state and national level, a law should be passed allowing families to decide what vaccines their children should receive, if any.
- Reverse the 1986 NCVIA to once again hold the pharmaceutical industry liable for childhood and adult injuries caused by adverse vaccines reactions, as it should be, just like any other business that pushes its product for financial gain.
- Require that VAERS adopt the recommendations of the Harvard Pilgrim study to convert from a passive reporting system to an active, automated tally of injuries in order to accurately identify adverse vaccine events.

- Take agencies that are beholden to the pharmaceutical industry, such as the CDC, FDA, and AAP, out of the decision-making process regarding what vaccines should be recommended, and create a neutral, nonpartisan committee based on current scientific research that includes the public sector's input.
- Revamp the Interagency Autism Coordinating Committee (IACC), which has been powerless in addressing the real issues surrounding autism. It has turned a blind eye to any connection between vaccines and autism for fear of the implications.
- If vaccinations are to occur, children should be screened carefully for any vulnerabilities, in order to rule out any contraindications related to health factors and family history.
- Reduce the number of vaccines children are receiving, realizing that common childhood diseases help to strengthen the immune systems of young children. There are more than 200 vaccines currently in the pipeline that Big Pharma would love for us to take because for them it is all about profits, not the welfare of society.
- For children who are vaccinated, spread out the vaccination schedule so that they do not receive multiple vaccines at one time and initiate the vaccination process after the child reaches a sensible age, such as 2 years or older. This will allow the child's body to mature to the point that they can fend off toxins more effectively.
- Arrange congressional hearings in a public forum, issuing subpoenas, if need be, with testimonies held under oath. Address previously withheld testimonies, as with Dr. William Thompson and other whistleblowers who have been silenced by the powers that be up to now.
- Form an impartial national committee to investigate biomedical interventions that have shown promise in helping heal autistic and other neurodevelopmentally

injured children. Reduce the monopoly that the medical establishment has largely held over alternative medical approaches that quite frankly have shown more promise. For example, rather than view autism as a genetic disease that can't change, look for the environmental triggers that can be addressed to improve the conditions of such vaccine-injured children.

APPENDIX A

UNETHICAL HUMAN EXPERIMENTATION IN THE UNITED STATES

This is a short list of some of the inhumane experiments done in the U.S. that were performed in most cases without the knowledge or consent of the test subjects or their guardians. It shows the kind of medically justified atrocities that have been committed in the name of science. It should raise concerns regarding the current trend in pushing for medical procedures, such as mandated vaccinations, without informed consent or the right of exemption.

- Between 1845 and 1849, J. Marion Sims, an Alabama physician, known as "the father of gynecology," performed a series of surgical experiments without anesthesia on enslaved black African women.
- In the 1880s, a California physician working at a Hawaiian hospital for lepers injected 6 girls under the age of 12 with syphilis.
- In 1895, Henry Heiman, a New York City pediatrician intentionally infected two mentally disabled boys (ages 4 and 16) by applying gonorrhea to their eyes as part of a medical experiment to see if it could spread like a germ.
- In 1896, Dr. Arthur Wentworth, a pediatrician trained at Harvard Medical School, performed spinal taps on 29

babies and young children at Children's Hospital in Boston, Massachusetts, without the knowledge or consent of their parents, to determine if the procedure was harmful.

- In 1906, 24 Filipino prisoners were intentionally infected with cholera under the guidance of Professor Richard Strong of Harvard University. The experiment was done without the patients' consent or understanding of what was being done to them, resulting in sickness, with 13 dying.

- In 1908, dozens of children were infected with tuberculin at the St. Vincent's House orphanage in Philadelphia by researchers resulting in painful lesions and inflammation of the eyes, and leading to permanent blindness in a number of the children.

- In 1911, 146 hospital patients, including children, were injected with syphilis at the Rockefeller Institute for Medical Research. The lead doctor, Hideyo Noguchi, was later sued by the parents of some of the child subjects, who ended up contracting syphilis as a result of his experiments.

- From 1913 to 1951, the chief surgeon at the San Quentin Prison, Dr. Leo Stanley, performed a wide variety of unethical experiments on hundreds of prisoners, ranging from sterilization to removing testicles from executed prisoners and surgically implanting them into live prisoners. In some cases, he even transplanted animal testicles from rams, goats, and boars into his captive subjects.

- Between 1932 and 1972, the U.S. Public Health Service experimented on 399 poor black males in Tuskegee, Alabama, who had syphilis. This was known as the "Tuskegee Syphilis Experiment," a clinical study in which the researchers did not tell the test subjects that they had syphilis and withheld treatment for the disease, in order to chart the progression of the disease.

- In 1930s and 1940s, Dr. William C. Black experimented on 23 children, injecting them with infected herpes virus. He wrote a report on one 12-month-old baby in 1941 who was "offered as a volunteer" and inoculated in order to monitor the symptoms caused by the herpes virus. His study was later published in the *Journal of Pediatrics* even though his medical experiment was viewed by some as an unethical abuse of power.

- In the early 1940s, the "Refrigeration" experiments were conducted by Harvard University and the University of Cincinnati, in which naked mental patients were exposed to freezing temperatures at 30 degrees Fahrenheit for up to 120 hours. This resulted in physical and psychological disorders as well as some deaths due to cardiac arrest. John Talbott, the Harvard psychiatrist leading the experiment, was later elected president of the American Psychiatric Association.

- In 1941, at the University of Michigan, virologists, including Jonas Salk, the creator of the polio vaccine, deliberately infected patients at mental institutions with the influenza virus by spraying the virus into their nasal passages.

- In 1942, U.S. Army and Navy doctors, as part of a military-sponsored research project, infected 400 prisoners at the Stateville Penitentiary in Illinois with malaria in order to test out experimental drugs, resulting in serious side effects.

- Between 1946 and 1947, the University of Rochester researchers injected uranium, plutonium, and polonium (all radioactive substances) into numerous subjects without their awareness to document the effects. The first subject was a healthy 53-year-old "colored man" who'd been hospitalized for a broken bone injury. The scientists cut samples from his bones and pulled 15 of his teeth to test for the plutonium content.

- Between 1946 and 1948, U.S. researchers conducted a study in Guatemala in which prostitutes were used to infect approximately 700 people (prison inmates, insane asylum patients, Guatemalan soldiers) with syphilis and other sexually transmitted diseases, in order to test the effectiveness of penicillin in treating STDs. Orphan children were also infected by inoculation of the syphilis bacteria.

- In 1952, a Sloan-Kettering Institute researcher, Chester M. Southam, injected live cancer cells into prisoners at the Ohio State Penitentiary. In addition, 300 healthy women were also injected with live cancer cells without being told even though the doctors knew at the time that the experiment would cause cancers.

- From the 1950s to 1972, the Willowbrook State School in Staten Island, New York, experimented on mentally disabled children by deliberately infecting them with viral hepatitis, telling parents they were being given a vaccine, when in fact it was an experiment to help discover a potential vaccine.

- From 1955 to 1960, mentally disabled children at Sonoma State Hospital were subjected to painful experiments, including spinal taps, without parental approval. CBS News reported that more than 1400 patients died.

- In 1963, the Jewish Chronic Disease Hospital in Brooklyn, New York, carried out experiments, led by Chester M. Southam once again, whereby 22 elderly patients were injected with live cancer cells. The researcher was subsequently placed on probation for a year by the medical licensing board due to his controversial methods. Ironically, two years later Southam was elected Vice President of the American Cancer Society.

- Between 1963 and 1973, Dr. Carl Heller, a leading endocrinologist, conducted experiments for the Atomic Energy Commission on prisoners in Oregon and Washington in which they had their testicles irradiated. Similarly, in 1963, the University of Washington researchers irradiated the testicles of 232 prisoners in order to see what effect extreme radiation exposure would have.

- During the Cold War period, the U.S. government funded numerous psychological experiments through the CIA and U.S. military in order to develop more effective torture and interrogation techniques. The School of the Americas trained Latin American paramilitary groups in these torture techniques to use in their own countries.

- From 1986 to 2000, children in a Catholic orphanage at the Incarnation Children's Center in New York City were used as subjects in HIV/AIDS drug and vaccine trials sponsored by the pharmaceutical industry and the federal government. The study was conducted on orphaned infants and children from poor families without parental consent. Referred to as the "Guinea Pig Kids," these children were forced to ingest dangerous toxic pharmaceuticals. If they refused, the drugs were surgically implanted in their abdomens through a tube.

- Between 1989 and 1994, the National Institute of Mental Health was funding experiments on inner-city poor black and Hispanic children with the drug, Fenfluramine, used for weight control. Though the diet drug was banned, the FDA gave permission to Columbia and Queen College for experimental research on children. The NIMH studies back in 1989 indicated that the drug had serious side effects and was deemed to have no therapeutic benefit whatsoever. Peter R. Breggin, MD, stated in a 1998 article, "The FDA has put the interests of drug companies and the psychiatric-research establishment ahead of those of America's children. It is time for the public and concerned professionals to take a stand against unethical pharmacological research on children."

- Between 1993 and 1995, a project was funded by the Environmental Protection Agency at the Kennedy Krieger Institute in which toddlers from low-income families were exposed to lead poisoning to test for blood lead levels. Johns Hopkins University was involved in the study.

- In 1997, the drug Propulsid was used to test a heartburn remedy on children, resulting in the death of a 9-month-old boy. The baby's parents signed a consent form that incorrectly claimed that the drug had been approved for infants. In 1993, the drug was approved for adults but ended up being associated with heart-rhythm abnormalities that caused 80 deaths, including 19 children.

- Thousands of human radiation experiments were performed by researchers in the U.S. in order to determine the effects of atomic radiation and radioactive contamination on the human body. Most subjects were poor, sick, or powerless, as in the case of solders serving in the military. Wikipedia summarized the human radiation experiments this way:

- Most of these tests were performed, funded, or supervised by the U.S. military, Atomic Energy Commission, or various other U.S. federal-government agencies. The experiments included a wide array of studies, involving things like feeding radioactive food to mentally disabled children or conscientious objectors, inserting radium rods into the noses of school children, deliberately releasing radioactive chemicals over U.S. and Canadian cities, measuring the health effects of radioactive fallout from nuclear bomb tests, injecting pregnant women and babies with radioactive chemicals, and irradiating the testicles of prison inmates among other things.

There is an obvious pattern across all of these experimental procedures, namely, the exploitation of the weak and vulnerable, those who have no say in the atrocities done to them. All of which is justified under the notion that it is advancing scientific knowledge for the benefit of the greatest number of people. This is the essential problem whenever an individual is forced to undergo a medical procedure against their will. What are the moral implications of experimenting with people, in these inhumane and cruel "scientific" experiments that are great for those who wield the power, but not for the health and well-being of those being experimented on.

HOW TO REPORT AN ADVERSE EVENT TO VAERS

(Vaccine Adverse Event Reporting System)

VAERS is a passive reporting system, jointly maintained by the CDC and FDA, that allows anyone to report adverse reactions to vaccines, including parents and patients.

Under the National Childhood Vaccine Injury Act (NCVIA), healthcare providers are required by law to report to VAERS:

- Any adverse event listed in the VAERS Table of Reportable Events Following Vaccination that occurs within a **three-year period** after vaccination.

- Serious adverse events include: death, a life-threatening adverse event, a persistent or significant disability or incapacity, a congenital anomaly or birth defect, hospitalization, or prolongation of existing hospitalization.

- An adverse event listed by the vaccine manufacturer as a contraindication to further doses of the vaccine.

Healthcare providers are encouraged to report to VAERS:
- Any adverse event that occurs after the administration of a vaccine, whether or not it is clear that a vaccine caused the adverse event

- Vaccine administration errors

Vaccine manufacturers are required to report to VAERS all adverse events that come to their attention.

There are 2 ways to submit a report to VAERS:

1. Submit a VAERS report online, or
2. Report using a Writable PDF Form (uploadFile/index.jsp)

If you need further assistance with reporting to VAERS, email info@VAERS.org or call **1-800-822-7967.**

The report should include:
- Patient information
- Information about the person submitting the form
- Contact information for healthcare professional
- Vaccine information (brand name, dosage)
- Date, time, and location administered
- Date and time when adverse event(s) started
- Symptoms and outcome of the adverse event(s)
- Medical tests and laboratory results (if applicable)
- Physician's contact information (if applicable)

AUTOIMMUNITY AND THE IMMUNE SYSTEM

The purpose of the immune system is to protect the body from invading microorganisms, such as bacteria and viruses, by producing antibodies that will recognize and destroy these foreign agents. Autoimmunity is an aberration that occurs when these antibodies end up attacking the body's own cells and tissues, causing a variety of autoimmune disorders. Numerous studies have demonstrated that the increasing use of vaccines with an overload of toxic chemicals has contributed to the dramatic rise in autoimmunity. As a matter of fact, the acronym for a relatively new autoimmune syndrome introduced in 2011, called **ASIA,** stands for **autoimmune/inflammatory syndrome induced by adjuvants.** This refers to "a spectrum of immune-mediated diseases triggered by an adjuvant stimulus" such as the most widely used vaccine adjuvant, aluminum.

Unfortunately, vaccines have had the effect of impeding the natural immune process that has evolved over millions of years. In order to better understand this turn of events, it is important to briefly highlight the complex nature of the immune process. The immune system is made up of cells, tissues, and molecules that are designed to protect the body from disease-causing microbes and toxins in the environment. The body's defense against these invaders falls into two categories: innate immunity and adaptive immunity. **Innate immunity** provides the first line of defense against infection due to viruses, bacteria, parasites, and the like. This includes: physical barriers, like the skin, the gastrointestinal and respiratory tracts; protective fluids, such as secretions, mucus, and saliva; and general immune system responses, such as inflammation, that is part of the healing process.

The **adaptive immune system,** also called acquired immunity, is activated against pathogens when the innate immune response is insufficient. It is composed of cell-mediated immunity and humoral immunity. **The cell-mediated immune system,** which operates within the cells, functions by sending white blood cells to areas of the body that have been invaded by foreign substances, creating the bodily experience of sickness in the form of a fever, rash, mucus, or a cough that is the body's attempt to rid itself of the disease and to restore health. The **humoral immune system** functions outside the cells involving any fluid-like substances that circulate in the body, such as blood, bodily secretions, and other fluids. The humoral response to an invading antigen is to release antibodies that are intended to provide a secondary defense when the first defense, cell-mediated immunity, is unable to contain the intruder.

Unfortunately, the cell-mediated immune system is bypassed as a result of vaccines that activate only the antibodies through the humoral immune system, creating an imbalance since both cell-mediated and humoral immune systems need to work in coordination. The common assumption is that simply activating antibodies due to the vaccine adjuvants equates to naturally acquired immunity is inaccurate, since antibodies, in and of themselves, do not guarantee immunity. For example, an individual who doesn't have sufficient antibody levels nevertheless may be protected from getting a disease, while one who has high levels of antibodies may still be susceptible to contracting the same disease. So, antibody levels alone do not necessarily determine one's protection from disease.

Infectious childhood illnesses, like measles, mumps, and chickenpox, cause an inflammatory response (fever, mucus, rash, etc.) that has been shown to strengthen the immune system so that children, in effect, become more resistant to future infections. This is in contrast to vaccines that can interfere with the immune process. For example, studies have shown that contracting the natural measles virus can protect against heart disease, allergies, and autoimmune diseases. While it is true that contracting the measles virus is not without risks, since it can cause ear infections, pneumonia, and in rare cases, encephalitis (inflammation of the brain), it is also true that vaccines can cause these same conditions. But by being exposed to these natural infectious diseases, the body learns to adapt to the virus and develop lifelong immunity, strengthening the immune system naturally.

In the past, when mothers, as children, normally contracted measles and other infectious diseases, they were protected for life and were able to transmit that protection to their offspring. But since vaccinations now interfere with the ability to acquire the natural disease, mothers are no longer able to pass on this naturally acquired immunity *in utero* and through breastfeeding. Consequently, infants today are more vulnerable to infection at an earlier age as a direct result of vaccinations.

In addition, studies have shown that the heavy metals in vaccines, like thimerosal and aluminum, are able to destroy glutathione, an antioxidant that prevents cell damage and depletes metallothionein (MT), a protein that binds with the heavy metals in order to excrete them from the body, making children more vulnerable to these toxins. As a result, these heavy metals contribute to demyelination, which is the breakdown of the myelin sheath of the nerve fibers, including those in the brain and spinal cord. The myelin sheath that covers the nerve fibers is analogous to the protective plastic coating around electrical wiring. When this causes nerve damage, neurological problems can occur, resulting in various medical problems, as in the case of multiple sclerosis, which is caused by the deterioration of the myelin sheath. In turn, this causes an active neuroinflammatory process referred to as an "immune activation event" in which the brain becomes chronically inflamed. This inflammation accounts for the "swollen" brains observed in autistic children who are noticeably in physical and emotional distress. This helps to explain many of the aberrant behaviors seen in autistic children: head banging, rocking back and forward, aggressiveness, crying, etc., all in an attempt to cope with this chronic inflammation of the brain.

But the toxins in vaccines can impact the "gut microbiome" as well, due to the brain's connection to the gastrointestinal system, which sends messages back and forth between the two. This is referred to as the "brain-gut connection" in which chemicals called neurotransmitters send messages that are impacted by the quality of the bacteria, viruses, and fungi that live in the gut. Though natural viruses are often viewed as dangerous, they also serve to strengthen the immune system, as stated above. Viruses are part of the human microbiome that is composed of trillions of microbial cells and genetic material from bacteria, fungi, and viruses that are on and in the body, including the nose, throat, gastrointestinal and urogenital tracts, and skin. Most of the human microbiome resides in the digestive tract, which is essential in fighting off diseases. Some researchers suggest that up to 90% of all diseases can be traced back to the gut and to the health of the microbiome. How the microbiome, viruses, and bacteria interact helps to determine what role they play in keeping us healthy or making us sick. Because autoimmune disease begins in the gut or gastrointestinal tract, the channel through which food travels, the way to treat autoimmunity is by restoring the microbiome. There are literally trillions of microbes that help govern nearly every function of the human body. Recent research indicates that current medical interventions, such as vaccinations and their toxic ingredients, can interfere with the health of the microbiome, causing numerous neurodevelopmental problems.

In 2000, Dr. Alessio Fasano, a leading authority in the field of immunology, discovered that intestinal hyperpermeability or "leaky gut" is a key factor in autoimmunity. This refers to perforations in the intestinal wall, allowing microorganisms, pathogens, toxins, bacteria, viruses, and food particles to leak across the intestinal wall into the bloodstream causing "leaky gut syndrome." This creates an excessive inflammatory response in the body that can cause gastrointestinal tract problems, such as chronic diarrhea, constipation and abdominal discomfort; autoimmune diseases; mood disorders; food allergies;

skin conditions such as eczema and psoriasis; thyroid disorders; celiac disease caused by gluten; and nutritional deficiencies, such as low levels of vitamin B12, digestive enzymes, and magnesium. In response, the body develops antibodies that end up mistakenly attacking the body's own cells, causing inflammation that then triggers autoimmunity. If the inflammation occurs in the joints, the individual can develop rheumatoid arthritis. If the pancreas is inflamed, pancreatitis can result, if the lining of the lungs is inflamed, asthma can develop.

Other factors, besides the toxins found in vaccines, can also adversely affect the gut microbiome, including: poor diet, the overuse of antibiotics; food grown under poor soil conditions; the poisons sprayed on crops, such as glyphosate; and the reliance on artificial baby formulas instead of the mother's own breast milk.

A BRIEF HISTORY OF POLIO

Historically, the polio virus was a benign condition that was rarely associated with paralysis. This started to change in the late 1800s and moving into the 1900s, when polio epidemics became prevalent during the period of industrialization. Industrial and agricultural pollution followed as a result of the innovation of pesticides that were freely used on crops and livestock in an attempt to get rid of insect-borne diseases of various kinds. One of the first modern polio epidemics occurred in Sweden in 1887, after the invention of DDT in 1874, used along with arsenic, and other poisons. Epidemics occurred in areas of the world where pesticides were widely used. With the introduction of DDT in the Philippines, for example, the first polio epidemic in the tropics took place. In the 1940s, the National Institute of Health (NIH) showed that DDT damaged the spinal cord, as did polio. However, DDT was later portrayed as harmless to humans, justifying the spraying of crops and animals and even on children at play. This was based on the false assumption that polio was spread by airborne insects like flies and that DDT would eliminate these pests safely.

In 1962, the U.S. biologist Rachel Carson, published *Silent Spring*, which warned of the dangers of DDT on insects and birds. For this discovery, she was ostracized by Monsanto, the producer of DDT, the AMA, government agencies, and the media. In 1972, DDT was finally prohibited in the U.S., 10 years after her seminal work was published. It should come as no surprise that polio cases followed the same pattern as pesticide production in the U.S. As DDT production decreased, so did polio cases.

Prior to 1954, polio was incorrectly over-reported by health officials based on a number of conditions that created polio-like paralytic diseases like DDT. Arsenic was another widely used poison in the past mimicking polio-like symptoms. It was sprayed on the sugarcane fields starting in 1913, to kill the weeds that made harvesting sugarcane difficult. The sudden rise of polio in the U.S. between 1916 and 1918 coincided with the spraying of sugarcane with arsenic. Arsenic was also sprayed on fruits and vegetables, prescribed by doctors to treat asthma, added to tobacco for smoking, used to destroy cholera, and applied to decayed teeth in order to kill nerve endings. Other conditions that could produce polio-like symptoms included congenital syphilis, transverse myelitis, GBS, limb paralysis based on a variety of vaccines, lead poisoning, and enteroviruses.

The polio epidemic in the U.S. reached its peak in 1952 and then rapidly declined prior to the introduction of the polio vaccine developed by Dr. Salk in 1955. Yet, in April of that year, Salk's vaccine was praised as one of the greatest achievements in modern medicine—the cure for polio. However, less than one month later, vaccinated children started coming down with polio, and on May 8, the U.S. government halted the production of the vaccine, due to the Cutter Incident, in which more than 200,000 were infected with the live polio virus, resulting in muscle weakness, some severe paralysis, and 10 deaths. Other polio vaccines from drug manufacturers, like Wyeth Pharmaceuticals, also caused paralysis, but only Cutter was blamed for the 1955 disaster. The number of reported cases of polio increased after the mass inoculations and the NIH was aware of the Salk vaccine causing polio, with some scientists describing the vaccine as being worthless. But pressure by the National Foundation for Infantile Paralysis and the vaccine companies, with their financial clout, coerced the U.S. Public Health Service to falsely claim that the vaccine was safe and effective.

After the polio vaccine was introduced, the criteria for diagnosis were deliberately changed, making it seem like the vaccine was eliminating polio. Before 1954, doctors diagnosed polio if the paralysis lasted for only a short period of time, which was often the case with polio. After the introduction of the vaccine, the criteria for diagnosis were changed to 60 days, so that any paralysis lasting less than 60 days was no longer classified as polio. In this way, the number of reported polio cases decreased dramatically, creating the perception that the vaccine was the reason. In addition, infectious diseases that were difficult to distinguish from polio, such as aseptic meningitis and Coxsackie virus, were mislabeled as paralytic poliomyelitis before the vaccine, but later excluded from polio diagnosis, creating once again the perception that polio diminished as a result of the vaccine itself.

The standard medical treatments used with paralytic victims actually exacerbated the recovery efforts by cutting children's tendons, straightening their legs and placing them in a plaster cast where they would be immobilized from a few months up to two years, causing atrophy of the limbs. Sister Elizabeth Kenny was a nurse from Australia who was able to effectively treat polio victims with the use of hot packs and physical therapy to correct the injurious conventional treatments of that time.

In the early 1950s, Jonas Salk used monkey kidneys in which to culture an abundant amount of polio viruses in order to mass produce the vaccine. But in 1960, Bernice Eddy, a government researcher responsible for testing vaccine safety, found that the monkey kidneys used to develop the polio vaccine contained a monkey virus that caused tumors in animal studies. The virus ended up being known as Simian Virus 40 (SV-40), which contaminated the polio vaccine, causing cancer. Though Eddy's superiors attempted to hide the evidence, she ended up presenting her data at a cancer conference and was subsequently demoted and lost her laboratory. In order to avoid a panic, the SV-40 debacle was kept from the public and the existing contaminated stocks continued to be used on 98 million Americans between 1955 and 1963. Despite denials by officials that there was no connection between polio vaccines and SV-40, cancer rates increased, with the SV-40 virus being detected in brain tumors, leukemia, mesothelioma and bone cancers. Some studies have even shown that the SV-40 virus can be passed on from mother to child *in utero*. For example, a 1988 study of 59,000 women found that the children of the mothers who got the Salk vaccine between 1959 and 1965 had brain tumors 13 times greater than those children of mothers who were not given the polio vaccine.

In 1963, Albert Sabin's oral "live-virus" polio vaccine replaced Salk's "killed-virus" vaccine, but this caused even more cases of polio, and eventually the U.S. medical authorities reverted back to the inactivated vaccine. However, the oral polio vaccine continues to be used today in developing countries around the world because it does not require refrigeration like the Salk vaccine does. Unfortunately, the oral dosage has been repeatedly given in an attempt to eradicate polio, causing an explosion in the related acute flaccid paralysis (AFP), as seen in India, where the wild poliovirus has declined, but the more virulent AFP form of polio has exploded, causing twice as many deaths as the wild poliovirus.

HOW TO IDENTIFY VACCINE REACTIONS

National Vaccine Information Center (NVIC) states that, if you or your child experiences any of the symptoms listed below in the hours, days, weeks, or months following vaccination, it should be reported to Vaccine Adverse Events Reporting System (VAERS).

- **Pronounced swelling, redness, heat, or hardness at injection site;**

- **Body rash or hives;**

- **Shock/collapse followed by unresponsive, deep sleep;**

- **High-pitched screaming or hours of persistent crying;**

- **Changes in sleep/wake pattern, and dramatic personality changes;**

- **High fever (higher than 103 F);**

- **Twitching or jerking of the body, arm, leg, or head;**

- **Weakness/paralysis of any part of the body;**

- Crossing of eyes, loss of eye contact or awareness, and social withdrawal;

- Loss of ability to roll over, sit up, or stand up;

- Head banging or unusual flapping, rubbing, rocking, spinning;

- Joint pain or muscle weakness;

- Disabling fatigue;

- Loss of memory;

- Onset of chronic ear or respiratory infections, breathing problems (including asthma);

- Severe/persistent diarrhea or chronic constipation;

- Excessive bruising, bleeding, or anemia.

APPENDIX F
BOGUS CANCER CHARITIES

Money interests often dictate outcomes whether we are talking about political decisions, corporate influence, or media coverage. It should not come as any surprise that charities as well can be influenced by financial considerations. Cancer charities in particular have engaged in unscrupulous practices for personal gain while preying on the generosity of a trusting public, as chronicled below.

In 2015, the Federal Trade Commission (FTC) and the Attorneys General of all 50 states filed charges alleging fraud on four cancer charities in the sum of $187 million taken from consumers. Instead of providing direct assistance to cancer patients, the "overwhelming majority" of the funds were used to enrich individuals associated with the organizations. The four charities are: Cancer Fund of America, Cancer Support Services, Children's Cancer Fund of America, and The Breast Cancer Society.

The Children's Cancer Fund of America and The Breast Cancer Society have folded as a result of these charges, and the individuals involved were banned from all fundraising activities in the future.

Cancer Fund of America spent about 97% of donations on themselves and fundraisers, while 3% went to cancer patients. It was listed as the second worst charity in America by the Center for Investigative Reporting in 2014.

The National Cancer Institute and the American Cancer Society were charged with the misappropriation of funds and of conflicts of interest through ties to pharmaceutical companies who manufacture cancer drugs, as well as pesticide industries and makers of mammogram equipment.

The American Cancer Society's 2014 Facts and Figures report deliberately spins their data to fraudulently fit their claim that "more Americans than ever are surviving cancer." ACS counted anyone diagnosed with cancer as a survivor, even those diagnosed yesterday. Although it is one of the largest cancer foundations in the world, it has done essentially nothing for childhood cancers, giving only one penny on every dollar raised in 2010, in spite of their claims that they were leading the fight against childhood cancers.

The extent of corruption is best exemplified by the fact that one of the cancer charities paid the company's president's son nearly $18 million over 8 years to solicit donations. But the number-one worst charity in America was the Kids Wish Network, which raised millions in donations in the name of dying children but spent less than 3% on actually helping kids. "The charity spends the majority of its donations on for-profit fundraisers, instead of directing that money to charitable works," as reported by CNN.

In December 2014, 8 out of the top 15 worst charities in the United States were listed as cancer organizations.

A BRIEF HISTORY OF THE PHARMACEUTICAL INDUSTRY'S INFLUENCE ON THE MEDICAL FIELD

John D. Rockefeller was considered the richest man in the world in the early 1900s, having refined approximately 90% of America's oil through his company, the Standard Oil Trust. In 1911, the U.S. Supreme Court found John Rockefeller and the Standard Oil Trust guilty of corrupt and illegal business practices under the Sherman Antitrust Act and was ordered to dismantle his oil corporation. In 1913, John Rockefeller established the Rockefeller Foundation, in which the petrochemical giant established a monopoly, similar to his oil business model, through the pharmaceutical investment business. As a result, much of Rockefeller's fortune at that time went toward "philanthropy," in the form of many charitable endeavors, including the funding of drug-based research through universities and medical schools in the U.S. and internationally. If institutions were not doing research that was drug-based, they would be refused funding and soon put out of business in favor of the lucrative pharmaceutical industry.

Around this same period, that the first vitamins were being discovered and proved to be effective, the drug-based model that

Rockefeller supported, came out against these alternative treatments to medicine. These non-pharmaceutical methods were portrayed as unscientific quackery and purposely excluded from medical schools that were taught to address health issues only through the use of sanctioned medical procedures and the exclusive use of drugs.

In the mid-1920s, Germany was establishing the first chemical/pharmaceutical cartel, led by I.G. Farben, the European competitor to the Rockefeller cartel. In the early 1930s, I.G. Farben, supported Hitler's rise to power who, in turn, assigned all chemical, petrochemical, and pharmaceutical industries over to the I.G Farben empire as he invaded and took over countries in Europe. In 1939, the Rockefeller empire and the German chemical company, I.G. Farben entered into an agreement called the "Drug Trust" alliance, creating the largest and extremely lucrative chemical and pharmaceutical monopoly in the world.

In Germany, during World War II, I.G. Farben assisted in the mass exterminations at Auschwitz. On April 14, 1941, Otto Armbrust, the I.G. Farben board member responsible for the Auschwitz project, stated to board members, "Our new friendship with the SS is a blessing. We have determined all measures integrating the concentration camps to benefit our company." I.G. Farben provided the poisonous gas that killed millions of Jews as well as other chemical agents used in human experiments. Concentration-camp prisoners were also used as subjects in testing I.G. Farben's patented pharmaceutical substances before being released to the public.

With the end of the Nazi regime in 1945, I.G. Farben was dismantled and the corporate shares of I.G. Farben went to the Rockefeller Trust in the U.S. and the Rothschild/J.P. Morgan organization in the U.K., thereby solidifying even greater profits and concentration of wealth. At the Nuremberg Tribunal in 1945–46, 24 I.G. Farben board members and executives were tried and convicted of mass murder, slavery, and other crimes. Incredibly, most of them had been released by 1951 and were reinstated with the German corporations, Bayer, BASF, and Hoechst, as part of the corporate restructuring. The public was not aware that many of the men from I.G. Farben who were responsible for Nazi atrocities were able to continue their work as executives in control of the large chemical and pharmaceutical companies. For almost three decades after the war, Bayer, BASF, and Hoechst (Aventis) filled their highest position, chairman of the board with former members of the Nazi regime. For example, Fritz Ter Meer, who was sentenced to 12 years but served only 7 years for his crimes at Auschwitz, ended up as Chairman of the Board of Bayer, Germany's largest pharmaceutical company, where he served until his retirement in 1964.

In 1945, the United Nations was founded, and its subsidiary organizations, the World Health Organization (WHO) and the World Trade Organization (WTO) became, over time, a political arm of the global oil and drug interests. In 1963, Dr. Matthias Rath stated, "Under the pretense of consumer protection, [the U.N.] launched a four-decade-long crusade to outlaw vitamin therapies and other natural, non-patentable health approaches in all member countries of the United Nations. The goal was to simply ban any and all competition for the multi-billion-dollar business in patented drugs."

Post WWII, the American Medical Association board members published a series of articles attacking alternative medical treatments as "quackery," coordinating their efforts through the Coordinating Conference on Health Information (CCHI). By 1964, the member organizations of the CCHI: the American Cancer Society, the American Pharmaceutical Association, the Food and Drug Administration, the Internal Revenue Service, the Attorneys General's Offices, the Office of Consumer Affairs, the National Health Council, the U.S. Postal Service, the Federal Trade Commission, the Arthritis Foundation, and the Council of Better Business Bureaus, were all involved in targeting and undermining alternative medical treatments.

In 1976, a number of chiropractors filed an antitrust lawsuit against the American Medical Association, contending that the AMA was attempting to destroy the chiropractic profession by depriving its practitioners of association with medical doctors and calling them "unscientific cultists." The judge's ruling came 11 years later in 1987, describing the conspiracy as "systematic, long-term wrongdoing and a long-term attempt to destroy a licensed profession." The movie *Undoctored* (2018), by Jeff Hays, goes into detail chronicling AMA's attempts to undermine the chiropractic profession over many years.

In 1978, the Congressional Office of Technology Assessment (COTA) released a report, *"Assessing the Efficacy and Safety of Medical Technologies,"* that acknowledged that U.S. medical-oriented trauma care was considered to be the best in the world. In contrast, it reported that allopathic-oriented drug medicine was only 15 to 20% effective as a medical approach. This finding by the COTA was in sharp contrast to the perception that allopathic medicine was the most effective approach to medical care. Alternative medical procedures that emphasized a non-drug, health-oriented model were portrayed with skepticism in the mainstream media, even though they were making inroads with a certain segment of the public who saw the disease-oriented model relying on pharmaceutical remedies as not providing lasting benefits.

In the 1980s, the Food and Drug Administration (FDA), intensified its attacks on alternative approaches to cancer, arthritis, and other food-supplement treatments using vitamins, minerals, enzymes, and laetrile that were proving to be effective alternatives to drugs. Disciplines utilizing chiropractic, homeopathy, naturopathy, acupuncture, chelation therapy, and holistic dentistry were "targeted for harassment, delicensing, or discrediting by the AMA."

Today, the U.S. and New Zealand are the only countries in the world that permit drug makers to advertise directly to consumers on TV and other news media. Up to 70% of advertising in the mainstream media comes from the pharmaceutical industry, which is clearly evident by simply turning on the TV. The drug companies obviously would not be spending the enormous amounts of money—in the billions of dollars—on advertisement if it were not a profitable endeavor.

The influence of the pharmaceutical industry on the medical community is best illustrated by the fact that in the U.S. today, out of 125 medical schools, only 30 programs require medical interns to take a nutrition course. In medical school, the average medical doctor spends 2.5 hours on nutrition education. Instead, interns in their medical training are strictly schooled on pharmaceutical remedies to address the patient's symptoms with essentially little or no emphasis on diet as a condition for maintaining good health.

PHARMACEUTICAL SETTLEMENTS

Between 2009 and 2014, Big Pharma paid out over $13,000,000,000 to the Dept. of Justice for fraudulent marketing practices including the promotion of medicines for uses that were not approved by the Food and Drug administration. One might think that these amount of fines would be prohibitive for the drug companies, but, in actuality, this is a small percentage of their total profits, which in essence is the "cost of doing business." Below is a summary of settlements, over a five-year period, as compiled by ProPublica.

Eli Lilly (Jan 2009)—fined $1.42 billion for off-label promotion of Zuprexa, an antipsychotic drug.

Pfizer (Sept 2009)—fined $2.3 billion for misbranding the painkiller Bextra and illegally promoting three other drugs, Geodon, Zyvox, and Lyrica.

AstraZeneca (April 2010)—fined $520 million for illegally promoting the antipsychotic drug Seroquel.

Merck (Nov 2011)—fined $950 million for the illegal promotion of Vioxx, for rheumatoid arthritis, a medication that was responsible for tens of thousands of heart attacks.

Abbott (May 2012)—fined $1.5 billion for marketing Depakote, for elderly dementia patients and schizophrenics, even though it was not approved for those purposes.

GlaxoSmithKline (July 2012)—fined $3 billion for misbranding the drug Paxil, for children under 18, and failing to disclose safety information for Avandia, a diabetes drug.

Boehringer Ingelheim (Oct 2012)—fined $95 million for promoting several drugs for nonmedical uses; the drugs included: Aggrenox, Atrovent, Combivent, and Micardis.

Sanofi-Aventis (Dec 2012)—fined $109 million for inflating the price of Hyalgan, an injection for knee pain, in which millions were paid in "kickback-tainted claims for Hyalgan."

Amgen (Dec 2012)—fined $762 million for illegally promoting Aranesp, a drug to treat anemia, at doses the FDA explicitly rejected and for off-label treatment.

Johnson & Johnson (Nov 2013)—fined $2.2 billion for illegally promoting Risperdal, Invega and Natrecor for use with elderly dementia patients while paying "kickbacks" to physicians.

Endo (Feb 2014)—fined $192 million for the illegal promotion of Lidoderm to healthcare providers.

HOW TO WIN THE VACCINE CREDIBILITY WAR

By Ted Kuntz, a psychotherapist, author, community activist, and father of a vaccine injured son. Below is a summarized version of his article that effectively captures the kind of propaganda used to convince others that diseases are bad and vaccines are good.

1. **Take All the Credit for Success**—Claim that vaccines are responsible for the decline in diseases, even though the mortality rates declined up to 99% before vaccines were introduced, as a result of improved living conditions.

2. **Tell a Good Story**—Vaccines are a miracle of modern medicine and vaccines have saved millions of lives, even though these claims are not supported by clinical or biological evidence.

3. **All for One and One for All**—"When you question the safety and effectiveness of any vaccine, you question the safety and effectiveness of all vaccines." Considering the impact of one vaccine is not allowed.

4. **Under Report Adverse Effects**—Do not keep accurate records of adverse effects from vaccine injuries. Out of

sight, out of mind. Say vaccine injuries are "one in a million" or simply deny vaccines cause injuries at all.

5. **Hear No Evil. See No Evil. Speak No Evil.**—Don't discuss any concerns about vaccine safety or effectiveness. Providing balanced reporting on vaccines is irresponsible—it would adversely impact the vaccine program and advertising revenues.

6. **Claim Consensus**—Everyone knows that vaccines are safe and effective. The science is settled. It is unethical to conduct clinical research with an unvaccinated population. Asking questions about vaccine effectiveness would be anti-science.

7. **Let the Money Speak for Itself**—Money is the best criterion for deciding the outcome of research. Money should decide which studies are published.

8. **Everyone Must Believe**—Everyone must be vaccinated for the greater good. Herd immunity means everyone must be vaccinated to be effective. Mandate vaccines if people aren't responsible enough to get vaccinated.

9. **Keep Everyone Afraid**—If everyone doesn't get vaccinated, diseases will return and kill us. Anyone who doesn't vaccinate is a danger to the community.

10. **Avoid Any Discussion**—It is best not to discuss the matter. It just confuses people. Everyone knows that vaccines are safe and effective. Anyone who disagrees should be discredited.

CENSORSHIP IN SCIENCE

Scientific evidence that does not fall in line with the conventional wisdom of the medical establishment and the financial interests of corporations is routinely ignored, discounted, reworked, and/or dismissed, and the scientists who dare to speak up are vilified, threatened, discredited, and /or fired by those who hold the purse strings. There are numerous cases of corruption in the medical-pharmaceutical-chemical industries that have been perpetuated throughout their history. The following examples are reflective of this corruptive influence:

Handwashing—Ignaz Semmelweis was a Hungarian physician who was considered an early pioneer of antiseptic procedures. He noticed that women giving birth under unsanitary delivery conditions resulted in a high death rate for the mothers. He proposed that doctors wash their hands with an antiseptic solution before delivery, but his view went against the prevailing medical opinions at the time, in spite of the fact that his approach reduced deaths by 90% from what was called, "Childbed Fever." He was viewed with contempt and ridiculed to such an extent that he left his practice in Vienna. The ongoing controversy gradually undermined his mental state, and, in 1865, he was unwittingly committed to an asylum by a colleague and subsequently beaten by the guards and died due to an infection from his wounds while incarcerated.

X-Rays—Alice Stewart, a British physician and epidemiologist, investigated the medical effects of radiation on health. In 1956, she made the association between X-rays of pregnant women and the high cancer rates in their children. Her findings went against the conventional wisdom at the time that X-rays were not harmful. This created an enormous backlash, in which she was berated by the medical establishment, the nuclear industry, and governmental agencies. It took more than two decades before her conclusions were finally accepted by the medical community.

Simian Virus 40—Dr. Bernice Eddy, a virologist and epidemiologist at the National Institute of Health, identified SV-40, a cancer-causing monkey virus that millions of children were exposed to from contaminated polio vaccines. When she attempted to warn the NIH officials, Eddy was banned from polio research, her findings were withheld from the public, and the contaminated vaccines continued to be used. In 1960, Eddy was invited to speak at a cancer society conference, where she addressed the problem with SV-40 and was subsequently reprimanded by her supervisor and from that point on, prevented from speaking publicly on the subject.

DDT—Rachel Carson, a marine biologist and conservationist, wrote a number of books, *Silent Spring* (1962) being the best known, which described the harmful effects of synthetic pesticides, especially DDT, responsible for the death of insects and birds, and its overall detrimental impact on the natural environment. She was attacked by Monsanto, the producer of DDT, and by the American Medical Association (AMA), governmental agencies, and the news media who dismissed her as an "hysterical woman" and "spinster."

Flu Vaccine—Dr. John Anthony Morris was the chief vaccine officer for the Bureau of Biological Standards at the NIH and later with the FDA, beginning his work in 1940. He argued that his research team found that there was no proof that vaccines were effective in preventing influenza and that, in fact, it could be potentially dangerous. FDA officials immediately demoted him, confiscated his research, and prevented him from publishing his work. Health and Human Services fired him in 1976 with the excuse that he failed to return library books on time. As it turned out, the swine-flu vaccine in 1976 caused 500 cases of Guillain-Barré syndrome, with 200 people paralyzed and 33 deaths.

Lead Poisoning—In 1979, Herbert Needleman, a researcher at University of Pittsburgh, discovered that exposure to lead, especially leaded gasoline and lead paint, caused neurodevelopmental damage that could adversely affect a child's IQ and learning abilities, and cause behavioral problems. The petroleum industry put pressure on the Environmental Protection Agency (EPA), the National Institute of Health (NIH), and other government agencies to silence Needleman and ultimately ruin his career.

Chickenpox Vaccine—Dr. Gary Goldman, a PhD computer scientist, conducted a large CDC-funded study in 1995 on the varicella vaccine, given to 300,000 residents in Antelope Valley, California. He found that the vaccine waned, causing dangerous chickenpox outbreaks in adults and increased cases of shingles in children who received the vaccine. The CDC would not allow the publication of the unfavorable results, so Goldman resigned from his employment in order to publish the results himself, stating that he did not want to be a part of what he "perceived as research fraud."

Juvenile Diabetes Epidemic—Dr. Bart Classen, an American immunologist, proposed in 1996 that vaccines, particularly the Hib vaccine, caused insulin-dependent diabetes mellitus, a serious condition mostly seen in juveniles. The FDA reacted swiftly, by silencing him and not allowing him to publish his findings. He was subsequently removed from government service.

Shaken Baby Syndrome—Dr. Waney Squier, a neuropathologist from John Radcliffe Hospital in Oxford, England, served as an expert witness in cases where babies died as a result of suspected abusive head trauma, referred to as Shaken Baby Syndrome. Squier testified that, in the cases that she represented, infant brain injuries were due to vaccines and not due to physical trauma as a result of abusive behavior. The Medical Practitioners Tribunal Service removed her from the medical register, but, on appeal to the High Court of England, the decision was reversed.

Corrupted Science—Peter Gotzsche, a Danish physician and researcher, who, in 1993, was the co-founder of the prestigious Cochrane Collaboration and headed the Nordic Cochrane Center in Copenhagen, Denmark, noted for its unbiased research. He became an outspoken critic within his own agency of the increasing corruption of published scientific studies financed and controlled by the pharmaceutical interests. He was particularly critical of the HPV vaccine which showed an increased risk of serious injury. This threatened to endanger pharmaceutical profits and in 2018, he was subsequently fired from the Cochrane Board that was dominated by industry representatives and controlled by Bill Gates.

Chronic Fatigue Syndrome—Dr. Judy Mikovits is a pioneer in discovering the association between human retroviruses and chronic fatigue syndrome (CFS). The retroviruses were also linked to blood cancers. Mikovits' research showed that the retrovirus seen in mice had been transported to humans by contaminated vaccines and that many of the female patients with the retrovirus had children with autism. The idea that retroviruses from animals could contaminate vaccines, threatened the financial interests of the entire pharmaceutical industry, which relies on animal cells in the development of vaccines. For her important discovery, Mikovits was put in jail without due process, all of her research was confiscated, and she was fired from her job. She was not charged with a crime, and yet she was unable to pursue legal actions against the government or her employer.

HOW TO REPORT AN INJURY FROM COVID-19 VACCINE FOR REIMBURSEMENT

The Countermeasures Injury Compensation Program (CICP), authorized under the Health Resources & Services Administration (HRSA), provides compensation for injures or death due to an adverse reaction if determined to be a direct result of vaccination and if the adverse event is reported within one year of inoculation. The CICP also states that they are the payer of last resort, meaning that they provide benefits or cover only expenses that are not provided by other third-party payers, such as health insurance or Workers' Compensation programs, and the like.

Summary of CICP Claims Process:

1. An individual submits a Request Package to the CICP (cicp@hrsa.gov).

2. The Package is reviewed by CICP medical staff to determine whether the requester is eligible for program benefits.

3. If eligible, the requester is asked to submit additional documentation to determine the type and amount of

compensation the requester may be entitled to receive. If ineligible, the requester is informed in writing of the disapproval.

4. If the requester is found to be entitled to program benefits, the requester is notified in writing, and payment is issued to the requester.

5. The requester may ask the HRSA to reconsider the program's eligibility or benefits determination. When a request for reconsideration is received, a qualified panel, independent of the program, is convened to review the program's determination.

6. The panel makes its recommendation to the Associate Administrator, who makes a final determination with regard to the specific issues(s), identified in the reconsideration request. Requesters may not seek review of a decision made on reconsideration.

Note:
- You need to fill out a separate form for each healthcare provider who treated you.

- The Request for Benefits forms should be sent via U.S Postal Service mail or a private courier. CICP does not accept forms via fax or email.

- You can download the necessary PDF forms (cicp@hrsa. gov) or call 1-855-266-2427 and request a paper copy.

- The CICP is not authorized to provide reimbursement for attorneys' fees. You may elect to use an attorney: however, you are responsible for any costs incurred from using one.

PHYSICIANS DECLARATION GLOBAL COVID SUMMIT— ROME, ITALY

International Alliance of Physicians and Medical Scientists
September 2021

We the physicians of the world, united and loyal to the Hippocratic Oath, recognizing the profession of medicine as we know it is at a crossroad, are compelled to declare the following;

WHEREAS, it is our utmost responsibility and duty to uphold and restore the dignity, integrity, art and science of medicine;

WHEREAS, there is an unprecedented assault on our ability to care for our patients;

WHEREAS, public policy makers have chosen to force a "one size fits all" treatment strategy, resulting in needless illness and death, rather than upholding fundamental concepts of the individualized, personalized approach to patient care which is proven to be safe and more effective;

WHEREAS, physicians and other healthcare providers working on the front lines, utilizing their knowledge of epidemiology, pathophysiology, and pharmacology, are often first to identify new, potentially life-saving treatments;

WHEREAS, physicians are increasingly being discouraged from engaging in open professional discourse and the exchange of ideas about new and emerging diseases, not only endangering the essence of the medical profession, but more importantly, more tragically, the lives of our patients;

WHEREAS, thousands of physicians are being prevented from providing treatment to their patients, as a result of barriers put up by pharmacies, hospitals, and public health agencies, rendering the vast majority of healthcare providers helpless to protect their patients in the face of disease. Physicians are now advising their patients to simply go home (allowing the virus to replicate) and return when their disease worsens, resulting in hundreds of thousands of unnecessary patient deaths, due to failure-to-treat;

WHEREAS, this is not medicine. This is not care. These policies may actually constitute crimes against humanity.

NOW THEREFORE, IT IS:

RESOLVED, that the physician-patient relationship must be restored. The very heart of medicine is this relationship, which allows physicians to best understand their patients and their illnesses, to formulate treatments that give the best chance for success, while the patient is an active participant in their care.

RESOLVED, that the political intrusion into the practice of medicine and the physician/patient relationship must end. Physicians, and all healthcare providers, must be free to practice the art and science of medicine without fear of retribution, censorship, slander, or disciplinary action, including possible loss of licensure and hospital privileges, loss of insurance contracts and interference from government entities and organizations—which further prevent us from caring for patients in need. More than ever, the right and ability to exchange objective scientific findings, which further our understanding of disease, must be protected.

RESOLVED, that physicians must defend their right to prescribe treatment, observing the tenet FIRST, DO NO HARM. Physicians shall not be restricted from prescribing safe and effective treatments. These restrictions continue to cause unnecessary sickness and death. The rights of patients, after being fully informed about the risks and benefits of each option, must be restored to receive those treatments.

RESOLVED, that we invite physicians of the world and all healthcare providers to join us in this noble cause as we endeavor to restore trust, integrity, and professionalism to the practice of medicine.

RESOLVED, that we invite the scientists of the world, who are skilled in biomedical research and uphold the highest ethical and moral standards, to insist on their ability to conduct and publish objective, empirical research without fear of reprisal upon their careers, reputations, and livelihoods.

RESOLVED, that we invite patients who believe in the importance of the physician-patient relationship and the ability to be active participants in their care, to demand access to science-based medical care.

IN WITNESS WHEREOF, the undersigned has signed this Declaration as of the date first written

GLOSSARY OF MEDICAL TERMS

Acupuncture—a complementary medical practice based on the belief in traditional Chinese medicine that disease is caused by disruptions to the flow of energy in the body. The procedure entails placing very thin needles under the skin at acupuncture points to stimulate the nerves that travel through channels called meridians. It helps to alleviate pain, nausea, and other health conditions.

Acute Flaccid Paralysis (AFP)—a rare strain of the poliovirus that has genetically mutated from the strain contained in the oral polio vaccine. The Global Polio Eradication Initiative solution is to "*immunize every child several times with the oral vaccine to stop polio transmission, regardless of whether the virus is wild or vaccine-derived.*" Unfortunately, this procedure of vaccinating multiple times has created AFP, a more severe form of polio-like symptoms that is twice as deadly.

Allergies—a condition in which the immune system reacts to a foreign substance, called allergens, that can include pollen, dust, animal hair, foods, drugs, etc. Symptoms can include: swelling, hives, nausea, congestion, runny nose, swollen eyes, and in severe cases, anaphylactic shock that can be life-threatening.

Allopathy—a system of medicine, referred to as conventional or Western medicine, that aims to combat disease by using remedies, such as drugs (e.g., antibiotics, pain medications, etc.), surgical procedures, and radiation treatments. Roughly, it refers to treating a symptom with its opposite, as in the example of using a laxative to treat constipation.

Alopecia—an autoimmune disorder in which the body attacks its own hair follicles that can cause hair loss anywhere on the body.

Alzheimer's disease—the most common form of dementia, in which nerve cells of the brain degenerate, causing a decline in thinking, memory, social and behavioral skills, and ultimately, the ability to function independently.

Anaphylaxis—a severe and potentially life-threatening allergic reaction associated with a food allergy (peanuts), an insect sting (bee), medications (like penicillin) or vaccinations as noted in the vaccine product inserts. Anaphylaxis can cause a skin reaction, lower blood pressure, nausea, vomiting, diarrhea, dizziness and a constriction of the airway by swelling of the tongue or throat causing wheezing and trouble breathing. In severe cases it can lead to death if not treated promptly.

Antibody-Dependent Enhancement (ADE)—a phenomenon in which antibodies enhance the entry of viruses into cells via vaccination, increasing viral infection that can cause inflammation and immunopathology.

Antioxidants—molecules that can prevent or slow damage to cells caused by free radicals. Examples include: certain fruits and vegetables, vitamins like C and E, selenium, etc.

Apnea—a sleep disorder in which breathing is repeatedly interrupted during sleep, reducing the amount of oxygen getting to the brain.

Arthralgia—joint pain due to injury, infection, illnesses (especially arthritis) or an allergic reaction to medications, including vaccinations. Like arthritis, it is associated with autoimmune disease.

Arthritis—inflammation of the joints, characterized by pain, swelling, stiffness, and redness. **Rheumatoid Arthritis** is the most severe type of arthritis, an autoimmune disorder, causing inflammation in which the body's immune system attacks and damages the joints, leading to deformity in severe cases.

Asperger's Syndrome—it is similar to autism in the sense that the child has deficits in social behaviors as it relates to the inability to engage in reciprocal conversation with others, preoccupation with specific topics of interest that are obsessive, lacking the ability to comprehend the nuances in conversation in spite of age-appropriate language development and self-help skills.

Asthma—a condition that inflames and narrows the airways of the lungs causing wheezing, coughing, and shortness of breath, making it difficult to breathe.

Ataxia—incoordination and clumsiness, affecting balance and gait, limb, and eye movements, swallowing, fine-motor tasks, and/or speech. Caused by injury to the brain or spinal cord as a result of nervous system degeneration, as in the case of a stroke, alcohol abuse, cerebral palsy, multiple sclerosis, etc.

Atrophy—a wasting away of a part of the body due to a breakdown of tissue as in the case of a loss of muscle mass due to inactivity, disease, or old age.

Autism—**or autism spectrum disorder (ASD)** is a neurological, medical, and behavioral condition that ranges from mild to very severe in which the child's development is disrupted by a regression in the ability to relate appropriately to others, suddenly withdrawing from social interactions, avoiding eye contact with others, losing previously acquired speech, learning, motor, and nonverbal communication skills, obsessing over ritualistic routines and self-stimulating behaviors, and reacting abnormally to sensory input, such as being hypersensitive to noises or being oblivious to what is going on around the child.

Autoimmune Disorders—caused by a reaction of the individual's immune system that attacks and destroys healthy body tissue by mistake. Examples: Rheumatoid arthritis, diabetes, lupus, Multiple Sclerosis, Hashimoto's thyroid disease, inflammatory bowel disease (Crohn's disease and ulcerative colitis), celiac disease, asthma.

Bacteria—germs or microscopic organisms that thrive both inside and outside of the body, living in a multitude of environments including soil, water, organic matter, and in the human body, especially the gut. Though some bacteria can cause food poisoning and infectious diseases, most are viewed as harmless, and many are seen as beneficial. Antibiotics are often used in treating bacterial diseases though the down side is in their ability to destroy healthy gut flora.

Bell's Palsy—paralysis of the facial muscles, usually one-sided and temporary, due to inflammation of a facial nerve in which the eyelid and corner of the mouth droop on one side of the face.

Bile—a fluid produced and secreted by the liver that carries away waste products formed in the liver and helps to break down fats in the intestines during digestion.

Carcinogen—any substance capable of causing cancer, including radiation, tobacco smoke, inhaled asbestos, synthetic materials, chemicals in food, and toxins such as arsenic, formaldehyde, benzene, cadmium, nickel, etc.

Celiac Disease—an immune reaction to eating gluten, a protein found in wheat, rye and barley, creating inflammation that damages the lining of the small intestines.

Cerebral Edema—a swelling in the brain caused by the presence of excessive fluid that can result from brain trauma, a stroke, or inflammation due to meningitis or encephalitis.

Cerebral Palsy (CP)—a form of paralysis causing involuntary movements and loss of coordination due to damage to the brain which may affect hearing, seizures, vision, speech, and/or cause retardation. CP may be due to encephalitis or meningitis (during infancy), injury to the brain, or a stroke.

Chelation—a treatment that uses specific drugs taken orally or intravenously that bind to toxic metals in the body such as lead, mercury, iron, and aluminum, which are removed through urination.

Chiropractic Medicine—healthcare dealing with the diagnosis and treatment of neuromuscular disorders by the manipulation of the spine to reduce back, leg, and neck pain, headaches, stress and anxiety, or a weakened immune system. Chiropractic treatment may include applied kinesiology (muscle testing) used to determine if certain foods, supplements, or other substances weaken or strengthen a patient.

Chronic Fatigue Syndrome (CFS)—characterized by extreme fatigue, exhaustion after physical or mental exertion, sleep disorders, cognitive impairment, etc. due possibly to a weakened immune system as a result of a viral infection.

Colitis—inflammation of the inner lining of the colon (large intestine) that can cause swelling of the colon, intense pain, diarrhea, bleeding ulcers, etc. Causes include inflammatory bowel diseases like Crohn's disease.

Congenital Rubella Syndrome—a condition that occurs in a baby whose mother is infected with rubella virus during pregnancy, usually in the first trimester, causing a miscarriage, stillbirths, or a severe birth defect.

Crohn's Disease—a chronic inflammatory bowel disease that can affect any part of the gastrointestinal tract and can cause abdominal pain, fatigue, and malnutrition. It is an autoimmune disease that may be due to abnormal allergic reaction from a bacterium or virus.

Croup—an infection of the upper airway that obstructs breathing due to inflammation, causing a barking cough, primarily in young children.

Cytokine Storm—a severe immune reaction in which the body releases too many cytokines into the blood too quickly as a result of an infection, autoimmune condition, or other diseases causing high fever, inflammation, fatigue and nausea. In severe conditions, it can be life threatening.

Dementia—a general decline in mental faculties affecting memory, thinking, and social behavior that interferes with the ability to live independently. Causes include: head injury, medication side effects, syphilis, alcoholism, etc.

Demyelination—the breakdown of the protective myelin sheath that surrounds and electrically insulates the nerve fibers of the brain, optic nerves, and the spinal cord. When the myelin sheath is damaged, the nerve impulses are short-circuited, causing loss of sensation and coordination to specific areas of the body.

Diabetes—a disorder in which the blood glucose is too high because the pancreas is unable to produce enough insulin or none at all. This can lead to excessive sugar in your blood that, in turn, can create serious health issues, such as heart disease, stroke, eye problems, nerve damage, etc.

DNA (deoxyribonucleic acid)—the genetic information found in the chromosomes of cells responsible for the development, functioning, growth, and reproduction of organisms.

Eczema—a condition that makes your skin red and itchy. It is common in children and can be caused by an autoimmune reaction, genetics, environmental factors or stress.

Encephalitis—inflammation of the brain usually caused by a viral infection, such as herpes simplex virus or by the immune system mistakenly attacking brain tissue.

Encephalomyelitis—inflammation of the brain and spinal cord, resulting in damage to the myelin sheath of the nervous system with symptoms that range from fever, confusion, and vomiting to seizures, paralysis, and coma. It often occurs after a viral or bacteria infection.

Encephalopathy—any disease or disorder affecting the brain, especially chronic degenerative conditions that can cause memory loss, personality changes, dementia, seizures, coma, or death.

Erythema multiforme—a skin reaction that can be triggered by an infection or medication; it is usually mild and disappears after a few weeks. However, there is a rare form that can affect the mouth, genitals, and eyes that can be life-threatening, referred to as erythema multiforme major.

Fibromyalgia—a chronic disorder characterized by widespread musculoskeletal pain, diffuse tenderness, fatigue, sleep, memory, and mood issues; like arthritis, it impairs the joints and/or soft tissues and causes chronic pain.

Free Radicals—unstable atoms that can damage cells and can cause a host of diseases through a process called oxidation. Cigarette smoke, air pollution, and other environmental toxins can be causative, in addition to being a byproduct of metabolism or oxidation.

Gain-of-Function (GOF) Research—a line of research in which scientists take viruses and study how they can be modified to become deadlier and more transmissible, in order to determine which viruses might threaten the public so that they can design countermeasures.

Gastroenteritis (stomach flu)—inflammation of the stomach and intestines that can be caused by any of a variety of viruses, bacteria, and parasites. It spreads through contaminated food or water or contact with an infected person.

Gastrointestinal tract (Gut)—the part of the digestive system that includes the mouth, esophagus, stomach, and intestines; it takes in food, digests it to absorb the nutrients for energy and eliminates the remaining waste as feces.

Genital Warts—a sexually transmitted disease caused by some types of human papillomavirus (HPV) that is different from those possibly causing cervical and anal cancers. It is contracted by skin-to-skin contact with an infected partner.

Glutathione—an antioxidant produced by the liver that is also found in plants, animals, fungi, and some bacteria that is capable of preventing damage to cells caused by free radicals, heavy metals, etc. It is critical in supporting immune function and reducing cell damage.

Guillain-Barré Syndrome—an autoimmune disease triggered by a bacterial or viral infection in which the body's immune system attacks part of the peripheral nervous system causing tingling and weakness in the legs, sometimes spreading to the arms and upper body. In severe cases, one may become paralyzed and have difficulty in breathing, leading to a life-threatening situation.

Hematoma (Subdural)—a clotting of the blood caused by a ruptured blood vessel under the skull and outside the brain due to an injury to the wall of the blood vessels usually associated with traumatic brain injury.

Hemorrhage (Intracranial)—bleeding inside the brain from a ruptured vessel most commonly from head trauma, untreated high blood pressure, or an aneurysm that can lead to a stroke.

Hepatitis (Types A, B, C)—an inflammation of the liver, with liver cell damage caused most frequently by viral infection, but also by certain drugs, chemicals, or poisons. The most obvious sign is jaundice with the most severe cases causing liver failure.

Homeopathy—a medical practice that emphasizes a holistic, natural approach to the treatment of the sick based on the belief that the body is able to cure itself. A thorough history of the patient is taken, including lifestyle, eating habits, temperament, personality, sleep patterns, and medical history, in order to determine the most appropriate medicine based on symptoms and one's level of health. Homeopathy operates on the principle of "likes cure likes," meaning that a patient suffering from symptoms can be treated with highly diluted medicines capable of producing similar symptoms in a healthy person.

Hypoglycemia—a condition in which a person's blood sugar (glucose) level is lower than normal. Treatment involves getting one's blood sugar level back to normal by ingesting foods or drinks with high sugar content or with medications.

Hypotonia—a symptom of decreased muscle tone as seen in babies born prematurely or with cerebral palsy or after a serious infection such as meningitis.

Immunogenicity—the ability of a foreign substance, such as an antigen used in a vaccine to provoke an immune response in the body.

Inflammatory bowel disease (IBD)—a chronic inflammatory disorder affecting the small or large intestine, such as Crohn's disease or ulcerative colitis.

Inoculation (Vaccination)—injecting a foreign substance for the purpose of stimulating the immune system to produce antibodies with the aim of protecting against future infections by bacteria or viruses.

Intussusception—a serious condition in which one part of the intestine telescopes inside of another, causing an intestinal blockage usually at the junction of the small and large intestines; usually requires emergency medical care.

Kawasaki Syndrome—an autoimmune disease-causing inflammation of the walls of the blood vessels in the body. It usually occurs in the first two years of life. It can cause a high fever, rash, swelling of hands and feet, joint pain, conjunctivitis, and swollen lymph nodes in the neck.

Leaky gut syndrome—a digestive condition that affects the lining of the intestines, creating gaps in the intestinal wall so that bacteria and other toxins can pass into the bloodstream associated with inflammation that triggers an autoimmune response that can affect different areas of the body.

Leukemia—several types of cancers in which there is an abnormal proliferation of white blood cells in the bone marrow that forces normal cells out from the marrow; causes cancers that can spread to other parts of the body.

Lou Gehrig's disease (Amyotrophic lateral sclerosis, ALS)—a condition that affects the neurons responsible for muscle movement, causing the muscles to weaken and the person to lose control throughout the body, eventually leading to death.

Lupus—an autoimmune disease in which the body's immune system can attack different areas of the body, such as connective tissue (tendons and cartilage), skin, kidneys, heart, and lungs causing inflammation, fever, headaches, painful joints, and swelling of the feet, legs, hands, and/or eyes.

Macrophagic Myofasciitis—a condition induced by aluminum hydroxide used in vaccines causing an adverse reaction characterized by demyelinating central nervous system problems that can precipitate chronic musculoskeletal pain, chronic fatigue, and cognitive disorders.

Meningitis—inflammation of the meninges (the membranes that cover the brain and spinal cord) that usually results from infection by a variety of microorganisms. Injuries, cancer, certain drugs, and other types of infections can also cause meningitis. Viral meningitis is relatively mild; bacterial meningitis is life-threatening and needs prompt treatment.

Metallothionein (MT)—a metal-binding protein that protects against oxidative stress and acts as a buffer against toxic heavy metals.

Microcephaly—a condition in which an infant's head is smaller than normal due to abnormal brain development that can be caused by exposure to drugs, alcohol, and toxic chemicals in the womb; chromosomal abnormalities, like Down's syndrome; decreased oxygen to the fetus; and infections.

Microglia—the primary immune cells of the CNS that are key regulators of brain development; they can affect both normal and pathological conditions within the brain.

Mitochondria—referred to as the "powerhouse of the cell"; generates most of the chemical energy needed to power the cell's biochemical reactions.

Multiple Sclerosis (MS)—a progressive disease of the central nervous system in which patches of myelin (the protective covering of nerve fibers) in the brain and spinal cord are destroyed. It is an autoimmune disorder that causes symptoms ranging from numbness and tingling in the limbs, tremors, lack of coordination, partial or complete loss of vision, slurred speech, and paralysis.

Mutation—a change in the genetic material, resulting in a divergent form of the chromosomes that can then be transmitted to subsequent generations of DNA.

Myelin—the insulating layer that forms around the nerves of the brain and spinal cord that allows the electrical impulses to move along the nerve cells quickly and efficiently.

Myelitis (Transverse)—inflammation of the spinal cord, often the result of a viral infection, such as poliomyelitis, measles, or herpes simplex; it can lead to eventual paralysis and sensory loss as in the case of multiple sclerosis.

Myocarditis—inflammation of the heart muscle that may affect the heart's ability to function, causing a rapid or abnormal heart rhythm. It can be caused by a viral infection, autoimmune diseases, toxins, and adverse reactions to medications. In its severe form, it can cause acute heart failure and sudden death, as in the case of sudden infant death syndrome (SIDS).

Narcolepsy—a sleep disorder characterized by excessive sleepiness during the day and sudden loss of muscle tone.

Naturopathy—a primary healthcare profession that emphasizes prevention, treatment, and optimal health in order to encourage the patient's self-healing process. Naturopathy is based on the healing power of nature, the identification and treatment of the underlying causes of the illness, avoiding the risk of harmful side effects, encouraging self-responsibility for one's health, treating the whole person, and emphasizing the prevention of disease.

Neuritis—inflammation of one or more nerves that can be caused by injury, infection, or autoimmune disease. Symptoms can include pain and tenderness, numbness, hypersensitivity, lack of strength, and/or abnormal circulation.

Neuropathy—a disease, inflammation, or damage to the peripheral nerves, which connect the central nervous system (brain and spinal cord) to the sense organs, muscles, glands, and internal organs. It can be caused by hereditary factors as well as acquired ones, including trauma, infections, autoimmune diseases, diabetes, medications, and toxins. Common symptoms include: numbness of the hands and feet, loss of coordination, muscle weakness, and abnormal blood pressure or heart rate.

Neutropenia—an unusually low number of white blood cells (neutrophils) which are important in fighting certain infections, especially due to bacteria.

Optic Neuritis—inflammation of the optic nerve that can cause a sudden loss of vision in some cases due to demyelination (destruction of the myelin sheaths) of the optic nerve fibers. It is linked to multiple sclerosis, and symptoms include: eye pain, loss of vision in one eye, and loss of side vision and color vision.

Orchitis—an inflammation of one or both testicles that can be caused by a bacterial or viral infection. Most men usually recover completely with no lasting effects.

Otitis Media—an inflammation or infection of the middle ear, causing ear pain, trouble hearing, loss of balance, and headache as a result of a cold, sore throat, or respiratory infection.

Oxidative Stress—an imbalance between free radicals (unstable molecules that can damage cells) and antioxidants (substances that can prevent damage to the cells). Over time, it can cause heart disease, cancer, arthritis, stroke, respiratory diseases, immune deficiency, and other inflammatory conditions.

Pancreatitis—inflammation of the pancreas often associated with alcohol abuse but also related to viral infection, such as mumps, gallstones, and certain drugs, such as tetracycline. Symptoms may include: abdominal pain, fever, nausea, vomiting, and loss of weight.

Paraesthesia—a sensation of tingling, pricking, burning, or numbing sensation on the skin caused by damage to peripheral nerves referred to as "pins and needles sensation." It may be associated with neuropathy.

Parkinson's disease—a disorder of the nerve cells of the brain with symptoms that include muscle tremors, rigid posture, awkward fine and gross motor movements, and difficulty with speech.

Pneumonia—an infection due to viruses, bacteria, and fungi that inflame the membrane lining of the lungs, which fill with fluid that causes coughing, fever, chills, fatigue, nausea, and difficulty breathing.

Poliomyelitis—an infectious disease caused by a virus which provokes no more than a mild reaction in most cases, though a more serious case, can attack the central nervous system (CNS) leading to paralysis and death.

Psoriasis—a skin condition characterized by thickened scaly patches of inflamed skin that are itchy and sometimes painful. It is related to an immune system malfunction of the white blood cells.

Pulmonary embolism—a condition in which one of the pulmonary arteries in the lung are blocked by a blood clot that travels to the lungs usually from the legs. Symptoms include shortness of breath, chest pain, and cough.

Purpura—bleeding under the skin, causing areas of discoloration due to thinning of the tissues supporting blood vessels, which rupture easily.

Retinal hemorrhage—bleeding that occurs in the light-sensitive tissue on the back wall of the eye. Symptoms can range from slight to severe vision problems.

Rhinitis (hay fever)—inflammation of the inside of the nose caused by an allergen, such as pollen, dust, mold, etc.

RNA (ribonucleic acid)—carries the inherited coded instructions within a cell that is responsible for regulation and expression of genes.

Seizures—a sudden episode of uncontrolled electrical activity in the brain that causes a seizure which may range from temporary confusion and a staring spell to uncontrollable jerking movements and loss of consciousness. It can be associated with a high fever, medications, head trauma, stroke, and abuse of alcohol or drugs.

Serum Sickness—a type of hypersensitive allergic reaction to a vaccine injection in which the immune system attacks an antigen, causing an itchy rash, fever, joint pain, and in severe cases, anaphylactic shock.

Shingles (herpes zoster)—an infection of the nerves causing a painful rash of a small, crusting blisters on different parts of the body due to the varicella-zoster virus, which also causes chickenpox. It can reappear later in life due to a weakened immune system.

Stevens-Johnson Syndrome—a rare skin condition characterized by severe blisters and bleeding in the mucous membranes of the lips, eyes, mouth, nasal passages, and genitals, usually caused by an adverse reaction to a medication or infection. It is a medical emergency usually requiring hospitalization.

Syncope—fainting or a temporary sudden loss of consciousness.

Thrombocytopenia—an autoimmune disease that reduces the number of platelet cells in the blood, which results in abnormal bleeding into the skin.

Tourette's syndrome (TS)—a disorder involving repetitive grimaces, erratic movements, or unwanted sounds (tics) that are difficult to control. Examples are repeated blinking of the eyes and blurting out unusual sounds or offensive words. The syndrome starts in childhood and is more common in males.

Vaginal lesions—female genital sores that cause bumps and lesions in and around the vagina. The sores may be tender, with painful itching, a burning sensation, bleeding and discomfort when urinating.

Vasculitis—inflammation of blood vessels leading to damage of the vessels, primarily due to the immune system attacking blood-vessel cells by mistake.

Viruses—a type of microorganism that can cause a variety of viral diseases, like the common cold, that can be spread from person to person. Most viruses are self-limiting in those with a healthy immune system.

BIBLIOGRAPHY

Books

A Shot in the Dark, Harris L Coulter and Barbara Loe Fisher (1991)

Altered Genes, Twisted Truth: How the Venture to Genetically Engineer Our Food Has Subverted Science, Corrupted Government, and Systematically Deceived the Public, Steven M. Druker (2015)

Bad Pharma: How Drug Companies Mislead Doctors and Harm Patients, Ben Goldacre (2012)

Béchamp or Pasteur? A Lost Chapter in the History of Biology, Ethel D. Hume (1923)

Dissolving Illusions: Disease, Vaccines, and the Forgotten History, Suzanne Humphries, MD; Roman Bystrianyk (2013)

Evidence of Harm: Mercury in Vaccines and the Autism Epidemic: A Medical Controversy, David Kirby (2005)

Healing and Preventing Autism, Jenny McCarthy and Jerry Kartzinel, MD (2009)

How to End the Autism Epidemic, J.B. Handley (2018)

How to Raise A Healthy Child…In Spite of Your Doctor, Robert Mendelsohn, MD (1984)

I Do Not Consent: My Fight Against Medical Cancel Culture, Simone Gold, MD, JD (2020)

In a Different Key: The Story of Autism, John Donvan and Caren Zucker (2016)

Jabbed: How the vaccine industry, medical establishment, and government stick it to you and your family, Brett Wilcox (2018)

Mandatory Vaccines: For Health or Profit? Brandy Vaughan, Learn the Risk.com

Master Manipulator: The Explosive True Story of Fraud, Embezzlement, and Government Betrayal at the CDC, James Ottar Grundvig (2016)

Miller's Review of Critical Vaccine Studies, Neil Z. Miller (2016)

NeuroTribes, The Legacy of Autism and the Future of Neurodiversity, Steve Silberman (2015)

Pasteur: Plagiarist, Imposter: The Germ Theory Exploded, R.B. Pearson (1942)

Plandemic: 100% Censored. 0% Debunked., Mikki Willis (2021)

Plague of Corruption: Restoring Faith in the Promise of Science, Dr. Judy Mikovits and Kent Heckenlively, JD; *CHD Books* (2020)

The Autism Book: What Every Parent Needs to Know About Early Detection, Treatment, Recovery, and Prevention, Robert W. Sears, MD, FAAP (2010)

The Autism Cover-Up: How and Why the Media Is Lying to the American Public, Anne Dachel (2014)

The Biology of Belief: Unleashing the Power of Consciousness, Matter, and Miracles, Bruce H. Lipton (2008)

The Longevity Paradox: How to Die Young at a Ripe Old Age, Steven R. Gundry (2019)

The Peanut Allergy Epidemic: What's Causing It and How to Stop It, Heather Fraser (2011)

The Poisoned Needle: Suppressed Facts about Vaccination, Eleanor McBean (1957)

The Real Anthony Fauci: Bill Gates, Big Pharma, and the Global War on Democracy and Public Health, Robert F. Kennedy Jr., (2021)

The Truth About COVID-19: Exposing the Great Reset, Lockdowns, Vaccine Passports, and the New Normal, Dr. Joseph Mercola, Ronnie Cummins, April 2021.

The Truth About the Drug Companies: How They Deceive Us and What to Do About It, Marcia Angell, MD (2005)

The Unvaccinated Child: A Treatment Guide for Parents and Caregivers, Judith Thompson, ND, Eli Camp, ND (2017)

Thimerosal: Let the Science Speak, Robert F. Kennedy, Jr., Editor (2014)

Vaccination Is Not Immunization, Tim O'Shea, 5th Edition (2017)

Vaccine Epidemic: How Corporate Greed, Biased Science, and Coercive Government Threaten Our Human Rights, Our Health,

and Our Children, Edited by Louise Kuo Habakus, MA, and Mary Holland, JD (2011)

Vaccines: Are They Really Safe and Effective? Neil Z. Miller (2018)

Vaccines, Autoimmunity, and the Changing Nature of Childhood Illness, Thomas Cowan, MD (2018)

Vaccine Primer: An Inoculation, Elliott Freed (2016)

Vaccine Whistleblower: Exposing Autism Research Fraud at the CDC, Kevin Barry, Esq. (2015)

Virus Mania: How the Medical Industry Continually Invents Epidemics, Making Billion-Dollar Profits at Our Expense, Torsten Engelbrecht, Dr. Claus Kohnlein, MD, Dr. Samantha Bailey, MD, Dr. Stefano Scoglio, BSc, PhD (2021)

What About Immunizations? Exposing the Vaccine Philosophy, Cynthia Cournoyer (2010)

Videos

Bought: Your Health Now Brought to You by Wall Street, a film by Jeff Hays (2014)

Do Vaccines Cause Autism? Rob Schneider, YouTube

Exposing the Vaccine Orthodoxy by Leon Canerot (2016)—YouTube

"Manufactured Consent" Part I & II, by Suzanne Humphries (2015)—YouTube

Silent Epidemic: The Untold Story of Vaccines and **Vaccine Nation,** two films by Gary Null available on YouTube

The Greater Good, a film by Leslie Manookian, Kendall Nelson, and Chris Pilaro (2011)

The Truth About Vaccines series, Ty Bollinger (2017)

Trace Amounts: Autism, Mercury, and the Hidden Truth, a film by Eric Gladen (2014)

Truth in Media: Video on "CDC, Vaccines, and Autism" (truthin-media.com)

Undoctored, Jeff Hays (2016)

Vaccines Revealed—Nine-part series, Patrick Gentempo, Beau Pierce, and Jeff Hays (2017)

Vaccine Secrets: COVID Crisis—Twelve-part series, Jonathan Otto (2021)

Vaxxed: From Cover-Up to Catastrophe, Del Bigtree, Polly Tommey, and Andrew Wakefield (2016)

Vaxxed: The People's Truth, Robert F. Kennedy Jr., Polly Tommey, Kay & Charles Chilton (2020)

Website Resources

A Comprehensive Review of Vaccines (www.visionlaunch.com/many-people-choosing-not-vaccinate)—An extensive and thorough 12-part series on vaccines, along with numerous resources.

Age of Autism: Daily Web Newspaper of the Autism Epidemic— Dan Olmsted, founder; provides current information on the autistic epidemic and its connection to environmentally induced illness that is treatable.

America's Frontline Doctors (americasfrontlinedoctors.com)— Advocates for more effective alternative medical protocols as opposed to the experimental COVID-19 vaccines.

AutismOne (autismone.org)—Ed Arranga, cofounder & president. A parent-driven organization that provides education and supports advocacy efforts for children and families affected by autism.

A Voice for Choice (avoiceforchoice.com), Christina Hildebrand, founder. An organization promoting people's rights to be fully informed regarding vaccines, the health effects of food and pharmaceutical products.

Children's Health Defense: Kennedy News & Views, Robert F. Kennedy, Jr., founder and chairman. An online newsletter covering a wide range of topics addressing autism and other neurodevelopmental disorders associated with toxins in vaccines and the environment.

Foundation for Autism Information & Research, Inc. (FAIR Autism Media) Provides autism information and education to support and improve the quality of life for individuals with autism and their families.

Generation Rescue (generationrescue.org)—J.B. and Lisa Handley, founders.—Provides information on how to treat the underlying symptoms of autism and advocates for those families impacted by autism.

Greenmedinfo.com—Compilation of vaccine studies by Sayer Ji, founder. Covers thousands of research articles on providing evidence-based natural medical information to increase consumer education.

Immunity Education Group (immunityeducationgroup.org)— Provides information on immunizations and infectious diseases, vaccination laws, and their impact on families. Emphasizes the importance of maintaining informed consent and medical freedom.

Informed Consent Action Network (ICAN) (icandecide.org), Del Bigtree, founder of the internet talk show, *The HighWire.* Investigates the safety of medical procedures, pharmaceutical drugs, and vaccines while supporting the public's right to informed consent.

LearnTheRisk (learntherisk.org), Brandy Vaughan, founder. An organization devoted to educating people worldwide on the dangers of pharmaceutical products, including vaccines, and unnecessary medical treatments.

National Vaccine Information Center (nvic.org), Barbara Loe Fisher, cofounder. An organization dedicated to preventing vaccine injuries and deaths by providing information on diseases and vaccine science, policy, law, and the ethical principle of informed consent.

Protection of the Educational Rights of Kids (PERK)—Amy Bohn, President & Founder. Advocates for the educational rights of children and supports legislation that will guarantee medical freedom and parental rights against vaccine mandates.

Religious Rights Coalition advocates for the protection of religious rights of families and individuals to make health decisions, without coercion, discrimination, or segregation, based on conscientious and religious beliefs, including exemptions from requird vaccines (religiousrightscoalition. org).

Stand for Health Freedom (SHF), Leah Wilson, cofounder. A nonprofit organization dedicate to protecting basic human rights, constitutional rights, and parental rights through direct contact with elected officials and others in positions of authority.

Steve Kirsch's newsletter-Substack—(stevekirsch. substack. com). A newsletter that covers information regarding COVID vaccine safety and efficacy, corruption, censorship, mandates, masking, and early treatments.

Stopmandatoryvaccination.com, Larry Cook, Founder and Director. A program that educates the public about the dangers of vaccines and advocates for stopping mandatory vaccinations.

The Dark Side of Vaccines (lukeyamaguchi.teachable.com). A 10-chapter curriculum on Vaccines that covers a wide range of topics such as: history, safety concerns, efficacy, manufactured science, and toxic metals in vaccines.

The National Health Federation (www.thenhf.com). Formed to protect the health rights and freedom of individuals and healthcare practitioners, to educate the consumers, and to provide expert representation on matters related to health.

Think Twice Global Vaccine Institute (thinktwice.com). Provides parents and others with educational resources enabling them to make informed vaccine decisions through the uncensored exchange of vaccine information, supporting every family's right to accept or reject vaccines.

Truth Will Prevail: 1200 studies that refute vaccine claims. Dr Alan Palmer (wellnessdoc.com/1200 studies). Extensive research on more than 1200 scientific studies in the form of a downloadable eBook covering the potential dangers of vaccines.

Vaccineinjury.info—A website that provides critical vaccine information and surveys parents on the side effects of vaccines, comparing the health outcomes between vaccinated and unvaccinated children.

Vaccines Uncensored: Your Right to a Critical View (pubmedinfo. org)—A website that encourages the public to question entrenched assumptions regarding the necessity and efficacy of vaccinations, quoting numerous doctors who are rarely covered in the news media.

Vaccine News from Dr. Mercola (vaccines.mercola.com)—Covers current news on vaccine research and the importance of fostering natural immunity through healthy lifestyle changes.

Vaccine Safety Research Foundation—Steve Kirsch's Newsletter (ste-vekirsch.substack.com) A newsletter that addresses issues regarding COVID vaccine safety and efficacy, corruption, censorship, mandates, and treatment options.

Vactruth.com—Website covers a range of topics related to studies and articles on adverse vaccine effects, and vaccine law and policy, provides access to the **vaccine package inserts** that are issued by the pharmaceutical companies.

ACKNOWLEDGMENTS

* There are a multitude of individuals who should be acknowledged for their work in exposing the vaccine orthodoxy. Pioneers in the field going back to the works of Antoine Béchamp, who laid the foundation for understanding the underlying conditions that allowed diseases to thrive. Other scientists of the 19th century, such as Alfred Russell Wallace and Dr. Walter Hadwen, who questioned the use of vaccinations from the beginning, raising concerns about the detrimental effects of vaccines.

* Dr. Robert Mendelsohn, one of the outspoken pediatricians who pushed for a sane approach to childcare, cautioning against vaccinations and the implications of their long-term use.

* The groundbreaking work of Harris Coulter and Barbara Loe Fisher, who questioned the pertussis vaccine and created a voice for those who witnessed their childrens' injuries, culminating in the informative work of the National Vaccine Information Center.

* Robert F. Kennedy Jr., a leading advocate for environmental health and a champion for those who have suffered vaccine injuries, working to inform and educate the public through the work of the Children's Health Defense, and his seminal book, *The Real Anthony Fauci.*

* Dr. Andrew Wakefield, who has been unjustly vilified in the mainstream media, for initially pointing out the danger of the MMR vaccine and its connection to gastrointestinal problems associated with autism.

* There are a number of medical editors, including Marcia Angell of the *New England Journal of Medicine;* Richard Horton, of the *Lancet;*

Richard Smith of the *British Medical Journal;* and Peter Gotzsche of the *Nordic Cochrane Center;* who have been vocal in their criticism of studies funded and controlled by the corrupting influence of the pharmaceutical industry.

* There are numerous other contributors who have reported on the legitimate vaccine research that has been largely censored in the mainstream media, showing the ill-effects of vaccination. They include: Del Bigtree of The High Wire, Dr. Sherri Tenpenny, Dr. Brian Hooker, Dr. Vijendra Singh, Dr. David Baskin, Dr. Jill James, Dr. Amy Holmes, William J. Walsh, Christina Hildebrand, Dr. Robert W. Sears, Sayer Ji, Dr. Paul Thomas, Ty and Charlene Bollinger, Anne Dachel, Jenny McCarthy and Jerry Kartzinel, MD, Heather Frazer, James Ottar Grundvig, Patrick Gentempo, Jeff Hays, and Gary Null, to name those I am most aware of in my own research.

* Specifically, in regards to COVID-19 research, the specialists that I am most familiar with include: Dr. Peter McCullough, Dr. Richard Fleming, Dr. Robert Malone, Dr. Paul Marik, Dr. Pierre Kory, Dr. Geert Vanden Bosche, Dr. Simone Gold, Dr. Valdimir Zelenko, Harvey A. Risch, and Luc Montagnier. They are some of the leading authorities in the world who have contributed to a greater understanding of the current coronavirus and have advocated for effective alternative treatments that avoid the dangers of the current experimental vaccine technology. Unfortunately, they have been systematically censored by the mainstream media, as with other voices attempting to sound the alarm regarding the inherent dangers of this most recent vaccine technology.

* Finally, I would like to thank a personal friend, Cheryl Ban, who has provided helpful feedback and suggestions on how to improve my manuscript throughout this process and my wife, Carmen, who has been my faithful companion, word editor, and sounding board since the very beginning of this project.

NOTES

1. Darold A. Treffert, MD. "Epidemiology of Infantile Autism", *Archives of General Psychiatry*, May 1970.
2. Qian Li, et al., "Prevalence of Autism Spectrum Disorder Among Children and Adolescents in the United States from 2019 to 2020." *JAMA Pediatrics;* July 5, 2022..
3. Adapted from Cynthia Cournoyer's book, *What About Immunizations? Exposing the Vaccine Philosophy* (2010).
4. From interview, Carol Krucoff, "The 6 O'Clock Scholar: Librarian of Congress Daniel Boorstin and His Love Affair with Books," *The Washington Post* (29 Jan 1984).
5. CDC, Vaccine Safety, "Vaccine ingredients do not cause autism," March 26, 2020.
6. *Bruesewitz et al. v. Wyeth LLC.*, Supreme Court of the United States, October Term, 2010.
7. Barbara Loe Fisher, " A Guide to Reforming Vaccine Policy & Law," National Vaccine Information Center, nvic.org. 2020.
8. Infant mortality rate—country comparison, www.cia.gov; Feb 2018.
9. U.S. Code Title 42. 300aa-22. Standards of responsibility. (b). Unavoidable Adverse Side Effects, Warnings (1). Cornell Law School.
10. Suzanne Humphries, "Smoke, Mirrors, and the Disappearance of Polio," International Medical Council on Vaccination, Nov 17, 2011.
11. "AMA Says Mature 12-year-olds Can Consent to Vaccination Without Parents— Taking Away the Last Barrier Protecting Innocent Children from Big Pharma." *Children's Health Defense; Jun 18, 2019*
12. Elliott Freed, Vaccine Primer: An Introduction" (2016).
13. Sofair and Kaldjian, "Eugenic sterilization and a qualified Nazi analogy: the United States and Germany, 1930–1945," *Annals of Internal Medicine* 132:4 (2000).
14. *Buck vs. Bell*, Justice Oliver Wendell Holmes Jr., *U.S. Supreme Court* ruling, 1927.
15. AMA Journal of Ethics, Opinion 8.08—*Informed Consent*, Jul 2012.
16. Brett Wilcox, "Jabbed: How the vaccine industry, medical establishment, and government stick it to you and your family." Chapter 19, Racism and the Vaccine Program: It's a Black-and-White Issue, p. 214.
17. Utilitarianism, *The American Heritage Dictionary of the English Language*, 1981.

18. "Autism Rates in California Schools Spike Up 17% Among Kindergartners Since SB 277 Bill Was Signed into Law," *circleofdocs.com*.

19. "Dr. Richard Pan Introduces SB 276 to Combat Fake Medical Exemptions that Put Children and Communities at Risk," *California State Senate*; March 26, 2019

20. Alix Mayer, MBA., "Health Committee Votes Yes to SB276, Pan's Labyrinth." *Children's Health Defense:* July 1, 2019.

21. *Ibid.*

22. Davis Taylor, "Texas Bill Would Increase Vaccine Safety, Reject Federal Narrative," *Tenth Amendment Center,* Apr 8, 2019.

23. "Vaccine Myths Debunked," *Public Health*. Oct 30, 2020.

24. *HHS.gov,* "Vaccines & Immunizations: National Adult Immunization Plan," June 10, 2019.

25. "21st Century Cures Act," *Wikipedia*.

26. Dr. Joseph Mercola, "US Surveillance Bill 6666: The Devil in the Details." *Articles. mercola.com*; Jan 5, 2022.

27. Philip J. Hilts, "Tobacco Chiefs Say Cigarettes Aren't Addictive." *New York Times*; Apr 15, 1994.

28. Mary Holland & Lou Conte, "Unanswered Questions from the Vaccine Injury Compensation Program: A Review of Compensated Cases of Vaccine-Induced Brain Injury." Pace Environmental Law Review, 2011.

29. E.J. Mundell, "Autism Largely Caused by Genetics, Not Environment." *WebMD*; July 17, 2019.

30. *Central Intelligence Agency* (CIA), Country comparison: Infant mortality rate, Feb 2018.

31. 2011–12, National Survey of Children's Health, *CDC National Center for Health Statistics*.

32. CDC, Asthma Surveillance Data, 2018.

33. Alexis Stoner, et al. "Ambient Air Toxics and Asthma Prevalence among a Representative Sample of US Kindergarten-Age Children," *PLoS One*, Sept 18, 2013.

34 "Understanding Learning and Attention Issues," *National Center for Learning Disabilities*, Jan. 24, 2017.

35. Rowland et al. "The prevalence of ADHD in a population-based sample." *Journal of Attention Disorders*, Sept 2015: 19(9): 741–754.

36. Corinne Keet and Robert A. Wood, "Food allergy in children: Prevalence, natural history, and monitoring for resolution." *UpToDate* website, Jun 2020.

37. Febrile Seizures Fact Sheet, *National Institute of Neurological Disorders and Stroke,* Sept 2015.

38. J.B. Handley, *How to End the Autism Epidemic*. 2018 p. 16.

39. "Autism New Jersey, Autism Prevalence," *Autism and Developmental Disabilities Monitoring (ADDM) Network,* 2016.

40. "Key Findings from the ADDM Network: A Snapshot of Autism Spectrum Disorder in 2016." *ADDM*; Oct 2, 2020.

41. Cynthia Nevison, PhD, "The 2020 ADDM Report on U.S. Autism Prevalence: Three Reasons Why the Popular Narrative Was Misleading." *Children's Health Defense;* Apr 21, 2020.
42. "Key Statistics for Childhood Cancers," *American Cancer Society*; Jan 8, 2020.
43. "What is Autism Spectrum Disorder?" *CDC: Autism Spectrum Disorder (ASD)*; Mar 25, 2020.
44. Beldeu Singh, "A Safer Approach in Vaccination—Can nanobiotechnology provide solutions to prevent adverse events following immunization by safely and rapidly removing heavy metals in vaccines?" *researchgate.net,* Jan 2016.
45. Becker & Schultz, "Similarities in features of autism and asthma and a possible link to acetaminophen use." *Medical Hypotheses.* Jan 2010.
46. See note 2.
47. Dr. Nicole Beurkens, "Glyphosate Exposure Affects Your Family's Health and Behavior." *Dr. Seneff interview*; 2020.
48. Dr. Alan Palmer, "Autism," *1200 Studies: To Vaccinate or Not to Vaccinate*, Mar 17, 2020 p. 145.
49. *Ibid.*, p. 195
50. "2018 Annual Report, America's Health Rankings: International Comparison." *United Health Foundation,* 2021.
51. Kristina Kristen, "Japan Leads the Way: No Vaccine Mandates and No MMR Vaccine = Healthier Children." *Children's Health Defense,* Apr 23, 2019.
52. Jason Glanz et al. "A Population-Based Cohort Study of Undervaccination in 8 Managed Care Organizations Across the United States." *JAMA, Pediatrics*, Mar 1, 2013; 167(3): 274-81.
53. Anthony R. Mawson et al. "Pilot comparative study on the health of vaccinated and unvaccinated 6- to 12-year-old U.S. children." *Journal of Translational Science*, Apr 24, 2017.
54. Hooker & Miller, "Health effects in vaccinated versus unvaccinated children, with covariates for breastfeeding status and type of birth." *Open Access Text (OAT),* June 12, 2021.
55. Dr. T. Obukhanych, "An Open Letter to Legislators Currently Considering Vaccine Legislation from Tetyana Obukhanych, PhD in Immunology." *www.aph.gov.au* Apr 17, 2015.
56. "Surveillance for Safety After Immunization: Vaccine Adverse Event Reporting System (VAERS)," *MMWR, CDC,* Jan 24, 2003.
57. Ross Lazarus, "Electronic Support for Public Health-Vaccine Adverse Event Reporting System (ESP: VAERS)," *Harvard Pilgrim Health Care, Inc., DHHS,* 12/1/07 to 9/30/10.
58. J.B. Handley, *How to End the Autism Epidemic*, Chapter 2, p. 41.
59. "Tripedia: Diphtheria and Tetanus Toxoids and Acellular Pertussis Vaccine Adsorbed." *Sanofi Pasteur Inc.* Dec 2005.
60. Del Bigtree, "ICAN vs. ID-IS: Key Legal Win Recasts Vaccine Debate." *Informed Consent Action Network*, Sept 14, 2018.

61. Mary Holland et al., "Unanswered Questions from the Vaccine Injury Compensation Program: A Review of Compensated Cases of Vaccine-Induced Brain Injury." *Pace Environmental Law Review*, (2011).

62. *Children's Health Defense blog*, entitled, "Congress Receives Vaccine Safety Project Details, Including Actions Needed for Sound Science and Transparency." Mar 13, 2018.

63. Goldman & Miller, "Relative trends in hospitalizations and mortality among infants by the number of vaccine doses and age, based on the Vaccine Adverse Event Reporting System (VAERS), 1990–2010." *Human & Experimental Toxicology*, Oct 2012.

64. Miller & Goldman, "Infant-mortality rates regressed against number of vaccine doses routinely given: Is there a biochemical or synergistic toxicity?" *Human and Experimental Toxicology*. Sept 2011.

65. Neil Z. Miller, *Miller's Review of Critical Vaccine Studies*, "Aluminum." 2016; p. 44–63.

66. Lyons-Weiler J, Ricketson R. "Reconsideration of the immunotherapeutic pediatric safe dose levels of aluminum." *Journal of Trace Elements in Medicine and Biology*, 2018; 48: 67–73.

67. Neil Z. Miller, *Miller's Review of Critical Vaccine Studies*, "Aluminum," 2016, p. 44–63.

68. Christopher Shaw, "Aluminum-Induced Entropy in Biological Systems: Implications for Neurological Disease." *Journal of Toxicology*. Volume 2014, Article ID 491316, PDF.

69. Nils Warfving, "Short Review of Aluminum Hydroxide Related Lesions in Preclinical Studies and Their Relevance," *International Journal of Vaccines & Vaccination*, Feb 27, 2017.

70. Gherardi et al., "Macrophagic myofasciitis lesions assess long-term persistence of vaccine-derived aluminuim hydroxide in muscle." *Oxford Academic, Brain: A Journal of Neurology*. Vol. 124, Issue 9, Sept 1, 2001.

71. Sealey, Hughes, et al., "Environmental factors in the development of autism-spectrum disorders." *Environment International*; Mar 2016; 88:288–298.

72. "Review of the Formaldehyde Profile in the National Toxicology Program 12th Report on Carcinogens," *NTP*, June l0, 2011.

73. *Studies: To Vaccinate or Not to Vaccinate?* "Formalin, AKA Formaldehyde." p. 101.

74. "Common Ingredients in U.S. Licensed Vaccines," *FDA*, 4/30/2018.

75. Dr. Sherri J. Tenpenny, "Formaldehyde in Vaccines." *Integrative Medical Center*, Jan 29, 2013.

76. *1200 Studies: To Vaccinate or Not to Vaccinate?* "Formalin, AKA Formaldehyde," p. 101–102.

77. Dana Scott, "Does Your Dog's Vaccine Contain Thimerosal (Even When It Says It Doesn't)? *Dogs Naturally Magazine;* Dec 12, 2021.

78. *House Congressional Record* Volume 149, Number 76, Wednesday, May 21, 2003.

79. Risher & Tucker, "Alkyl Mercury-Induced Toxicity: Multiple Mechanisms of Action." *Reviews of Environmental Contamination and Toxicology*. 2017; 240:105–149.

80. Hooker, Kern, et al. "Methodological isssues and evidence of malfeaseance in research purporting to show thimerosal in vaccines is safe." *BioMedical Research International* 2014; article ID 247218.

81. "Robert F. Kennedy Jr.: Q&A About Vaccine Safety." *Healthline*, Aug. 22, 2018.

82. David Kirby, *Evidence of Harm, p. 295.*

83. "Toxicological Profile for Mercury", *DHHS*. March 1999.

84. Tomljenovic, Dorea, et al. "Commentary: A link between mercury exposure, autism spectrum disorder, and other neurodevelopmental disorders? Implications for thimerosal-containing vaccines." *Journal of Developmental Disabilities*. 2012; 18(1): 34–42).

85. Stephan Bose-O'Reilly, et al. "Mercury Exposure and Children's Health." *Current Problems Pediatric Adolescent Health Care*, Sept 2010.

86. Bernard et al. "Autism: A novel form of mercury poisoning." *Medical Hypotheses*, 2001, 56(4), 462–471).

87. Rishma Parpia, "Polysorbate 80: A Risky Vaccine Ingredient," *The Vaccine Reaction*, Jan 7, 2016.

88. "Polysorbate 80 Risks," *Vaccine Choice Canada*, Dec, 9, 2013.

89. Carlson, Jansson, et al. "The Endogenous Adjuvant Squalene Can Induce a Chronic T-Cell Mediated Arthritis in Rats," *American Journal of Pathology*, 2000 Jun; 156(6): 2057–2065.

90. "A Glimpse into the Scary World of Vaccine Adjuvants," *Vaccine Choice Canada*. Sept 30, 2008.

91. Gary Matsumoto, *Vaccine A: The Covert Government Experiment That's Killing Our Soldiers—and Why GT's Are Only the First Victim*, August 10, 2010.

92. "1200 Studies: To Vaccinate or Not to Vaccinate?" p. 107, *wellnessdoc.com*.

93. Russell Blaylock, *Excitotoxins: The Taste That Kills*, July 1, 1994.

94. Kamal Niaz, et al. "Extensive use of monosodium glutamate: A threat to public health?" *EXCLI Journal*, 2018; 17: 273–278.

95. Westcott & Wang, "Number of faulty children's vaccines in China surges to over 900,000." *CNN*, Aug 16, 2018.

96. Thomas Cowan, MD, *Vaccines, Autoimmunity, and the Changing Nature of Childhood Illness*, 2018, pg. 26.

97. Tsumiyama et al., "Self-Organized Criticality Theory of Autoimmunity," *PLoS One*, 2009.

98. Suzanne Humphries, MD, and Roman Bystrianyk, *Dissolving Illusions: Disease, Vaccines, and the Forgotten History* (2013), pg. 35–36.

99. "Annual Summary of Vital Statistics: Trends in the Health of Americans During the 20th Century." *Pediatrics*. Dec 2000.

100. Walter Hadwen, MD, *The Case Against Vaccination*. (1896), en.wikisource.org.

101. Humphries & Bystrianyk, *Dissolving Illusions: Diseases, Vaccines, and the Forgotten History*; 2013 p. 59.

102. Walter Hadwen, MD, *The Case Against Vaccination*. (1896), en.wikisource.org.

103. Alfred Russel Wallace, *Vaccination: A Delusion* S536: 1898.

104. J.T. Biggs, *Leicester: Sanitation Versus Vaccination*, 1912.

105. Mahatma Gandhi, *A Guide to Health*, Chapter VI, 1921.

106. Dr. William Howard Hay Addresses the *Medical Freedom Society*, June 25, 1937.

107. Roman Bystrianyk on the Measles Vaccine. *International Medical Council on Vaccination*. Mar 8, 2017.

108. R.B. Pearson, *Pasteur: Plagiarist, Impostor—The Germ Theory Exploded*. Chapter 7, Are Biologicals Injurious? p. 57.

109. George Bernard Shaw, a letter to the *Irish Times*, 1944.

110. R.R. Porter, "The Contribution of the Biological and Medical Sciences to Human Welfare." Ivan Illich, *Medical Nemesis*. Chapter 1—The Epidemics of Modern Medicine, NY: Bantam Books, 1976.

111. Richard Moskowitz, M.D, "The Case Against Immunizations." *Journal of the American Institute of Homeopathy*, Mar 1983.

112. Ramiel Nagel, *Vaccine Truth—Healing Our Children*. Dr. Albert Sabin MD, lecture to Italian doctors in Piacenza, Italy, Dec 7, 1985.

113. Dr. Glen Dettman, "Doctors Warn Against Vaccination (Immunisation)," Australia, 1992.

114. Dr. Boyd Haley, "What doctors say about vaccination, To Vaccinate or Not To," encognitive.com (2001).

115. Gerhard Buchwald, MD, quote from *The Vaccination Nonsense*, 2005.

116. Dr. Russell Blaylock, "Truth About Tetanus Infection and the Vaccine," *Steemit*, 2013.

117. Robert Mendelsohn, MD, *How to Raise A Healthy Child …. In Spite of Your Doctor*, "Chapter 19: Immunization Against Disease: A Medical Time Bomb?" (pg. 231–2).

118. Robert F. Kennedy, "Read the Fine Print: Vaccine Package Inserts Reveal Hundreds of Conditions Linked to Vaccines," *Children's Health Defense*; Apr 14, 2020.

119. Mooi FR, van Loo IH, et al., "Bordetella pertussis Strains with Increased Toxin Production Associated with Pertussis Resurgence." *Emerging Infectious Diseases Journal,* Aug. 2009; 15(8): 1206–1213.

120. Verstraeten, Thomas MD, *NIP, Division of Epidemiology and Surveillance, Vaccine Safety and Development Branch*, 1999.

121. Russell Blaylock, "Immunology primer for neurosurgeons and neurologists part 2: Innate brain immunity." *Surgical Neurology International*; Sept 18, 2013.

122. Mary Holland, et al., "Unanswered Questions from the Vaccine Injury Compensation Program: A Review of Compensated Cases of Vaccine-Induced brain Injury," *Pace Environmental Law Review,* Jan 2011, Vol. 28.

123. J.B. Handley, *How to End the Autism Epidemic*. 2018 p. 178.

124. "83 Cases of Autism Associated with Childhood Vaccine Injury Compensated in Federal Vaccine Court." *Safe Minds*; May 10, 2011.

125. Nevison and Parker, "California Autism Prevalence by County and Race/Ethnicity: Declining Trends Among Wealthy Whites," *Journal of Autism and Developmental Disorders*, 19 March 2020.

126. Brandon Turbeville, "The Antibody Deception." *Brandon Turbeville website*; Jan 14, 2014.

127. Jeremy R. Hammond, "Paul Offit Unwittingly Exposes Scientific Fraud of FDA's Vaccine Licensure." *Children's Health Defense*; July 31, 2019.

128. Dr. Peter Patriarca, Director of the Viral Products Division of the FDA Center for Biological Evaluation, "FDA Acknowledged That Vaccine Technology Outpacing Ability to Predict Adverse Events," *Children's Health Defense*, Lyn Redwood, April 9, 2018.

129. William J. Walsh, "New Research Suggests Cause of Autism," press release, PRNewswire, May 10, 2001.

130. Kubota, Iso, et al. "Association of measles and mumps with cardiovascular disease: the Japan Collaborative Cohort (JACC) study." *Atherosclerosis,* Jun 18, 2015.

131. Rosenlund, et al. "Allergic Disease and Atopic Sensitization in Children in Relation to Measles Vaccination and Measles Infection." Pediatrics Vol 123, Number 3, March 2009.

132. Vadala et al. "Vaccination and autoimmune diseases: Is prevention of adverse health effects on the horizon? *EPMA Journal,* Sept 2017.

133. "PediNeuroLogic Exam, Developmental Anatomy: Myelination and Development." *University of Utah;* May 2020.

134. Adam Hadhazy, "Think Twice: How the Gut's 'Second Brain' Influences Mood and Well-Being." *Scientific American;* Feb 12, 2010.

135. Olga Vera-Lastra, et al. "Autoimmune/inflammatory syndrome induced by adjuvants (Shoenfeld's syndrome): Clinical and immunological spectrum." *Expert Review of Clinical Immunology;* Apr 2013.

136. "Dr. Fasano on Leaky Gut Syndrome and Gluten Sensitivity," *Gluten Free Society,* 2011.

137. "Update: Vaccine Side Effects, Adverse Reactions, Contraindications, and Precautions." *CDC MMWR Report,* Sept 6, 1996; Vol 45: No. RR-12.

138. "How the Institute of Medicine Helped Suppress Questions About Vaccine Safety." *Children's Health Defense;* July 2, 2019.

139. Miller NZ, Goldman GS. "Infant mortality rates regressed against number of vaccine doses routinely given. Is there a biochemical or synergistic toxicity?" *Human Experiment Toxicology* 2011; 30(9) 1420–28.

140. Selected Discontinued U.S. Vaccines, Appendix B, *CDC Epidemiology and Prevention of Vaccine-Preventable Diseases,* May 2019.

141. Alter and Hadler, et al. "The changing epidemiology of hepatitis B in the United States," *Journal of the American Medical Association* 1990; 263:1218–1222.

142. *Subcommittee on Criminal Justice, Drug Policy, and Human Resources of the Committee on Government Reform,* "U.S. House of Representatives RE: Hepatitis B Vaccine," June 14, 1999.

143. Michael Belkin, "Hepatitis B Vaccine," *Vaccine Safety Manual*, think.twice.com, 1999.

144. "Hepatitis B Virus: A Comprehensive Strategy for Eliminating Transmission in the United States Through Universal Childhood Vaccination: Recommendations of the Immunization Practices Advisory Committee (ACIP)," *CDC, MMWR*, Nov 22, 1991.

145. Miller, Neil Z. "The Hepatitis B Vaccine: Do Doctors Think It is Necessary?" *Vaccines: Are They Really Safe and Effective?* Hepatitis, pg. 51.

146. Cynthia Cournoyer, "Hepatitis B," *What About Immunizations?* pg. 181-182.

147. Neil Z. Miller, *Vaccine Safety Manual*, New Atlantean Press, 2008, p. 288.

148. Le Houezec, D. "Evolution of multiple sclerosis in France since the beginning of hepatitis B vaccination." *Immunologic Research*, 2014 Dec; 60(2-3):219-25.

149. Neil Z. Miller, "Hepatitis B," *Miller's Review of Critical Vaccine Studies*, 2016, pg. 166-170.

150. David Geier and Mark Geier, "A case-control study of serious autoimmune adverse events following hepatitis B immunization," *Autoimmunity*. 2005 Jun; 38(4): 295–301.

151. Souayah N. Nasar A, et al. *Journal of Clinical Neuromuscular Disease*, Sept 2009.

152. Carolyn Gallagher & Melody Goodman, "Hepatitis B triple series vaccine and developmental disability in US children aged 1–9 years," *Toxicological and Environmental Chemistry*, 13 Nov 2008.

153. Gallagher and Goodman, "Hepatitis B vaccination of male neonates and autism diagnosis, NHIS 1997–2002," *Journal of Toxicology and Environmental Health*, 2010; 73(24):1665-77).

154. Paul Thomas, MD, "Episode 2: What's in a Vaccine?" *The Truth About Vaccines Transcript; p.49.* (FDA's Code of Federal Regulations, CFR, Title 21, Volume 4).

155. Miller, Neil Z., *Vaccine Safety Manual*. New Atlantean Press, 2008. p. 315.

156. *CDC Recommended Child and Adolescent Immunization Schedule for ages 18 years or younger*, United States, 2020).

157. Jennifer Hyman, "Children at Risk: The DPT Dilemma," *The Democrat and Chronicle*, 1987.

158. Harris L. Coulter & Barbara Loe Fisher, "The Search for a Safer Vaccine," *A Shot in the Dark*, 1985; p. 205-212.

159. Hurwitz, et al. "Effects of diphtheria-tetanus-pertussis or tetanus vaccination on allergies and allergy-related respiratory symptoms among children and adolescents in the United States," *Journal of Manipulative and Physiological Therapeutics*, Vol. 23, Issue 23, Feb 2000.

160. Amanda Seitz, "Autism is not listed as a side effect of vaccines on federal agency's website." *apnews.com;* May 6, 2019.

161. Mogensen et al., "The Introduction of Diphtheria-Tetanus-Pertussis and Oral Polio Vaccine Among Young Infants in an Urban African Community: A Natural Experiment," *PubMed.gov*, PMC 5360569, Feb. 1, 2017.

162. Humphries and Bystrianyk, *Dissolving Illusions: Disease, Vaccines, and the Forgotten History*. 2013, p. 203.

163. Robert Mendelsohn, M.D., *How to Raise a Healthy Child in Spite of Your Doctor*, 1984, p. 245.

164. Adams et al., "Summary of Notifiable Infectious Diseases and Conditions—United States," Aug 11, 2017 /64(53); 1–143, *CDC MMWR*.

165. Humphries & Bystrianyk, *Dissolving Illusions: Disease, Vaccines, and the Forgotten History*, 2013, p. 294.

166. Coulter and Fisher, *A Shot in the Dark* (1991).

167. "Pertussis (Whooping Cough) Disease & Vaccine Information," *National Vaccine Information Center*.

168. Steinman et al "Murine model for pertussis vaccine encephalopathy: Linkage to H-2." *Nature* Vol. 299, Oct. 1982.

169. Christie et al. "The 1993 epidemic of pertussis in Cincinnati. Resurgence of disease in a highly immunized population of children." *New England Journal of Medicine*. Jul 1994.

170. "Pertussis Mutations," *Miller's Review of Critical Vaccine Studies*. 2016; p. 85–104.

171. Alberto E. Tozzi et al., "Clinical presentation of pertussis in unvaccinated and vaccinated children in the first six years of life." *Pediatrics,* Nov 2003 Vol. 112.

172. Dr. David Witt, "Whooping Cough Vaccination Fades in 3 Years," *Associated Press*, Sept 19, 2011.

173. Hegerle N, et al. "Evolution of French Bordetella pertussis and Bordetella parapertussis isolates: increase of Bordetellae not expressing pertactin." *Clinical Microbiological Infections*, Sept. 2012).

174. "Pertussis Outbreaks," *CDC*, Nov. 18, 2019.

175. Human Vaccine Inserts, Vaccine Information: 2017, "Tetanus (Tdap)," *vactruth. com.*

176. Barbara Loe Fisher, "Pertussis Microbe Outsmarts the Vaccines As Experts Argue About Why" *National Vaccine Information Center*, March 27, 2016.

177. "Can Pertussis Vaccine Cause Injury and Death?" *National Vaccine Information Center*, nvic.org.

178. *CDC Morbidity and Mortality Weekly Report (MMWR);* Tetanus Surveillance - Untied States, 2001–2008, April 1, 2011/60(12); 365–369.

179. *CDC Pink Book*, "Epidemiology and Prevention of Vaccine-Preventable Diseases, Tetanus, Chapter 21, Secular Trends in the United States," 2015.

180. *National Vaccine Information Center*." Tetanus Vaccine and Disease Information," nvic.org.

181. Skudder, McCarroll. "Current status of tetanus control: importance of human tetanus-immune globulin." *Journal of American Medical Association* 1964; 188: 624–627.

182. Peltola et al. "Haemophilus influenzae Type b Capsular Polysaccharide Vaccine in Children: A Double-Blind Field Study of 100,000 Vaccinees 3 Months to 5 Years of Age in Finland," *Pediatrics*, Nov 1977, 60 (5) 730–737.

183. Osterholm, et al. "Lack of efficacy of Haemophilus b Polysaccharide Vaccine in Minnesota," *JAMA*; 1988; 260(10): 1423–1428.

184. Sood, Daum. "Disease caused by Haemlophilus influenzae type b, in the immediate period after homologous immunization." *Pediatric* 1990 Apr, 85(4 Pt 2): 698–704.

185. Adam, Richardson, et al., "Changing epidemiology of invasive Haemophilus influenzae in Ontario, Canada: evidence for herd effects and strain replacement due to Hib vaccination." *Vaccine*, May 28, 2010; 28(24):4073–78.

186. David C. Classen, "Association between type 1 diabetes and Hib vaccine: Causal relation is likely." *British Medical Journal*, Oct 23, 1999; 319(7217): 1133.

187. Neil Z. Miller, "Haemophilus Influenzae Type B (HIB)." *Vaccines: Are They Really Safe and Effective?* 2018, p. 57.

188. Dworkin et al. "The changing epidemiology of invasive Haemophilus influenzae disease, especially in persons> or= 65 years old." *Clinical Infectious Disorders*, Mar 15 2007; 44(6): 810–16.

189. Moro et al., "Adverse events following Haemophilus influenzae type b (Hib) vaccines in the Vaccine Adverse Event Reporting System (VAERS)." *Journal of Pediatrics*, Apr 2015, 166(4); 992–997.

190. *CDC, MMWR,* "Withdrawal of Rotavirus Vaccine Recommendation." Nov 5, 1999 / 48(43); 1007.

191. Miller, Neil Z. *Vaccine Safety Manual.* Santa Fe, NM: New Atlantean Press, 2008 p. 353.

192. Timo Vesikari, MD, et al., "Safety and Efficacy of a Pentavalent Human Bovine Reassortant Rotavirus Vaccine." *NEJM*, Vol 34, Jan 2006.

193. Margaret M. Cortese, MD, "Prevention of Rotavirus Gastroenteritis Among Infants and Children. Recommendations of the Advisory Committee on Immunization Practices (ACIP)." *CDC MMWR*; Feb. 6, 2009.

194. 2007 *Physicians Desk Reference (PDR),* 61st Edition.

195. Neil Z. Miller, *Miller's Review of Critical Vaccine Studies.* 2016, p. 119–126.

196. Norton, Stanek, et al. "Routine pneumococcal vaccination of children provokes new patterns of serotypes, causing invasive pneumooccal disease in adults and children." *American Journal of Medical Science*, Feb 2013; 3345(2): 112–20.

197. Ricketson, Wood, et al. "Trends in asymptomatic nasopharyngeal colonization with Streptococcus pneumoniae after introduction of the 13-valent pneumococcal conjugate vaccine in Calgary, Canada." *Pediatric Infectious Disease Journal*, July 2014; 33(7): 724–30.

198. *Vactruth.com*, Human Vaccine Inserts, "Prevnar 13." July 2019.

199. "Polio Disease in-Short," *Centers for Disease Control and Prevention, Dept. of Health and Human Services,* www.cdc.gov/ vaccines/ vpd-vac/ polio/ in-short-both. htm, accessed June 17, 2013.

200. Humphries & Bystrianyk, *Dissolving lllusions: Disease, Vaccines, and the Forgotten History*, 2013, "Chapter 12: The Disappearance of Polio," p. 232–234.

201. *Ibid.* p. 265

202. Paul A. Offit, "The Cutter Incident: How America's First Polio Vaccine Led to a Growing Vaccine Crisis." *Journal of the Royal Society of Medicine*; Vol 99; Mar 2006.

203. Bookchin, D. & Schumacher, J. "The Virus and the Vaccine," *The Atlantic Monthly*, Feb 2000 issue.

204. Humphries & Bystrianyk, *Dissolving Illusions: Disease, Vaccines, and the Forgotten History*. 2013, p. 230–255.

205. *Ibid*. p. 243–250.

206. Dan Olmsted, "The Age of Polio. Explosion." *Age of Autism*.

207. Humphries, Bystrianyk, 2013, p.251.

208. *ibid*. p.237–240).

209. Miller, Neil Z. *Vaccine Safety Manual*, New Atlantean Press, 2008, p.61–62.

210. "Jonas and Darrell Salk, Creators of the Salk Polio Vaccine." *Science*; Mar 4, 1977.

211. Albert Sabin Dec. 7, 1985 lecture to Italian doctors in Piacenze, Italy, *Healing Our Children*. 2012.

212. Vashisht & Puliyel, "Polio programme: let us declare victory and move on." *Indian Journal of Medical Ethics* Apr–Jun 2012; 9(2): 114–7.

213. Rachana Dhiman et al. "Correlation between Non-Polio Acute Flaccid Paralysis Rates with Pulse Polio Frequency in India." *International Journal of Environmental Research and Public Health*. Aug 2018; 15(8): 1755.199.

214. Robert Roos, "Efficacy of flu shots in children under 2 questioned," *Center for Infectious Disease Research and Policy*, Feb 25, 2005.

215. Bodewes, Kreijtz, Rimmelzwaan, "Yearly influenza vaccinations: a double-edged sword?" *The Lancet Infectious Disease*, 2009 Dec 9(12): 784–8.

216. Simonsen, et al. "Impact of influenza vaccination on seasonal mortality in the US elderly population." *Archives of Internal Medicine*. 2005 Feb 14: 165(3): 265–72.

217. Jefferson, Rivetti et al. "Vaccines for preventing influenza in healthy children." *Cochrane Database System Review*. Feb 2018.

218. Ayoub, Yazbak, "Influenza Vaccination During Pregnancy: A Critical Assessment of the Recommendations of the Advisory Committee on Immunization Practices (ACIP)," *Journal of the American Physicians and Surgeons*. 2006 Summer; 11(2) :41-47.

219. Paul Forster, "To Pandemic or Not? Reconfiguring Global Responses to Influenza, Introduction," *STEPS Centre*, 2012 p. 2.

220. Goldman G, "Comparison of VAERS fetal-loss reports during three consecutive influenza seasons," *Human Environmental Toxicology Journal*, 2013 May; 32(5): 464–475.

221. Cowling, Fang et al., "Increased risk of non-influenza respiratory virus infections associated with receipt of inactivated influenza vaccine," *Clinical Infectious Disorders*, 2012 June 15; 54(12): 1778–83.

222. John Anthony Morris, MD (1919–2014), *Alliance for Human Research Protection*, Sept 27, 2014.

223. Human Vaccine Inserts, *Vaccine Information*: 2017, "Flulaval," vactruth.com.

224. "Influenza Quick Facts." *National Vaccine Information Center.* July 31, 2020.

225. *Human Vaccine Inserts,* Vaccine Information: 2017, M-M-R II Adverse Reactions.

226. "Japan: Why Japan banned MMR vaccine." *Vaccine Confidence Project; May 11, 2019.*

227. Trier & Ronne, "Duration of immunity and occurrence of secondary vaccine failure following vaccination against measles, mumps, and rubella." *Ugeskr Laeger;* July 13, 1992.

228. "Every 2 Hours Another Child Suffers a Seizure;" *Physicians for Informed Consent.* Nov 24, 2019.

229. Shira Miller, MD, "The unofficial vaccine educators: Are CDC funded non-profits sufficiently independent?" *British Medical Journal;* Nov 7, 2017.

230. Dr. Edward Yazbak, "An Autism & Vaccine Link." *Planet Chiropractic.* April 13, 2001.

231. Kubota, Iso, et al. "Association of measles and mumps with cardiovascular disease: The Japan Collaborative Cohort OACC) Study," *Atherosclerosis,* 2015 Aug; 241(2): 682–6.

232. Rosen, Rota, et al. "Outbreak of measles among persons with prior evidence of immunity, New York City, 2011," *Clinical Infectious Diseases,* Vol 58, Issue 9, 2014 May, 1205–1210.

233. Wang, Yan, et al., "Difficulties in Eliminating Measles and Controlling Rubella and Mumps: A Cross-Sectional Study of a First Measles and Rubella Vaccination and a Second Measles, Mumps, and Rubella Vaccination." *PLoS One;* Feb 20, 2014.

234. Deisher, Doan, et al., "Impact of environmental factors on the prevalence of autistic disorder after 1979." *Journal of Public Health Epidemiology,* Sept 2014.

235. Corrigan, S, "Former science chief: 'MMR fears coming true." *Mail Online,* 22 May 2016.

236. Mendelsohn, Robert. *How to Raise a Healthy Child ... In Spite of Your Doctor,* Chapter 19, Measles, 1984 p. 237.

237. *Ibid.* p. 238.

238. Sencer, et al., "Epidemiologic basis for eradication of measles in 1967." *Public Health Reports;* Mar 1967.

239. Poland and Jacobson, "Failure to reach the goal of measles elimination. Apparent paradox of measles infections in immunized persons," *Archive of Internal Medicine,* 1994 Aug 22; 154(16): 1815–1820.

240. Mark Papania, et al. "Increased Susceptibility to Measles in Infants in the United States," *Pediatrics,* Nov 1999.

241. Rosen, Rota, et al., "Outbreak of measles among persons with prior evidence of immunity, New York City, 2011." *Clinical Infectious Disease;* May 2014.

242. *Human Vaccine Inserts,* "Vaccine Information: Measles"; 2017; vactruth.com.

243. Gaston De Serres, et al., "Largest measles epidemic in North America in a decade—Quebec, Canada, 2011: contribution of susceptibility, serendipity, and superspreading events." *Journal of Infectious Diseases;* Mar 15, 2013.

244. See Note 231.

245. Albonico, et al. "Febrile Infectious Childhood Diseases in the History of Cancer Patients and Matched Controls," *PubMed.gov.* 1998 Oct.

246. Peter Aaby, et al. "Low mortality after mild measles infection compared to uninfected children in rural West Africa," *Vaccine.* Nov 22, 2002; 21(1-2): 120–6.

247. *Physicians Desk Reference;* 55th edition, Montvale, NJ: Medical Economics, 2001.

248. Shilavy, Brian, "ZERO U.S. Measles Deaths in 10 Years, but Over 100 Measles Vaccines Deaths Reported," *Health Impact News,* Jan 30, 2015.

249. Fawzi W. et al. "Vitamin A supplementation and Child Mortality: A Meta-Analysis," *Journal of the American Medical Association,* Feb 17, 1993, p. 901.

250. Mendelsohn, Robert. *How to Raise a Healthy Child in Spite of Your Doctor,* Mumps. 1984, p. 234–36.

251. Matson, et al. "Outbreak of Measles in Fully Vaccinated School Population," *Pediatric Infectious Diseases,* 12:292, 1993.

252. "Mumps Cases and Outbreaks," *CDC.* Jan 25, 2020.

253. Cynthia Cournoyer, *What About Immunizations? Exposing the Vaccine Philosophy.* 2010, p. 122.

254. Albonico & Klein et al., "The immunization campaign against measles, mumps and rubella—coercion leading to a realm of uncertainty: medical objections to a continued MMR immunization campaign in Switzerland." *Semantic Scholar;* 1992

255. Maclaren & Atkinson, "Is Insulin-Dependent Diabetes Mellitus Environmentally Induced?" *New England Journal of Medicine;* July 30, 1992; 327:348–349.

256. *Physician's Desk Reference* (PDR); 55th edition. 2001, p. 778.

257. "Mumps Overview," *National Vaccine Information Center;* nvic.org.

258. Mendelsohn, Robert. *How to Raise a Healthy Child in Spite of Your Doctor,* 1984 p. 240.

259. Cynthia Cournoyer, *What About Immunizations? Exposing the Vaccine Philosophy.* 2010, p. 132.

260. Ibid. p. 133.

261. Neil Z. Miller, *Vaccines: Are They Really Safe and Effective?* 2018, p. 36.

262. *Physician's Desk Reference* (PDR); 55th edition. 2001, p. 1966.

263. Mendelsohn, Robert S. "More Vaccine Arguments." *The People's Doctor Newsletter* 8.12. Print.

264. Thomas Cowan, MD. *Vaccines, Autoimmunity, and the Changing Nature of Childhood Illnesses.* 2018 p. 77.

265. "Varivax, Varicella Virus Vaccine Live," *Human Vaccine Inserts,* 2017.

266. Yih, et al., *British Medical Council of Public Health,* Article number 68, June 2005.

267. Colleen Chun, et al. "Laboratory Characteristics of Suspected Herpes Zoster in Vaccinated Children," *Pediatric Infectious Disease Journal,* Aug 2011—30(8): 719–721.

268. Goldman, G.S. and King P.G., "Review of the United States universal varicella vaccination program: Herpes zoster incidence rates, cost-effectiveness, and vaccine efficacy based primarily on the Antelope Valley Varicella Active Surveillance Project data." *Vaccine.* Mar 25, 2013.

269. See Note 265.

270. Wise, R.P. "Postlicensure safety surveillance for varicella vaccine." *Journal of the American Medical Association*, Sept. 13 2000: 1273. 232.

271. "Zostavax: Zoster Vaccine Live," *Human Vaccine Inserts*, vactruth.com, 2017.

272. Neil Z. Miller, *Miller's Review of Critical Vaccine Studies*; 2016 p. 162.

273. Cynthia Cournoyer, *What About Immunizations? Exposing the Vaccine Philosophy.* "HPV" p. 213-214.

274. *Ibid.* p. 215.

275. Dr. Diane Harper talk, *4th International Public Conference on Vaccination.* Oct 2009.

276. Sharyl Attkisson, "Gardasil Researcher Speaks Out." *cbsnews.com*; Aug 19, 2009.

277. "Top Ten Facts for Consideration Regarding the Health Impacts of HPV Vaccination in Children." *Children's Health Defense*; July 3, 2020.

278. Tomljenovic & Shaw, "Human papillomavirus (HPV) vaccine policy and evidence-based medicine: are they at odds?" *Annals of Medicine*, 2013 Mar; 45(2):182–93.

279. "Can HPV Vaccine Cause Injury and Death?" *National Vaccine Information Center*, nvic.org.

280. Tomljenovic and Shaw, "Who Profits from Uncritical Acceptance of Biased Estimates of Vaccine Efficacy and Safety?" *American Journal of Public Health*, Sept 2012 102(9).

281. Dr. Bernard Dalbergue, "Merck's Former Doctor Predicts Gardasil to Become the Greatest Medical Scandal of All Time," *Global Possibilites*, 2013.

282. Geier, Kern, Geier, "A cross-sectional study of the relationship between reported HPV vaccine exposure and the incidence of reported asthma in the U.S." *SAGE Open Medicine*, Jan 2019.

283. Liu, X.C. et al. "Adverse events following HPV vaccination, Alberta 2006–2014," *Vaccine.* Apr 4, 2016; 34(15): 1800–5.

284. Robert F. Kennedy, Jr. *Children's Health Defense*, "25 Reasons to Avoid the Gardasil Vaccine," May 21, 2019.

285. "Human Papillomavirus (HPV) Disease and Vaccine Information," *National Vaccine Information Center*, nvic.org.

286. *Children's Health Defense*, 25 Reasons to Avoid the Gardasil Vaccine, May 21, 2019.

287. *Ibid.*

288. *Ibid.*

289. *Ibid.*

290. Claire P. Rees et al., "Will HPV vaccination prevent cervical cancer?" *Journal of the Royal Society of Medicine*, Jan 21, 2020.

291. Coulter & Fisher, *A Shot in the Dark.* 1991; p. 11–12.

292. "Vaccines have not been shown to cause sudden infant death syndrome (SIDS)," *CDC Vaccine Safety*; Aug 14, 2020.

293. Coulter & Fisher, *A Shot in the Dark: Why the P in the DPT vaccination may be hazardous to your child's health*, "Adverse Reactions: An Afterthought?" Chapter Two, p. 26–57.

294. Brogan & Ji, "Is the Epidemic of Sudden Infant Deaths a Medically Induced 'Syndrome'?" *GreenMedInfo*; June 13, 2014.

295. Neil Z. Miller, "Sudden Infant Syndrome (SIDS)" *Vaccines: Are They Really Safe and Effective?* p. 43.

296. Miller NZ & Goldman, "Infant-mortality rates regressed against number of vaccine doses routinely given: Is there a biochemical or synergistic toxicity?" *Human and Experimental Toxicology*, 2011 Sept; 30(9): 1420–1428.

297. Zinka B, Rauch E, et al. "Unexplained cases of sudden infant death shortly after hexavalent vaccination." *Vaccine* 2006; 24(31-32): 5779–80.

298. Heather Fraser, *The Peanut Allergy Epidemic: What's Causing it and How to Stop It.* 2011 p.122.

299. *Ibid.* p. 106.

300. "Shaken Baby Syndrome: Rotational Cranial Injuries–Technical Report," *Pediatrics* July 2001, 108(1) 206–210.

301. Coulter, H L and Fisher, B L, *A Shot in the Dark: Why the P in DPT vaccination may be hazardous to your health.* p. 46–48.

302. "Gulf War Veterans' Medically Unexplained Illnesses," U.S. Department of Veterans Affairs. *Publichealth.va.gov.*

303. "Research Advisory Committee on Gulf War Veterans' Illnesses Government Report (RACGWVI)." *Vaccine Syndrome movie, YouTube*, 2017.

304. Landee Martin, "Is There a Vaccine-Cancer Connection?" *The Truth About Vaccines*, June 2, 2015.

305. Rosa FW, et al., "Absense of antibody response to simian virus 40 after inoculation with killedpoliovirus vaccine of mother's offspring with neurological tumors." *New England Journal of Medicine*, 1988; 318: 1469.

306. Garcea & Imperiale, "Simian Virus 40 Infection of Humans." *Journal of Virology*; May 2003.

307. Leslie, Kobre, et al. "Temporal Association of Certain Neuropsychiatric Disorders Following Vaccination of Children and Adolescents: A Pilot Case-Control Study, Yale Child Study Center," *Frontiers in Psychiatry*, 19 Jan 2017.

308. "Fortune 500 company average annual gains," *Fortune Magazine*, 2015.

309. Justin McCarthy, "Big Pharma Sinks to the Bottom of U.S. Industry Rankings." *Gallup News*, Sept 3, 2019.

310. Beth Mole, "Big Pharma shells out $20B each year to schmooze docs, $6B on drug ads." *ARS Technica*; Jan 11, 2019.

311. Marcia Angell, MD, *The Truth About the Drug Companies: How They Deceive Us and What to Do about It.* 2004, p. 219.

312. Potter, W. "Opinion: Big Pharma's Stranglehold on Washington," *The Center for Public Integrity*, Feb 11, 2013.

313. Ray Moynihan et al., "Commercial influence in health: from transparency to independence," *British Medical Journal*, 2019.

314. David H. Freedman, "Lies, Damned Lies, and Medical Science." *The Atlantic*. Nov 2010.

315. Robert F. Kennedy Jr., "Vaccine debate with Harvard law professor Alan Dershowitz," *You Tube,* Jul 24, 2020.

316. Joseph Mercola, DO, "Sit Down Science," *www.mercola.com*, Jan 25, 2017.

317. "Close Ties and Financial Entanglements: The CDC-Guaranteed Vaccine Market." *Children's Health Defense;* June 6, 2019.

318. "Hearing–Committee on Government Reform," *House of Representatives, 106 Congress,* June 15, 2000.

319. "Congress Receives Vaccine Safety Project Details, Including Actions Needed for Sound Science and Transparency," *Children's Health Defense,* Mar 13, 2018.

320. *Immunization Action Coalition*, IAC Mission Statement.

321. "Is Doctors' Cash Incentive Sidelining the Hippocratic Oath?" *Children's Health Defense;* Sept 19, 2019.

322. "Congress slams NIH, CDC reps for evading vaccine/autism evidence," *The Canary Party*, Nov 30, 2012.

323. J.B. Handley, *How to End the Autism Epidemic*, 2018, p. 98.

324. *FDA,* "Center for Biologics Evaluation and Research, About CBER," 2/6/2018.

325. U.S. House Committee on Oversight and Government Reform, *106th Congress;* June 15, 2000.

326. "Survey: FDA Scientists (2006)," *Union of Concerned Scientists.* July 11, 2008.

327. Donald W. Light et al. "Institutional Corruption of Pharmaceuticals and the Myth of Safe and Effective Drugs," *Journal of Law, Medicine, and Ethics* (JLME); Fall 2013; 41(3): 590–600.

328. Steven M. Druker, *Altered Genes, Twisted Truth.* 2015.

329. Darrow, Avorn, & Kesselheim, "FDA Approval and Regulation of Pharmaceuticals, 1983–2018," *JAMA,* 2020; 323(@2):164–176.

330. "Rubber Stamping:The FDA and Vaccines—Conflicts of Interest Undermine Children's Health: Part IV." *Children's Health Defense;* May 29, 2019.

331. "Constitutional Attorney on US Federal Drug Administration (FDA) Corruption, Disinformation, and Cover Up of Health Dangers." *Global Research;* Feb 9, 2015.

332. Sharyl Attkisson, "How Independent Are Vaccine Defenders?" *CBS news*, July 25, 2008.

333. "The Pharmaceutical Industry's Front Men." *Children's Health Defense;* July 23, 2019.

334. Jeremy R. Hammond, "American Academy of Pediatrics Refuses to Back Vaccine Claims with Science." *Children's Health Defense;* May 3, 2017.

335. "Richard Gale & Gary Null, PhD, on the Myth of Settled Science." *The Vaccine Reaction;* June 27, 2016.

336. Frank A. Chervenak, et al., "Professional Responsibility and Early Childhood Vaccination." *The Journal of Pediatrics;* Nov 25, 2015.

337. Eric Lipton, "The Chemical Industry Scores a Big Win at the E.P.A." *New York Times*, June 7, 2018.

338. "Glyphosate: Interim Registration Review Decision Case Number 0178." *Environmental Protection Agency.* Jan 2020.

339. "Monsanto Roundup & Dicamba Trial Tracker: Bayer's Monsanto headache persists," *US RTK* Oct 1, 2020.

340. Mogensen, Aaby, et al. "The Introduction of Diphtheria-Tetanus-Pertussis and Oral Polio Vaccine Among Young Infants in an Urban African Community: A Natural Experiment," *EBioMedicine.* 2017 Mar; 17: 192–198.

341. Jeremy Hammond, "WHO Experimenting on African Children without Informed Consent," *Foreign Policy Journal*, Mar 1, 2020.

342. Dr. Joseph Mercola, "New Documentary Exposes WHO's 'Diabolical' Plan to Use Vaccines to Reduce Global Population." *Children's Health Defense;* July 11, 2022.

343. Jeff Stier, "Stop Funding WHO Until It Cleans Up Its Act: U.S. taxpayer funding of scandalplagued World Health Organization needs strings attached." *National Review*, June 14, 2017.

344. "Robert Mugabe's WHO appointment condemned as an insult." *BBC News*, Oct 21, 2017.

345. Marcia Angell, MD, *The Truth About the Drug Companies,* published in the *New York Review of Books,* 2005, p. xxv–xxvi.

346. Geoffrey Spurling et al. "Pharmaceutical company advertising in *The Lancet*," July 2, 2011.

347. Meryl Nass, MD, "The Elephant in the Auditorium—Big Pharma Profiteering on the Bodies of Children," *Alliance for Human Research Protection*, Jan 24, 2020.

348. David L. Lewis, PhD. Science for Sale: How the US Government Uses Powerful Corporations and Leading Universities to Support Government Policies, Silence Top Scientists, Jeopardize Our Health, and Protect Corporate Profits," *Simon & Schuster;* June 3, 2014.

349. Light & Lexchin, "Pharmaceutical research and development: what do we get for all that money?" *British Medical Journal*, Aug 7, 2012; 345.

350. Richard Smith, "Medical Journals: An Extension of the Marketing Arm of Pharmaceutical Companies?" *Health Watch;* Newsletter no. 56: Jan 2005.

351. Peter Gotzsche, *Deadly Medicines and Organized Crime* (2013).

352. Brendan Pierson, "Merck accused of stonewalling in mumps-vaccine antitrust lawsuit," *Reuters*, June 4, 2015.

353. "Joseph Mercola—Wakefield Interview, 4/10/2010," *mercola.com.*

354. Anderson Cooper, *CNN interview of Andrew Wakefield*, Jan 2011.

355. Judy Mikovits, PhD, *Plague, One Scientist's Intrepid Search for the Truth About Human Retroviruses and Chronic Fatigue Syndrome, Autism, and Other Diseases,* Apr 14, 2011.

356. Brandy Vaughan, Founder/Executive Director at Learn The Risk, *Linkedin.com.*

357. Brandy Vaughan, "The post I wish I didn't have to write…" *Facebook,* Dec 1, 2019.

358. Kevin Barry, Esq. *Vaccine Whistleblower: Exposing Autism Research Fraud at the CDC* (2015).

359. Ethan A. Huff, "Secret government documents reveal vaccines to be a total hoax." *Natural News;* Jan 8, 2013.

360. Almashat, Lang, et al. "Twenty-Seven Years of Pharmaceutical Industry Criminal and Civil Penalties: 1991 Through 2017," *Public Citizen*, Mar 14, 2018.

361. Gary G. Kohls, MD, "Why You Can't Trust the FDA, the WHO, the CDC, the AAP, Merck, GlaxoSmithKline, Sanofi, or Pfizer." *Reader News & Articles*; Dec 12, 2019.

362. "Humira, TV commercial statement regarding adverse effects."

363. Ray Moynihan and Alan Cassels, *Selling Sickness: How Drug Companies Are Turning Us All Into Patients* (2005).

364. "Drug Industry, Sen. Frist, and the White House Conspired to Obtain Broad Liability Shield for Lawsuits Related to Pandemic Illnesses." *Public Citizen*; May 4, 2006.

365. Dan Olmsted, "Age of Autism Awards 2010: Dr. Paul Offit, Denialist of the Decade." *Age of Autism*, Dec 29, 2010.

366. Paul Offit, et al. "Addressing parents' concerns: do multiple vaccines overwhelm or weaken the infant's immune system?" *Pediatrics* 2002; 109(1): 124–129.

367. Marco Caceres, "Dr. Offit Quotes: Top 10 List." *Opinion*; Mar 26, 2017.

368. "Dr. Paul Offit's Aluminum Deceptions and Academic Misconduct," *Vaccine Papers*, Feb 13, 2015.

369. Kawahara & Kato-Negishi, "Link between Aluminum and the Pathogenesis of Alzheimer's Disease: The Integration of the Aluminum and Amyloid Cascade Hypotheses." *International Journal of Alzheimer's Disease*. Mar 8, 2011.

370. Robert F. Kennedy, Jr., "Merck's Vaccine Division President Julie Gerberding Sells $9.1 Million in Shares–Is She Jumping Ship?" *Children's Health Defense*; Feb 5, 2020.

371. Lee Fang, "When a Congressman Becomes a Lobbyist, He Gets a 1,452 Percent Raise (On Average)." *RepublicReports.org*. Mar 14, 2012.

372. Chris Mills Rodrigo, "Schiff calls out Facebook, Google over anti-vaccination information." *The Hill*, 2/14/2019.

373. "Bayer Division Sold Hemophilia Drug with HN Risk to Asia, Latin America in 1980s." *Kaiser Health News*; May 23, 2003.

374. Robert F. Kennedy Jr., "Gates Globalist Vaccine Agenda: A Win-Win for Pharma and Mandatory Vaccinations." *Children's Health Defense*; Apr 9, 2020.

375. Rachana Dhiman, et al., "Correlation between Non-Polio Acute Flaccid Paralysis Rates with Pulse Polio Frequency in India." *International Journal of Environmental Research and Public Health*; Aug 15, 2018.

376. See note 374.

377. "India Holds Bill Gates Accountable for His Vaccine Crimes." *Reseau International*, Oct 9, 2014.

378. *Ibid.*

379. Jose Solis, "Vaccine Coverage in Mainstream Media—Variations on a Theme of Propaganda. *Children's Health Defense*, July 3, 2019."

380. Nathan Shasho, "Perspective: Making Sense of It All." *Outskirts Press*; Sept 29, 2015.

381. Ted Kuntz, "How to Win the Vaccine Credibility War." *The Vaccine Reaction*, Jan 2, 2020.

382. 'TED Talk: Sharyl Attkisson Discusses Astroturf's Role in Media Manipulation." *The Daily Scholar*, Feb 6, 2015.

383. Steve Silberman, *NeuroTribes: The Legacy of Autism and the Future of Neurodiversity*. 2015, p. 470.

384. Donvan & Zucker, *In a Different Key: The Story of Autism*, 2016.

385. Michael Fitzpatrick, "The Cutter Incident: How America's First Polio Vaccine Led to a Growing Vaccine Crisis." *Journal of the Royal Society of Medicine*; Mar 2006; 99(3): 156.

386. Torsten Engelbrecht, Claus Kohnlein, MD, Samantha Bailey, MD, Dr. Stefano Scoglio, BSc PhD, *Virus Mania*, 2021, pg. 11.

387. World Health Organization, "Bangul Definition" (1986); *Virus Mania*, 2021, pg. 103.

388. Torsten Engelbrecht, et al., *Virus Mania*, 2021, pg. 130.

389. Venters, George, "New variant Cruetzfeldt-Jakob disease: the epicemic that never was, *British Medical Journal*, Oct 13, 2001, p. 858–861.

390. Grippe-Pandemie: Uno rechnet mit 150 Millionen Tote, *Spiegel Online*, 30 September 2005.

391. Siegel, Marc, "Why we shouldn't fear bird flu." *Ottawa Citizen*, Sept 19, 2005, p. A15.

392. Rokuro, Hama et al., Oseltamivir and early deterioration leading to death: a proportional mortality study for 2009A/H1N1 influenza, *International Journal of Risk and Safety in Medicine*, 2011, pg. 201–215.

393. "CDC Concludes Zika Causes Microphaly and Other Birth Defects." *CDC Newsroom*, Apr 13, 2016.

394. "Report from Physicians in the Crop-Sprayed Town regarding Dengue-Zika, microcephaly, and massive spraying with chemical poisons." *Red Universitaria de Ambiente Y Salud*. Feb 9, 2016.

395. Claire Robinson, "Argentine and Brazilian doctors suspect mosquito insecticide as cause of microcephaly." *Ecologist: The Journal for the Post-Industrial Age*. Feb 10, 2016.

396. "Emergency Use Authorization for Vaccines Explained/FDA." www.fda.gov, Nov.20, 2020.

397. Patrick Delaney, "Former Pfizer VP: No need for vaccines, the pandemic is effectively over." *LifeSiteNews*, Nov 23, 2020.

398. Robert F. Kennedy Jr., "New Docs: NIH Owns Half of Moderna Vaccine." *Children's Health Defense*; July 7, 2020.

399. Public Health Emergency, "Public Readiness and Emergency Preparedness Act." *U.S. Dept. of Health & Human Services;* Dec 3, 2020.

400. "How Billions in COVID Stimulus Funds Led to Dangerous, Tyrannical Policies in U.S. Schools." *Children's Health Defense Team,* Jan 20, 2022.

401. "The Truth About Lockdowns." *Rational Ground—Clear Reasoning on National Policy for COVID-19.* July 6, 2021.

402. Paul Elias Alexander, "More Than 400 Studies on the Failure of Compulsory Covid Interventions." *Brownstone Institute,* Nov 30, 2021.

403. Geert Vanden Bossche, DMV, PhD., "Letter to the WHO," *geertvandenbossche.org;* Mar 6, 2021.

404. Megan Redshaw, "More than 1.3 Million Adverse Events Following COVID Vaccines Reported to VAERS, CDC Data Show." *Children's Health Defense,* July 11, 2022.

405. Dr. Joseph Merdola, "People Injured by COVID-19 Jab Share Their Horror Stories" *Articles.mercola.com, Oct 5, 2021.*

406. Whistleblower Testimony, "America's Frontline Doctors, et al., vs. Xavier Becerra, Secretary of the U.S. DHHS, et al." Preliminary Injunction, *Civil Action No. 2:21-cv-00702-CLM,* Filed 07/19/21

407. Nikolai Eroshenko et al., "Implications of antibody-dependent enhancement of infection for SARS-CoV-2 countermeasures." *Nature Biotechnology;* June 5, 2020.

408. James Lyons-Weiler, "Pathogenic priming likely contributes to serious and critical illness and mortality in COVID-19 via autoimmunity." *Journal of Translational Autoimmunity;* Apr 9, 2020.

409. "Media Hypes Moderna's COVID Vaccine, Downplays Risks." *Children's Health Defense; Nov 17, 2020.*

410. Dr. Joseph Mercola, "COVID-19 'Vaccines' Are Gene Therapy." *Articles.mercola .com,* Mar 16, 2021.

411. "Components of mRNA Technology "Could Lead to Significant Adverse Events in One or More of Our Clinical Trials," says Moderna." *Children's Health Defense;* Aug 6, 2020.

412. Dr. Joseph Mercola, "The Many Ways in Which COVID Vaccines May Harm Your Health." *Articles.mercola.com,* June 13, 2021.

413. Brock & Thornley, "Spontaneous Abortions and Policies on COVID-19 mRNA Vaccine Use During Pregnancy." *Science, Public Health Policy, and the Law;* Volume 4:130–143, Nov 2021.

414. Katharine Lee, et al., "Investigating trends in those who experience menstrual bleeding changes after SARS-Co-2 vaccination." *Science Advances;* July 15, 2022, Vol 8, Issue 28.

415. Steven R. Gundry, "Abstract 10712: MRNA COVID Vaccines Dramatically Increase Endothelial Inflammatory Markers and ACS Risk as Measured by the PULS Cardiac Test: a Warning." *Circulation,* Nov 8, 2021.

416. Dr. Joseph Mercola, "Why Aren't We Investigating Surge in Sudden Deaths of Athletes?" *Children's Health Defense;* Feb 18, 2022.

417. Michael Nevradakis, PhD, "COVID Vaccine Mandate for Pilots Violates Federal Law, Puts Passengers at Risk, Citizen Group Warns." *Children's Health Defense;* Apr 18, 2022.

418. "15 Embalmers Confirm 'New" Fatal Strange Clots Since 2021 Vaccine Roll-Out."
     True Democracy Party; June 12, 2022.

419. "COVID-19: The Science We Should Know." *The National Heallth Federation,*
     thenhf.com/resources/covid-19-the-science-we-should-know, Nov 17, 2021.

420. Steve Kirsch, "All you need to know about COVID vaccine safety." *www.skirsch.io;*
     Oct 17, 2021.

421. Mikki Willis, 'Plandemic: 100% Censored. 0% Debunked." 2021, p. 26.

422. Dr. Joseph Mercola & Ronnie Cummins, *The Truth About COVID-19: Exposing the
     Great Reset, Lockdowns, Vaccine Passports, and the New Normal;* 2021, p. 78.

423. Dr. Joseph Mercola, "Are the COVID Shots Working?" *Articles.mercola.com,* Oct
     13, 2021.

424. Henry Ealy, et al., "COVID-19 Data Collection, Comorbidity & Federal Law: A
     Historical Retrospective." *Science, Public Health Policy, and The Law, Volume 2:4–
     22, Oct 12, 2020.*

425. Sharyl Attkisson, "Counting Covid," *Full Measure,* Sinclair Broadcasting Network,
     Sept 20, 2021.

426. Hilda Labrada Gore, "Frontline Nurses Speak Out," *Weston A. Price Foundation;*
     Apr 12, 2021.

427. Andrew Mark Miller, "CDC director acknowledges hospitals have a monetary
     incentive to overcount coronavirus deaths." *Washington Examiner,* Aug 1, 2020.

428. Michelle Rogers, "Fact check: Hospitals get paid more if patients listed as COVID-
     19, on ventilators." *USA Today Network,* Apr 24, 2020.

429. Shiyi Cao et al., "Post-lockdown SARS-CoV-2 nucleic acid screening in nearly ten
     million residents of Wuhan, China." *Nature Communications,* Nov 20, 2020.

430. Dr. Robert Malone, "The Hidden Gateway podcast Episode 43: Speaking Truth to
     Power: A Scientific Odyssey," Oct 7, 2021.

431. Paul E. Alexander, et al., "Early Multidrug Outpatient Treatment of SARS-CoV-2
     Infection (COVID-19) and Reduced Mortality Among Nursing Home Residents."
     medRXiv, Feb 1, 2021.

432. Simone Gold, MD, JD "White Paper on Hydroxychlorquine" I Do Not Consent,
     Bombardier Books, 2020, p. 84.

433. Dr. Vladimir Zelenko, "Two New Studies Test Quercetin and COVID Outcomes."
     Articles.mercola.com, Oct 14, 2021.

434. Dr. Joseph Mercola, "Journal of Medicine Says HCQ + Zinc Reduces COVID
     Deaths." *Articles.mercola.com,* Feb 1, 2021.

435. Pierre Kory, MD, et al., "Review of the Emerging Evidence Demonstrating the
     Efficacy of Ivermectin in the Prophylaxis and Treatment of COVID-19." *FLCCC
     Alliance,* Dec 7, 2020.

436. The 2015 Nobel Prize in Medicine—Press release regarding Ivermectin, Oct 5, 2015.

437. Dr. Peter A. McCullough, et al., "Pathophysiological Basis and Rationale for Early
     Outpatient Treatment of SARS-Co-2 (COVID-19) Infection." *American Journal of
     Medicine.* Jan 2021.

438. Jon Cohen & Kai Kupferschmidt, "The 'very, very bad look' of remdesivir, the first FDA-approved COVID-19 drug." *Science,* Oct 28, 2020.

439. Gain of Function Research, *National Institute of Health, Office of Science Policy.* May 15, 2019.

440. Luc Montagnier interview on CNews, "French Nobel prize winner: Covid-19 made in lab." *The Connexion: French news and views.* Sept 19, 2020.

441. Robert Redfield, MD, "Former CDC Director Believes Coronavirus Came from Lab in China."1*CNN interview with Sanjay Gupta,* Mar 26, 2021.

442. Fred Guterl, "Dr. Fauci Backed Controversial Wuhan Lab with Millions of U.S. Dollars for Risky Coronavirus Research." *Newsweek*, Apr 28, 2020.

443. Dr. Joseph Mercola, "Wuhan Lab Caught Deleting Files Proving Fauci Funding." *Articles.mercola.com,* May 26, 2021.

444. Hub staff report, "Public health experts condemn 'dangerous' research funded by government." *Johns Hopkins University*, Feb 28, 2019.

445. Nikolas Lanum, "Chinese Whistleblower Exposes COVID-19's origins." Tucker Carlson interview, *foxnews.com,* June 30, 2021.

446. "Top 5 Myths about the Immunization Infrastructure Modernization Act." *Stand for Health Freedom,* Dec 10, 2021.

447. "Biden: 'Patience wearing thin with unvaccinated Americans'—video." *The Guardian,* Sept 10, 2021.

448. "Vaccine Passports: Your Ticket to a New Social Control System." *Citizen's Journal;* Jan 26, 2022.

449. Dr. Joseph Mercola, "Pfizer Admits Israel Is the Great COVID-19 Vaccine Experiment." *Articles.mercola.com,* Sept 21, 2021.

450. Martin Kulldorff, "A Review and Autopsy of Two COVID Immunity Studies." *The Vaccine Reaction,* Nov 7, 2021.

451. Sivan Gazit et al., "Comparing SARS-CoV-2 natural immunity to vaccine-induced immunity: Reinfections versus breakthrough infections." *MedRxiv, BMJ Yale,* Aug 25, 2021.

452. "Pfizer Admits Israel Is the Great COVID-19 Vaccine Experiment—History Repeating Itself?" *Total Health Matters,* Sept 25, 2021.

453. Subramanian & Kumar, "Increases in COVID-19 are unrelated to levels of vaccination across 68 countries and 2947 counties in the United States." *European Journal of Epidemiology,* Sept 30, 2021.

454. Seth Hancock, "FDA Should Need only '12 Weeks' to Release Pfizer Data, Not 75 Years, Plaintiff Calculates." *Children's Health Defense; Dec 17, 2021.*

455. Mimi Nguyen Ly, "Judge Gives FDA Just Over 8 Months to Produce Pfizer's Safety Data." *The Epoch Times;* Jan 8, 2022.

456. Dr. Joseph Mercola, "Breaking—Japan Puts Warnings on COVID Jabs." *Articles. mercola.com*, Dec. 29, 2021.

457. John Elflein, "COVID-19 deaths worldwide as of January 03, 2022, by country." *Statista.com,* Jan 7, 2022

458. "The Great Barrington Declaration," *gbdeclaration.org;* Oct 4, 2020.

459. The Rome Declaration, "Thousands of Physicians and Medical Scientists Sign 'Rome Declaration' in Protest, Launch New Information Platform." *International Allliance of Physicians and Medical Scientists,* Sept 23, 2021.

460. Florence Nightingale, "Notes on Nursing, 1st ed., 1860, p.32; taken from Béchamp or Pasteur? A Lost Chapter in the History of Biology; 1923, p.13.

461. "The Great Hippocrates, Father of Modern Medicine." *The Health Moderator,* Jan 14, 2013.

462. Bruce H. Lipton, PhD, *The Biology of Belief Unleashing the Power of Consciousness, Matter, & Miracles;* 2008 p. 78.

463. Jay L. Hoecker, MD, "Autism treatment: Can chelation therapy help?" *Mayo Clinic,* Nov 23, 2016.

464. Jeffery Bradstreet, et al. "Biomarker–guided interventions of clinically relevant conditions associated with autism spectrum disorders and attention deficit hyperactivity disorder." *Alternative Medical Review,* Apr 2010.

INDEX

21st Century Cures Act, 11

A
AAP (American Academy of Pediatrics), pharmaceutical industry and, 142–143
ACIP (Advisory Committee on Immunization Practices), 138
acute flaccid paralysis (AFP), 109
acute infections, 51
adaptive immunity, 52–54
ADDM (Autism and Developmental Disabilities Monitoring) Network, 23–24
ADE (antibody-dependent enhancement), 101, 183
ADHD (attention deficit/hyperactive disorder), 20, 28
adjuvants, 78
    ASIA (autoimmune/inflammatory syndrome induced by adjuvants), 86
administration site conditions, 68
adverse effects
    anaphylaxis, 84
    autoimmune disorders, 85–86
    demyelination, 84–85
    DNA alteration, 82
    heavy metals, 83
    immune system suppression, 82
    immunogenicity, 83

infectious diseases, 83
IOM (Institute of Medicine) and, 87–88
leaky gut syndrome, 86–87
live-virus vaccinations, 83
microbiome disorders, 85–86
mucous membranes, 82
myeline sheath and, 82
AHA (American Heart Association), 185
allergen free diet, 213
allopathic model of medicine, 206–208
aluminum, 38–40, 72–73
Alzheimer's disease, 38, 41, 47, 72, 73, 151
AMA (American Medical Association)
    Code of Medical Ethics, xvii, 3
anaphylaxis, 68, 83–84, 87, 88, 101, 111, 115, 117, 118, 120, 182, 184, 186
anthrax vaccine, 46
anti-vaxxer term, xix–xxi
antibiotics, 46–47, 79
antibodies, 78–79
antigens, 77–78, 79
apnea, 34, 68, 105, 125
arthralgia, 68, 117, 119
arthritis, 46, 68, 72, 86, 87, 88, 94, 101, 111, 117, 153, 166
artificial immunity, 49

ASD (autism spectrum disorder), 8,
   21–24, 28, 40, 75
   Applied Behavioral Analysis, 211
   Astroturf movement, 163–165
   as autoimmune disorder, 70
   biomedical treatment options,
      209–214
   chelation therapy, 71
   connection, 19–20
   glutathione and, 71
   increase in, 70
   leaky gut syndrome and, 71
   metallothionein (MT), 71
   rates, 22–24, 221–222
   vaccine-induced, 72–74
ASIA (autoimmune/inflammatory
   syndrome induced by adjuvants), 86
assumptions
   autism, 67–76
   disease elimination, 55–66
   effectiveness, 48–54
   neurological disorders, 67–76
   risks, 31–47
   safety and benefits, 31–47
asthma, 20, 29, 30, 47, 68, 86–87, 96,
   108, 122, 165, 215
Astroturf movement, 163–165
ataxia, 111, 115
atrophy, limbs, 115
autism. *See* ASD (autism spectrum
   disorder)
autoimmune disorders, 21, 38–39,
   46, 185
   ASIA (autoimmune/
      inflammatory syndrome
      induced by adjuvants), 86
   autism as, 70
   GWS (Gulf War Syndrome) and,
      127

microbiome and, 85–86
Avian Flu (H5N1), 172–173

B
bacteria
   antibiotics and, 79
   antigens, 79
   autoimmunity and, 86
   cholera and, 56
   diphtheria and, 97
   dysentery and, 56
   germ theory and, 205
   Hib and, 101–102
   inactivated vaccines and, 90
   innate bacteria and, 52
   microbiome and, 85, 212–213
   pertussis (whooping cough) and,
      98
   pneumococcal disease and, 104
   probiotics and, 214
   scarlet fever and, 56
   tetanus (lockjaw) and, 100–101
   toxoid vaccines and, 91
   typhoid fever and, 56
bacterial meningitis, 102
BBB (blood brain barrier), polysorbate
   80 and, 45
Béchamp, Antoine
   host theory, 206
   Pasteur and, 206–207
Bell's Palsy, 68, 118
Bentham, Jeremy, 5
Bernays, Edward, 162
Big Pharma. *See also* pharmaceutical
   industry
   vaccine orthodoxy and, 19–20
Big Tobacco, 18–19
Biggs, J.T., 60
blood and lymphatic system disorders,
   68

BMGF (Bill and Melinda Gates Foundation), 145, 160–161
brachial neuritis, 87, 101
brain damage, mercury and, 71
BSE (Bovine Spongiform Encephalopathy), Mad Cow Disease, 171–172

C
CA Senate Bill 277, 6–7
cancers, vaccine-induced, 128–129
cardiac disorders, 68
casein-free diet, 213
casual deniers, xviii
CDC (Centers for Disease Control)
    data manipulation, 139
    pharmaceutical industry and, 137–139
    vaccine recommendations, 24–25
cell culture media, 79–80
cell-mediated immune system, 52, 54
censorship, 201–203, 223
cerebral edema, shaken baby syndrome (SBS), 126
Cervarix (HPV), 120
CHD (Children's Health Defense), 37
chelation therapy, 71, 210–212
chemokines, 73
chickenpox (varicella-zoster virus) vaccine, 53, 118–119
children
    childhood cancers, 21, 128–129
    childhood diseases, 16, 218–219
    childhood health in the 1950s versus 1980s, 17–18
    chronic conditions, 20
    COVID-19 vaccine, 178
chiropractic medicine, 210
cholera, 56
chronic conditions, 51

chronic illnesses in children, 20
CNS (central nervous system), microglia, 73
coercion, government and, 201–203
conjugate vaccines, 91
contagious (zymotic) diseases, 60–61
conventional medicine, 207–208
Coronavirus (SARS-CoV-2), 175–203. *See also* COVID-19 vaccine
    acquired immunity, 180
    COVID-19 Early Treatment Fund, 186
    data falsification, 190–192
    GOF (gain of function) research, 192–194
    lockdown impact, 178–179
    mutations, 180
    origins, 192–195
    risk, relative *versus* absolute, 181–182
    SARS-Co-2 spike protein, 184–185
    treatment options, 187–189
cost of vaccinations, 89
court cases
    Buck vs. Bell, 2–3
    Jacobson v. Massachusetts, 2
    medical experiments, 2–3
Couter, Harris L., 17–18
COVID-19 Early Treatment Fund, 186
COVID-19 vaccine, 10, 92
    ADE (antibody-dependent enhancement), 183
    adverse reactions, 182–187
    American Heart Association (AHA), 185
    boosters, 179–180
    deaths, 182–183
    disease enhancement, 183
    effectiveness, 179–181

EUA (Emergency Use Authorization), 175
government enticement, 176
Great Barrington Declaration, 199–200
immune enhancement, 183
immune system dysregulation, 184–185
Israeli Experiment, 196–198
Japan, vaccination policies, 198–199
Moderna, 177
mRNA vaccines, 184
mutation emergence, 180–181
National Health Federation studies, 186
Operation Warp Speed, 175
pregnant women, 185
Rome Declaration, 200–201
schoolchildren, 178
transmissibility, 192
vaccine passports, 195–196
whistleblower testimony, 183
Creutzfeldt-Jakob disease, 171–172
cytokines, 73

D
dementia, 38, 73
demyelination, 22, 71–72, 84–85, 94
detoxification treatment, 211–212
DHHS (Dept. of Health and Human Services), 32–33
diabetes, 47, 72, 86, 95, 102, 105, 116, 125, 166, 191
Dick-Kronenberg, Letitia, 205
diphtheria, 57, 95–98
discontinued vaccines, 33, 92
disease
    history, 55–56

living conditions and, 55–56, 217–218
disease enhancement, 183
DNA (deoxyribonucleic acid), 79, 82, 91, 151, 220
DNA alteration, 82
DPT (diphtheria-pertussis-tetanus) shot, 17–18
DTP (diphtheria, tetanus toxoid, pertussis), 87
DuBeau, Gretchen, 48
dysentery, 56

E
ear and labyrinth disorders, 68
eczema, 28, 87
encephalitis, 68, 84, 95, 108, 111, 115, 116, 117, 118, 121
encephalomyelitis, 46, 86, 98, 101
encephalopathy, 24, 36, 68, 74, 87, 98, 111, 117, 170
ENGERIX-B (Hepatitis B Vaccine [Recombinant]) product insert, 67–69
EPA (Environmental Protection Agency), pharmaceutical industry and, 144–145
erythema multiforme, 68, 103
ethics, pharmaceutical industry and, 167–168
evidence of harm, 69–72
evolution of man, 15–16
evolutionary immune process, 53–54
excipient ingredients, 78
excitotoxins, 73
eye disorders, 68

F
false claims about viruses, 169–170
Fasano, Alessio, 86–87

Fauci, Anthony, NIAID (National Institute of Allergy and Infectious Diseases), 193

FDA (Food and Drug Administration)
  EUA (Emergency Use Authorization), 176
  GMOs (genetically modified organisms), 141
  Pfizer documentation, 198
  pharmaceutical industry and, 139–141

fears about vaccine safety, dismissal, xv

fetal cells, 79–81

FOIA (Freedom of Information Act), 70

food allergies, 20–21

forced sterilization, 2–3

formaldehyde, 40–41

free radicals, 73
  antioxidants, 214
  ozone therapy, 212

functional medicine, 208–209

G

Gandhi, Mahatma, 61

Gardasil (HPV), 119–123

gastrointestinal disorders, 68, 70

gastrointestinal tract (gut), 39
  autoimmune diseases, 85–86
  immune system, 82

GAVI (Global Alliance for Vaccines and Immunization) and, 160

genital warts, 120

germ theory *vs.* host theory, 205–216

glutathione, 22, 83, 211, 212, 214

glutathione antioxidant capacity, 44, 71

gluten-free diet, 213

GMOs (genetically modified organisms), FDA and, 141

GOF (gain of function) research, 192–194

grass roots organization, 223–227

Great Barrington Declaration, 199–200

Guillain-Barre Syndrome, 68, 101, 111, 121, 170

Gulf War Syndrome (GWS), 46, 127–128

H

H5N1 (Avian Flu), 172–173

Hayflick, Leonard, 80–81

Health Medicine Division of the National Academies of Sciences, Engineering, and Medicine, 88

heavy metal chelation, 211–212

Hedrich, A.W., 49–50

hematoma (subdural), 126

Hemophilus influenzae Type B meningitis (HiB), vaccine study, 101–103

hemorrhage, retinal, 126

hepatitis, autoimmune, 121

hepatitis, 81, 90, 130
  hepatitis B, 22, 91
    Hexavalent, 125
    vaccine, 24, 26, 67–68, 88
    vaccine study, 92–95

herd immunity, 49–51, 220

Hib vaccine, 87, 101–102

Hippocrates, 207

Hitler, Adolf, 131

HIV/AIDS (Human Immunodeficiency Virus/Acquired Immunodeficiency Syndrome), 170–171

homeopathic doctors, 210
homeopathy, low dose
  immunotherapy (LDI), 212
host theory, 206
human papilloma virus (HPV)
  vaccine study, 119–123
Humira, 153–154
humoral immune system, 52–54
Humphries, Suzanne, 77
hyperbaric oxygen, 212
hypotonia, 34, 105

I
IAC (Immunization Action
  Coalition), 138
ignorance, xiii–xiv
immune activation events, 72
immune enhancement, 183
immune system, 52
  ASIA (autoimmune/
    inflammatory syndrome
    induced by adjuvants), 86
  disorders, 68
  evolutionary immune process,
    53–54
  innate immunity, 52
  suppression, 82
immunity
  acquired, 180
  adaptive
    cell-mediated immune system,
      52, 54
    humoral immune system,
      52–54
  artificial immunity, 49
  herd immunity, 49–51
  innate immunity, 52
  natural immunity, 48–49

Immunization Infrastructure
  Modernization Act (H.R. 550),
  195–196
immunogenicity, 83
inactivated vaccines, 90
infant mortality rates, 20
infectious diseases, 83, 84
influenza (flu), vaccine study, 109–111
informed consent, 3
infrared sauna, 212
ingredients, Chinese, 47–48
injury potential, 12–13
innate immunity, 52
inoculation theory, 77–79
institutional racism, 4
intentional deniers, xviii
intervention, treatment and, 209
intussusception, 104
IOM (Institute of Medicine), adverse
  reactions to vaccines, 87–88
Israeli Experiment, COVID-19
  vaccine, 196–198

J
JAMA Psychiatry, on autism, 19
Japan, rates of vaccine, 25–26
Jenner, Edward, 58

K
Kawasaki Syndrome, 86, 119
Kennedy, Robert F., Jr., 37, 43, 141

L
leaky gut syndrome, 70, 71, 86–87, 206
learning disabilities, 20
legislation
  21st Century Cures Act, 11
  CA Senate Bill 277, 6–7
  HR 2232 (Vaccinate All Children
    Act), 9

HR 2527 (Vaccinate All Children Act of 2019), 9
HR 6666, Testing, Reaching, and Contacting Everyone (TRACE) Act, 11–12
SB 2350 (Texas), 9
SB 276 (California), 7–8
leukemia, 95, 128, 151, 184
Litton, Bruce, 15
live attenuated vaccines, 90
live-virus vaccinations, 83
living conditions, disease and, 55, 217–218
   cholera, 56
   dysentery, 56
   scarlet fever, 56
   tuberculosis (TB), 56
   typhoid fever, 56
   typhus fever, 56
   yellow fever, 56
lobbying money, pharmaceutical industry, 132–133
Lou Gehrig's disease, 38, 47
low dose immunotherapy (LDI), 212
lupus, 38, 46, 72, 86, 94, 121

M
macrophagic myofasciitis (MMF), 38, 40
Malcolm X, 217
mandatory vaccines, 4–7
measles
   mortality rates, 57
   mumps, rubella (MMR), vaccine study, 111–113
measles (rubeola) vaccine study, 113–116
media messaging, 221–222
medical experiments. *See also* ethics
   early court decisions, 2–3

history, 1–2
   institutional racism and, 4
   medical school, vaccine information, xvi–xvii
Medicare, pharmaceutical industry and, 133–134
Mendelsohn, Robert, 64–65
meningitis, 68, 83, 87, 95, 96, 103, 104, 116, 117, 118, 130, 146, 161
   bacterial, 102
   Hib (Hemophilus influenzae Type B Meningitis), 101–102
   viral, 102
mercury
   brain damage and, 71
   thimerosal (ethylmercury), 41–45
metallothionein (MT), 71, 83
methylation, 212
microbiome, 85–87
microcephaly, Zika virus and, 173–175
microglia, 73
Mill, John Stuart, 5
misinformation, government and, 201–203
mitochondria, 74, 211
MMR vaccine, 87
Moderna, COVID-19 vaccine, 177
money in politics, 131–132
morbidity *versus* mortality, 65–66
mortality rates
   diphtheria, 57
   disease in the U.S., 57
   infant mortality, 20
   measles, 57
   scarlet fever, 57
   typhoid, 57
   whooping cough, 57
mortality *versus* morbidity, 65–66
mouse toxicity test, 124
mRNA (messenger RNA) vaccines, 91

American Heart Association
(AHA), 185
COVID-19 vaccine, 184
Polyethylene glycol (PEG), 184
MSDS (Material Safety Data Sheet), 44
MSG (monosodium glutamate), 47
Multiple Sclerosis (MS), 38, 68, 86
mumps, vaccine study, 116–117
mutation, 68, 82, 166, 180, 221
mutations of vaccine, 69
myelin
    demyelination, 84–85
    methylation and, 212
myelin sheath, 22, 46, 71, 82, 94
myelitis (transverse), 68, 103, 107, 111,
    118, 121
myocarditis, 101, 178, 182, 186, 198

N
NAIP (National Adult Immunization
    Plan), 10–11
narcolepsy, 46, 86, 173
natural immunity, 48–49
naturopathic doctors, 210
NCVIA (National Childhood Vaccine
    Injury Act), 32, xv
NDD (neurodevelopmental disorder),
    8, 22, 28
neomycin, 46–47
nervous system disorders, 68
neuritis, 46, 68
    brachial neuritis, 87, 101
    ocular neuritis, 111
    optic neuritis, 68, 94, 115, 119, 121
    polyneuritis, 117
neuropathy, 34, 68
    polyneuropathy, 117
NIAID (National Institute of Allergy
    and Infectious Diseases), 193
Nightingale, Florence, 205

Nuremberg Trials, 3–4
NVIC (National Vaccine Information
    Center), xiv
    influenza (flu), 111
    mumps, 117
    pertussis (whooping cough), 100
NVICP (National Vaccine Injury
    Compensation Program), 32
    Vaccine Court, 34–36

O
Obsessive-Compulsive Disorder
    (OCD), 129–130
Omnibus Autism Proceeding (OAP),
    73–74
Operation Warp Speed, 175
optic neuritis, 68, 94, 115, 119, 121
OPV (oral polio vaccine), 87
orchitis, 116
otitis media, 28, 104
oxidative stress, 211, 212
ozone therapy, 212

P
Pan, Richard, 7–9
pancreatitis, 87, 111, 121
Parkinson's disease, 38, 73, 86, 115,
    151, 186
Pasteur, Louis
    Béchamp and, 206–207
    germ theory and, 205
pathogenic priming, 183
peanut allergies, 126
pertussis (whooping cough), vaccine
    study, 98–100
pharmaceutical industry, 13–14,
    220–221
    AAP (American Academy of
        Pediatrics) and, 142–143
    Bernays, Edward, 162

Big Pharma, 19–20
BMGF (Bill and Melinda Gates
    Foundation) and, 160–161
CDC (Centers for Disease
    Control) and, 137–139
criminal conduct cases, 136
critics
    Angell, Marcia, 147
    Gotzsche, Peter, 149
    Horton, Richard, 147
    Krahling, Stephen, 149
    Lewis, David, 148
    Mikovits, Judy, 151
    Nass, Meryl, 147–148
    Smith, Richard, 148–149
    Tomljenovic, Lucija, 152–154
    Vaughan, Brandy, 151–152
    Wakefield, Andrew, 149–150
    Wlochowski, Joan, 149
defenders
    Fauci, Anthony, 155–156
    Frist, Bill, 156
    Gerberding, Julie, 158–159
    Offit, Paul, 156–158
    Reuben, Scott, 156
    Schiff, Adam, 159
    Tauzin, Billy, 159
EPA (Environmental Protection
    Agency) and, 144–145
ethics and, 167–168
FDA (Food and Drug
    Administration) and, 139–141
GAVI (Global Alliance for
    Vaccines and Immunization)
    and, 160
Humira, 153–154
illness definition and, 154
legal settlements, 153
lobbying money, 132–133
Medicare and, 133–134

pricing and, 133–134
regulations, 132
study funding, 134–137
study reporting, 135–136
WHO (World Health
    Organization) and, 145–147
pneumococcal disease (PCV7/PCV13/
    PPSV23), vaccine study, 104–105
pneumonia, 28, 84, 102, 104, 105, 111,
    119
Poling, Hannah, 74–76
poliomyelitis (polio), vaccine study,
    105–109
Polyethylene glycol (PEG), 184
polysorbate 80, 45
preservatives, 79
prevention of illness, 209
pro-vaxxer term, xix–xxi
purpura, 34, 121
Pythagoras, 169

Q
QR codes (Quick Response Code),
    vaccine passports, 195–196

R
racism, institutional racism, 4
recombinant vaccines, 91
reporting system, 32–33
respiratory, thoracic, and mediastinal
    disorders, 68
retinal hemorrhage, 126
rhinitis (hay fever), 28
RNA (ribonucleic acid), 190
Rockefeller Foundation Population
    Council, 4
Rome Declaration, COVID-19
    vaccine, 200–201
rotavirus, vaccine study, 103–104
rubella (German measles), 117

S

Sabin, Albert, 63, 108

safety, assumptions, 31–47

Salk, Jonas, 108

SARS (Severe Acute Respiratory Syndrome), 172

SARS-Co-2 spike protein, 184–185

scarlet fever, 56–57

seizure disorders, 21

seizures, 20, 46, 47, 68, 95, 101, 102, 103, 104, 105, 111, 112, 115, 117, 118, 215

serum sickness, 68

shaken baby syndrome (SBS), vaccine-induced, 126–127

Shaw, George Bernard, 62

shingles (herpes zoster), 53, 81, 83, 118, 119, 158, 186

shingles vaccine (Zostavax), 119

SIDS (sudden infant death syndrome), 8, 124–125

Simpsonwood Conference, 69–72

Sinclair, Upton, 67

sleep disorders, 70

smallpox, 58–66

vaccine early critics, 58–66

speech disorders, 70

squalene, 46

stabilizers, 79

Stevens-Johnson Syndrome, 111, 118

streptomycin, 46–47

studious deniers, xviii

subunit (acellular) vaccines, 91

swine flu, 170, 173

syncope, 68, 111

T

tetanus (lockjaw), vaccine study, 100–101

thimerosal (ethylmercury), 41–45, 71

thrombocytopenia, 87, 94, 103, 111, 117, 118, 125, 184

Tourette's syndrome, 127, 165, 215

toxins

antigens, 79

environmental, 52

ASIA and, 86

excitotoxins, 73

host theory of disease, 206

microbiome and, 86–87

in vaccines, 8, 16

aluminum, 38–40, 157–158

autism and, 69

demyelination, 71, 85

formaldehyde, 40–41

monosodium glutamate (MSG), 47

myelin sheath damage, 82

neomycin, 46–47

polysorbate 80, 45

squalene, 46

streptomycin, 46–47

thimerosal (ethylmercury), 41–45

vitamin K shot, 24

toxoid vaccines, 91

Tripedia, discontinuation, 33–34

tuberculosis (TB), 56

scarlet fever and, 56

Tuskegee Syphilis Experiment, 2

typhoid, mortality rates, 57

typhoid fever, 56

typhus fever, 56

U

UCS (Union of Concerned Scientists), 140

utilitarianism, mandatory vaccines and, 4–5

V

vaccinated vs. unvaccinated children, 27–30
vaccination (inoculation)
  cost, 89
  description, 16
  pressure, xvii
vaccine choice, 1–14
Vaccine Court, 34–36
vaccine ingredients
  adjuvant, 78
  aluminum, 38–40
  antibiotics, 79
  antibodies, 78–79
  antigens, 79
  cell culture media, 79–80
  excipient, 78
  formaldehyde, 40–41
  MSG (monosodium glutamate), 47
  neomycin, 46–47
  polysorbate 80, 45
  preservatives, 79
  squalene, 46
  stabilizer, 79
  streptomycin, 46–47
  thimerosal (ethylmercury), 41–45
vaccine orthodoxy, 221
  Big Pharma and, 19–20
  reinforcement, xiv
vaccine passports, 195–196
vaccine rates
  increase in use, 24–27
  Japan, 25–26
vaccine safety science flaws, 165–167
vaccine schedule for children, xv
  aluminum and, 38
  CDC (Centers for Disease Control), 24–25

vaccine studies
  chickenpox (varicella-zoster virus), 118–119
  diphtheria, 95–98
  Hemophilus influenzae Type B meningitis (HiB), 101–103
  hepatitis B, 92–95
  human papilloma virus (HPV), 119–123
  influenza (flu), 109–111
  measles, mumps, rubella (MMR), 111–113
  measles (rubeola), 113–116
  mouse toxicity test, 124
  mumps, 116–117
  pertussis (whooping cough), 98–100
  pharmaceutical industry and, 134–137
  pneumococcal disease (PCV7/PCV13/PPSV23), 104–105
  poliomyelitis (polio), 105–109
  rotavirus, 103–104
  rubella (German measles), 117
  shingles vaccine (Zostavax), 119
  tetanus (lockjaw), 100–101
vaccine-induced conditions. *See also* ASD (autism spectrum disorder)
  brain damage, 19
  cancers, 128–129
  Gulf War Syndrome (GWS), 127–128
  Obsessive-Compulsive Disorder (OCD), 129–130
  peanut allergies, 126
  shaken baby syndrome (SBS), 126–127
  sudden infant death syndrome (SIDS), 124–125

vaccines
    ADE (antibody-dependent
      enhancement), 183
    chickenpox, 53
    classifications, 90–92
    discontinued, 33, 92
    disease enhancement, 183
    early inoculation, 58
    immune enhancement, 183
    inactivated vaccines, 90
    Jenner, Edward, 58
    live attenuated vaccines, 90
    mRNA (messenger RNA)
      vaccines, 91
    subunit (acellular) vaccines
      conjugate vaccines, 91
      recombinant vaccines, 91
      toxoid vaccines, 91
    viral vector vaccines, 92
VAERS (Vaccine Adverse Event
   Reporting System), 32–33
    COVID-19 vaccine, 182
    Hemophilus influenzae Type B
      meningitis (HiB), 103
    hepatitis B vaccine, 93
    human papilloma virus (HPV),
      120–121
    pertussis (whooping cough), 100
varicella zoster virus, 53
vascular disorders, 68
vasculitis, 68, 94, 111, 121
Verstraeten, Tom, 70
viral meningitis, 102
viral vector vaccines, 92
viruses
    BSE (Bovine Spongiform
      Encephalopathy), Mad Cow
      Disease, 171–172
    Coronavirus (SARS-CoV-2),
      175–203

    Creutzfeldt-Jakob disease,
      171–172
    false claims, 169–170
    H5N1 (Avian Flu), 172–173
    HIV/AIDS (Human
      Immunodeficiency Virus/
      Acquired Immunodeficiency
      Syndrome), 170–171
    SARS (Severe Acute Respiratory
      Syndrome), 172
    swine flu, 170, 173
    Zika virus, 173–175
VSD (Vaccine Safety Datalink), 70

W
Wakefield, Andrew, 70
Wallace, Alfred Russell, 60
WHO (World Health Organization),
   pharmaceutical industry and,
   145–147
whooping cough
    increased cases, Bordetella
      pertussis strain, 69
    mortality rates, 57

X–Y–Z
yellow fever, 56
Zika virus, 173–175
Zimmerman, Andrew, 74–76
zymotic (contagious) diseases, 60–61

ABOUT THE AUTHOR

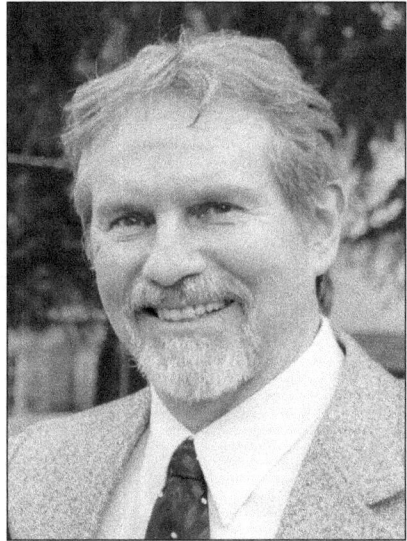

Leon Canerot is a retired school psychologist with 35 years of experience, who worked with special-needs children at the preschool and elementary through high school, and postsecondary levels. It was during the early 1990s that he first became aware of the autistic epidemic, while working in Head Start and later in the elementary school system, specifically, as part of a diagnostic team evaluating children with autism. This unprecedented rise in autism coincided with the dramatic increase in the number of vaccines that children were being given during that period. His investigation focused on numerous scientific studies that led to the controversial, yet undeniable, conclusion that vaccines were associated with autism and other neurodevelopmental disorders, which ultimately led to *The Unfortunate Truth About Vaccines.*

www.ingramcontent.com/pod-product-compliance
Lightning Source LLC
Chambersburg PA
CBHW062114020426
42335CB00013B/964